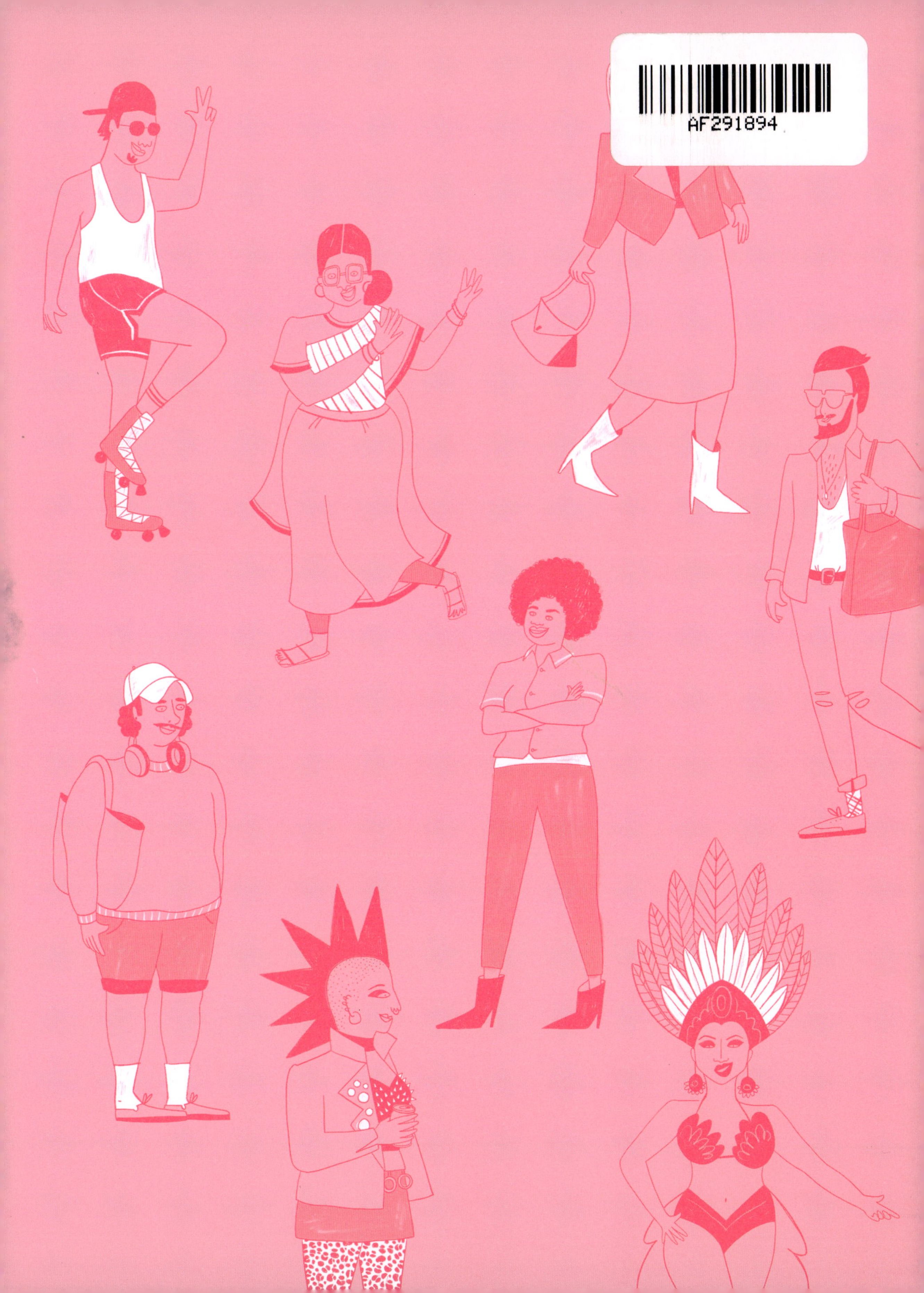
AF291894

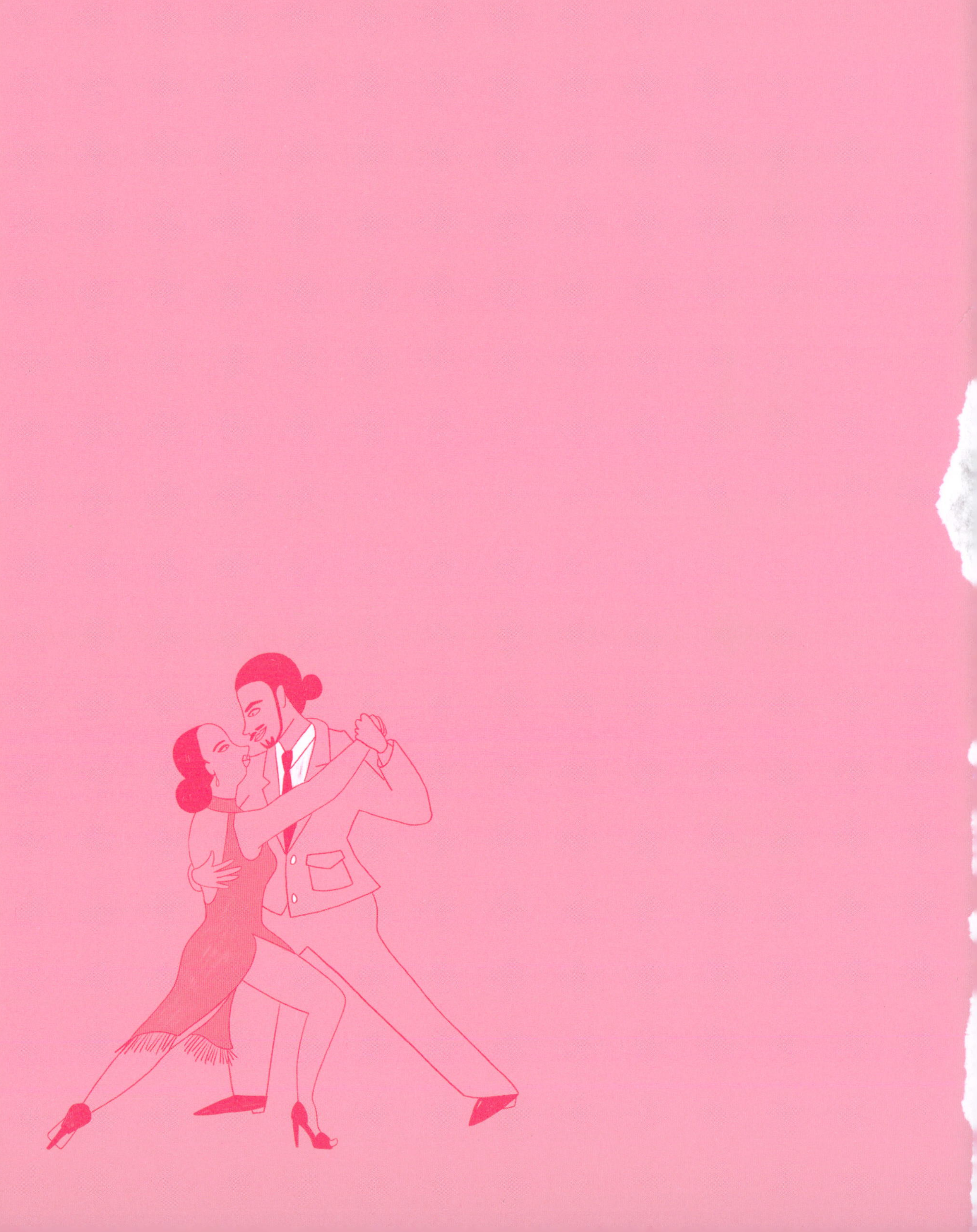

DRAW HAPPY

PEOPLE & FACES

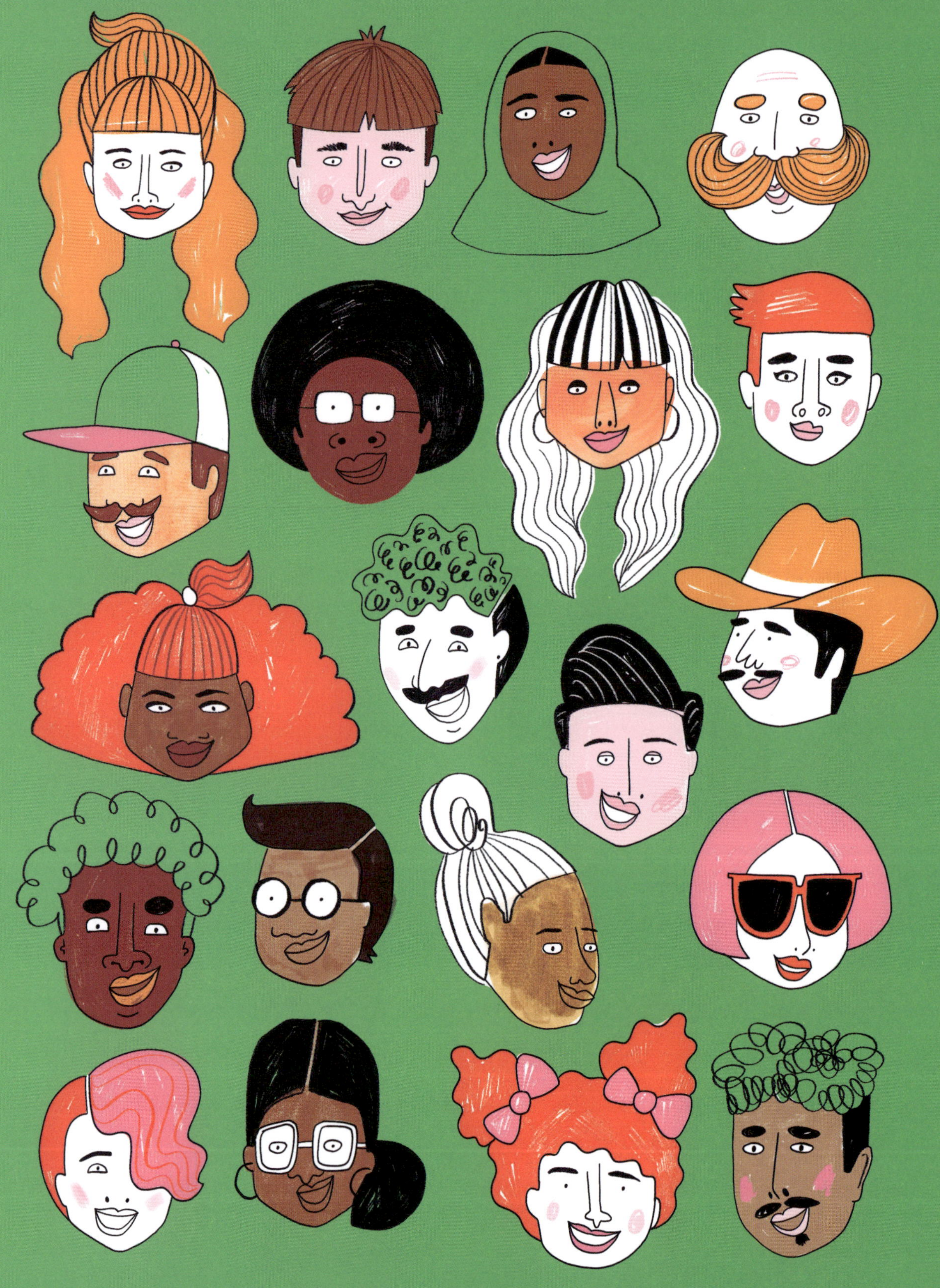

DRAW HAPPY

PEOPLE & FACES

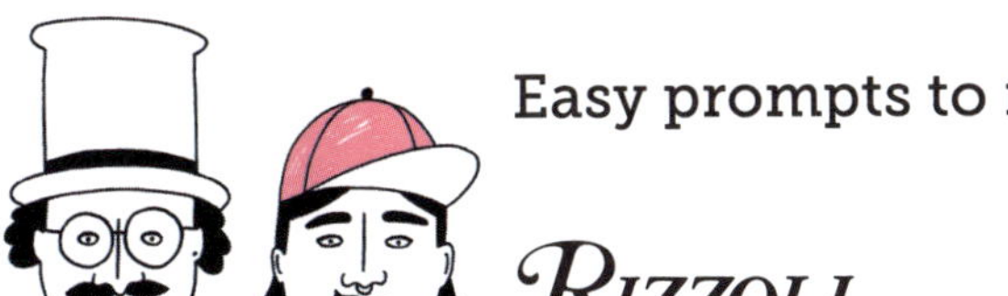

Easy prompts to find joy through creativity

RIZZOLI UNIVERSE

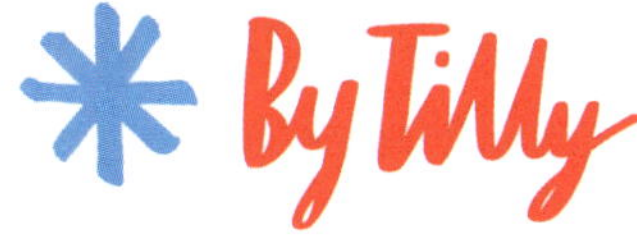

By Tilly

INTRODUCTION

In this book you will find over 100 prompts and exercises designed to help you explore drawing people. You will learn some foundations in drawing techniques, such as drawing people in proportion and in movement; develop your drawing skills from observation and without looking at the page; and practice using your imagination to develop your own characters. This book is a space to create and experiment, taking the pressure of the blank page away, and serving as a source of inspiration. A family of people are ready and waiting to welcome you!

One of the most important things in life is our relationship with others and drawing them is a wonderful way to connect. Think of your pencil as a tool for your characters to communicate with each other and the viewer. Give them a voice by showing how they feel and want to be seen by the world around them.

I could sit at a window and watch people wander by all day long. You can gather a lot of information from a person by observing their body language and gestures; they offer a snippet into a person's life, like a quick sketch. You can then use your imagination to finish the narrative of that person's story. I call these characters my "made-up friends." It's a great way to develop your skills in character building and it can also be lots of fun! Next time you're in a coffee shop or out and about, try it; use those observations in your drawings!

You don't have to create realistic portraits to be good at drawing people; perhaps you are brilliant at conveying emotion and expression, or maybe you are great at visualizing a character's personality. Move the goal post—instead of creating the perfect portrait give yourself permission to play. It will help you learn and develop as an artist. You might just discover moments of creativity and joy along the way.

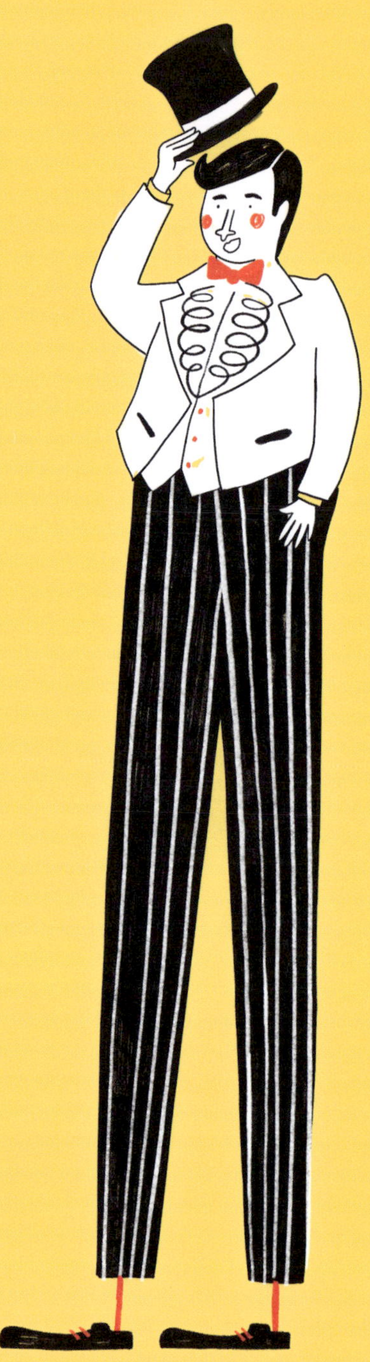

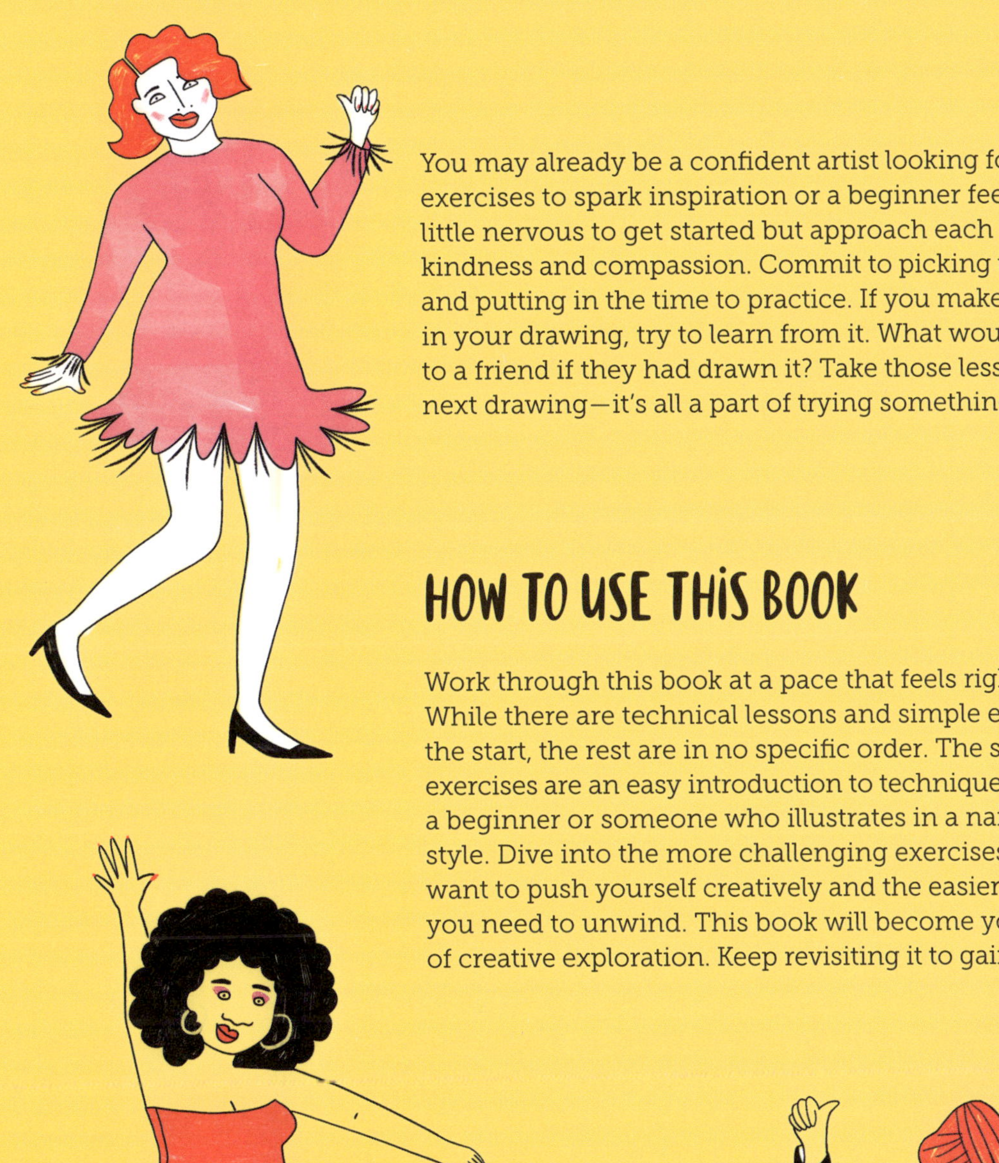

You may already be a confident artist looking for drawing exercises to spark inspiration or a beginner feeling a little nervous to get started but approach each page with kindness and compassion. Commit to picking up a pencil and putting in the time to practice. If you make a "mistake" in your drawing, try to learn from it. What would you say to a friend if they had drawn it? Take those lessons to the next drawing—it's all a part of trying something new.

HOW TO USE THIS BOOK

Work through this book at a pace that feels right to you. While there are technical lessons and simple exercises at the start, the rest are in no specific order. The step-by-step exercises are an easy introduction to techniques, which suit a beginner or someone who illustrates in a naive drawing style. Dive into the more challenging exercises when you want to push yourself creatively and the easier ones when you need to unwind. This book will become your archive of creative exploration. Keep revisiting it to gain inspiration.

FINDING INSPIRATION

There may be times when you're feeling uninspired or find yourself in a creative block. Instead of sitting at your desk, take a break and spend time being creative in a different way. Use the ideas here as an opportunity to look closer at the everyday to find inspiration.

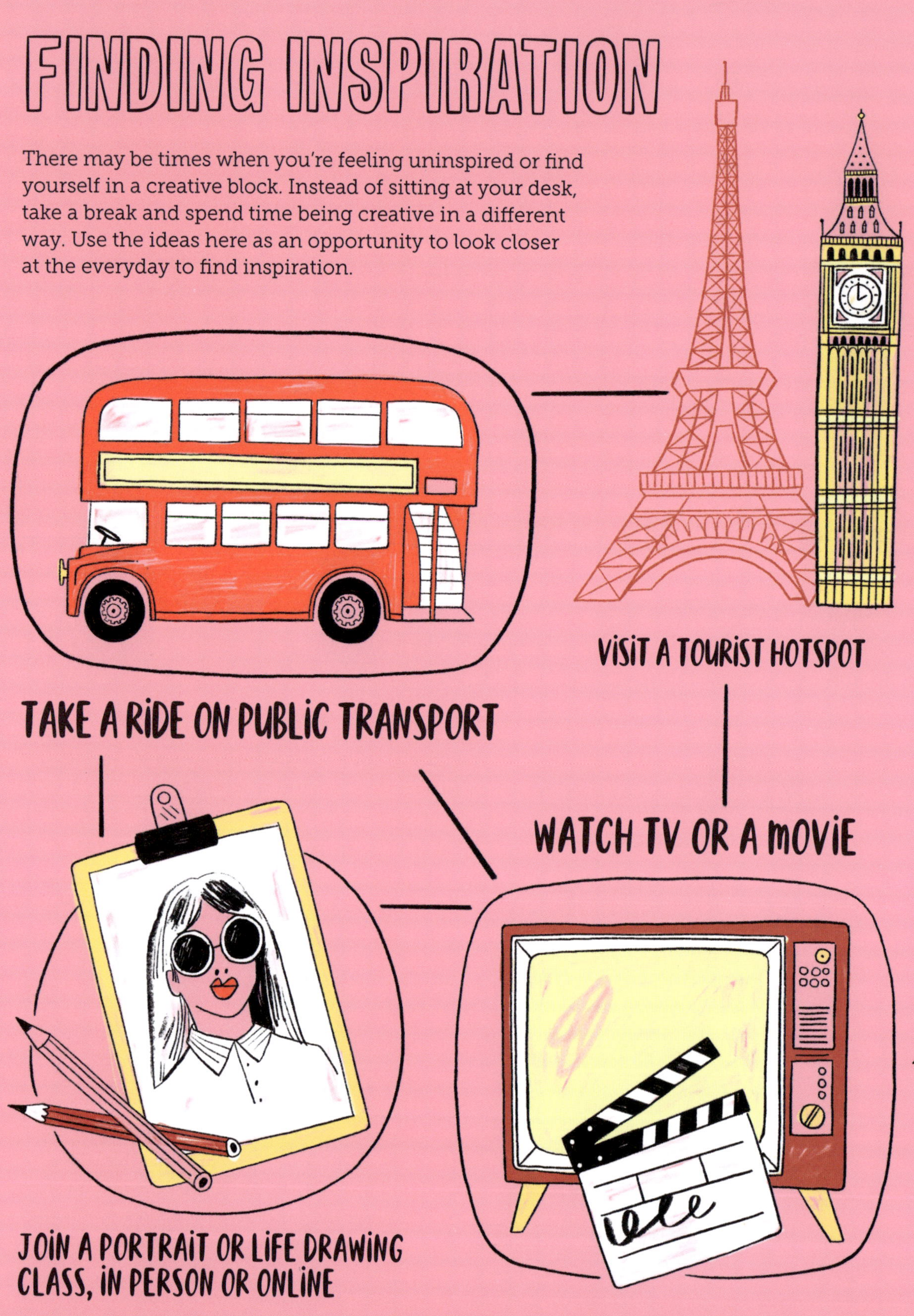

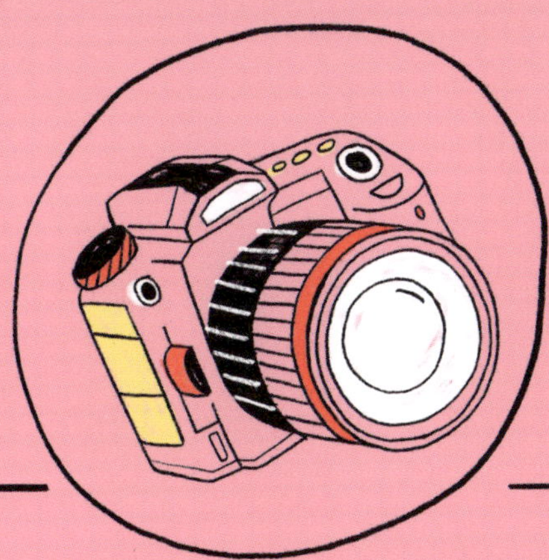

USE A CAMERA AS YOUR TOOL INSTEAD OF A PENCIL

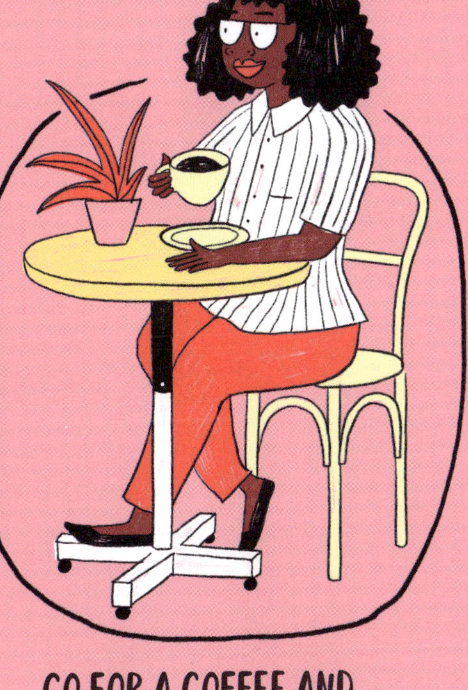

GO FOR A COFFEE AND SIT IN THE CAFÉ WINDOW WATCHING PASSERSBY

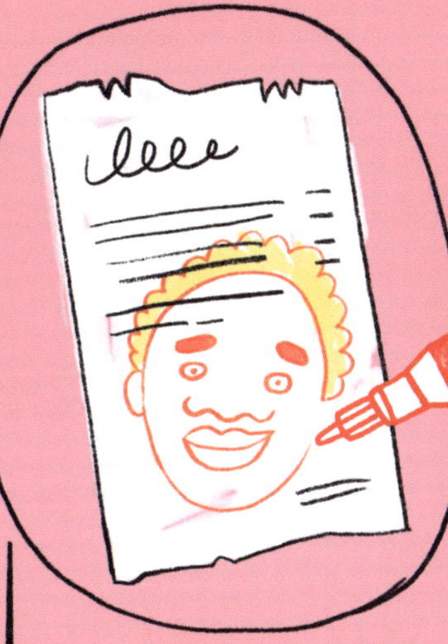

WANT TO DRAW? DO IT ON SCRAP PAPER LIKE A RECEIPT, THEN THROW IT AWAY!

GO TO THE THEATER

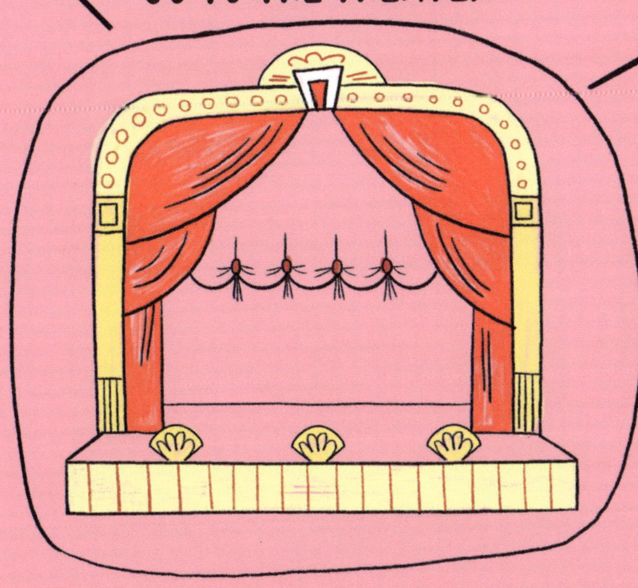

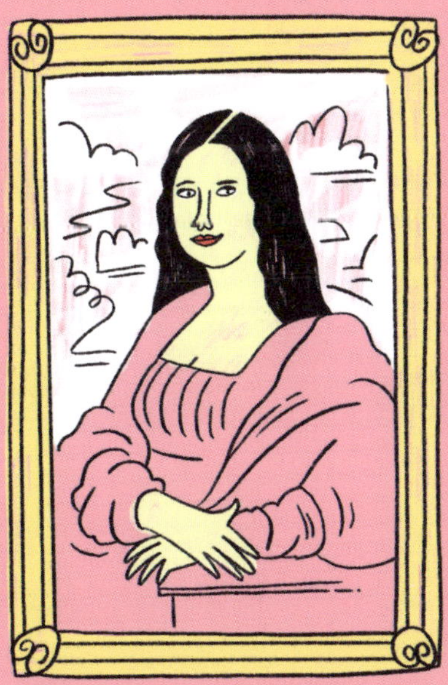

VISIT A NATIONAL OR LOCAL PORTRAIT GALLERY

MATERIALS

Here is a collection of materials to get you started in building your own creative toolbox. Drawing is incredibly accessible and buying the best you can afford is always worthwhile. However, you can make a great drawing with just a biro or pencil, so don't feel any pressure to purchase expensive tools.

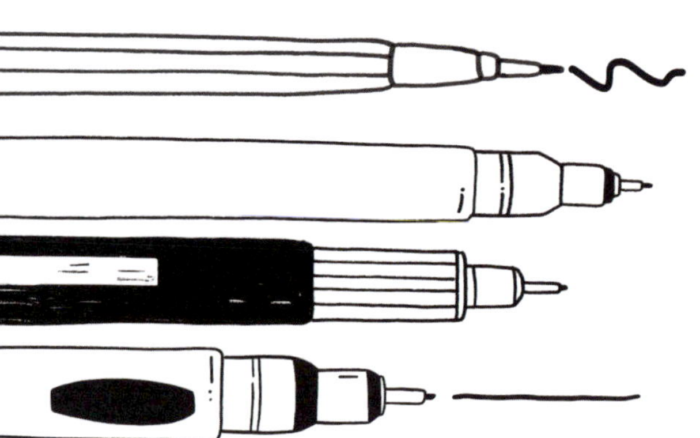

FINELINERS

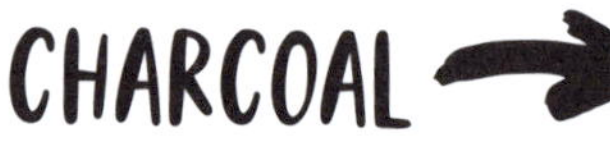

My most trusty tool. With a solid line that dries quickly, they are great for detailed drawing. They come in various line widths, from 0.05mm for a super skinny line to a 0.8mm for a bold, chunky line. My personal favorite is the Staedtler brand.

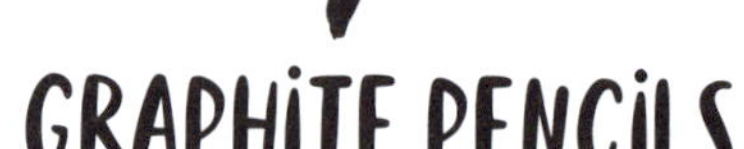

GRAPHITE PENCILS

An essential in every artist's toolbox, they range from H, which makes a hard, light line, to 9B for soft dark marks. You could also try a mechanical pencil, which is fancy but refillable. Some even come with a hidden sharpener. My favorite is the Koh-i-noor brand.

CHARCOAL

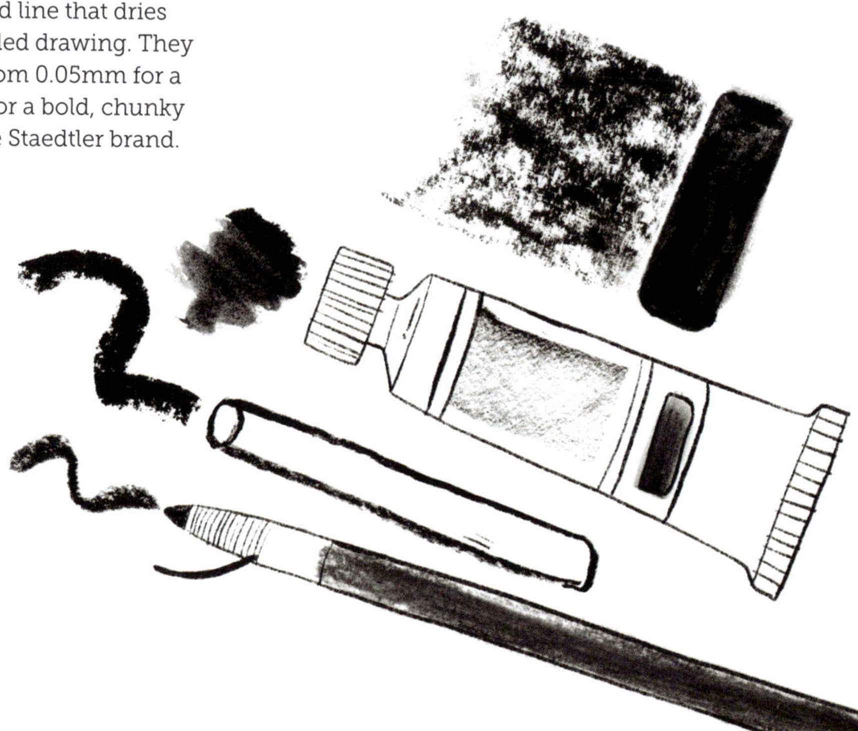

A great way to create texture, charcoal comes in a traditional stick form, or as a solid block, liquid, or pencils, which are a lot less messy! Make sure you use a fixative when you have finished to prevent your artwork from smudging.

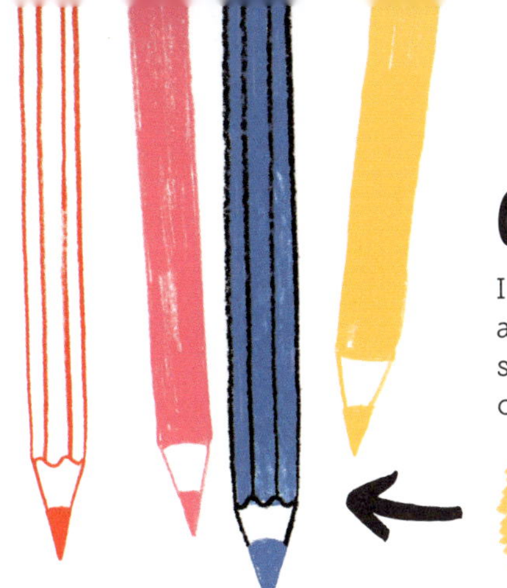

COLORED PENCILS

I would suggest buying the best ones you can afford. Faber-Castell and Caran d'Ache are exceptional. The better the quality, the smoother the blending, but a basic grocery store coloring pencil can still do the job.

WATERCOLOR PENCILS

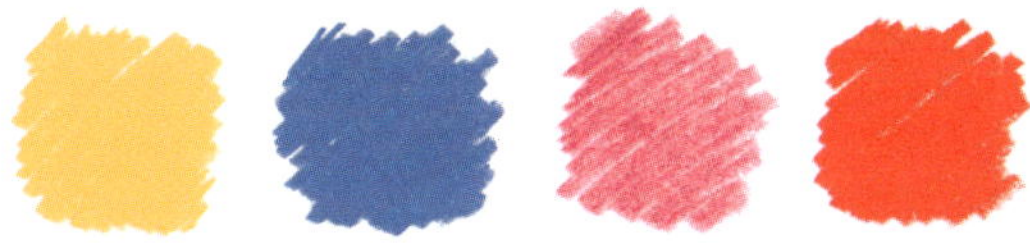

What's better than a material that can be used in multiple ways? If you love drawing with colored pencils and want to explore painting, these are a great stepping stone. They are also handy when you are drawing on location and don't want to carry lots of paint tubes.

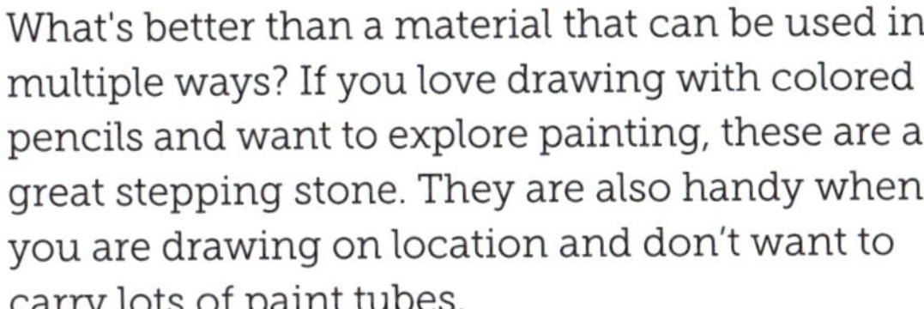

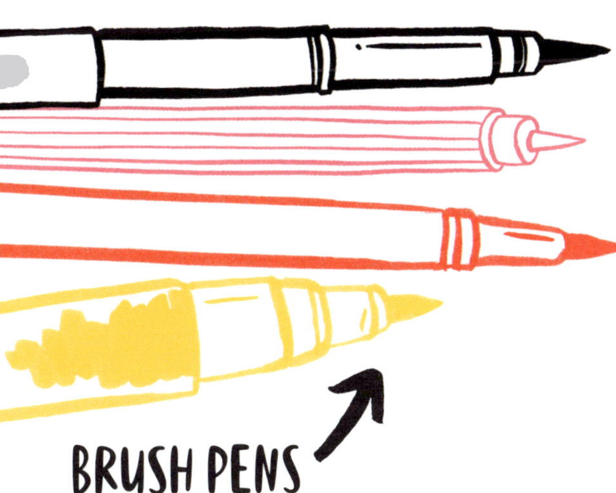

BRUSH PENS

The brush tip has a lovely, soft quality and feels similar to working with a paintbrush; you can also find them as dual tips with another harder standard pen nib the other end. Both options are great for mark making. Tombow and Ecoline are top choices for my pencil case.

MARKER PENS AND FELT TIPS

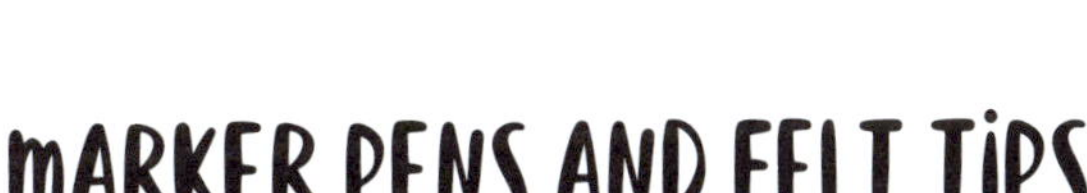

Marker pens are perfect for getting large areas of color down fast, and come in standard or a flat chisel nib. You can also find a colorless blender pen, which is a helpful tool for easier shading and blending. Winsor & Newton offer excellent markers, but I also always keep a cheap felt tip in my toolbox, which creates a fantastic texture.

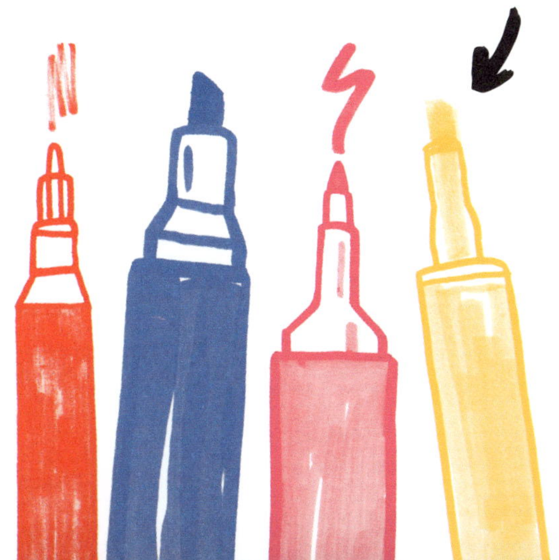

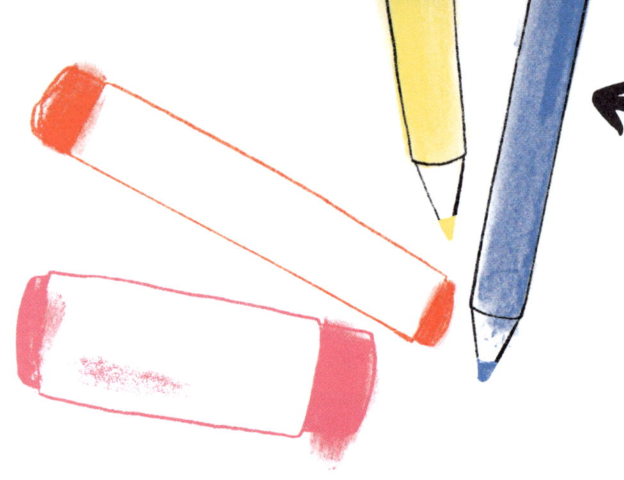

CHALK PASTELS

If you want to create a soft texture then pastels are perfect. You can use a brush to blend, but it's fun to use your fingers, plus you will have more control. They are also available as pencils, which are really convenient and allow for finer detail. Use a fixative to prevent your artwork from smudging. Derwent and Faber-Castell have some great affordable sets.

OIL AND WAX PASTELS

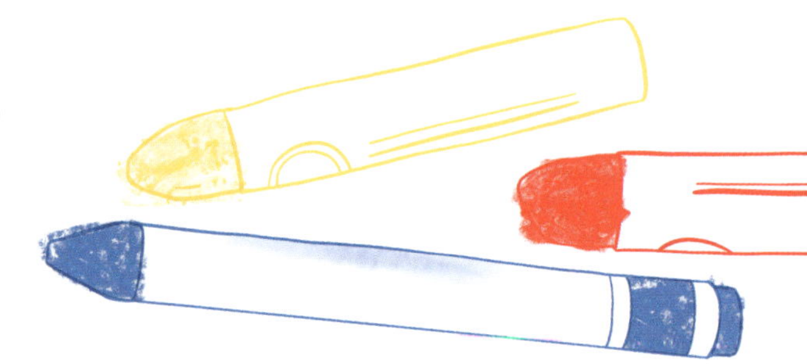

Oil pastels have a creamy, thick consistency that allows you to slowly build up the layers and marks. If you are after top quality, Sennelier's range, created in collaboration with Pablo Picasso himself, are incredible and come as sets and individual pastels. Wax pastels are closer to a traditional crayon and are also available as water-soluble.

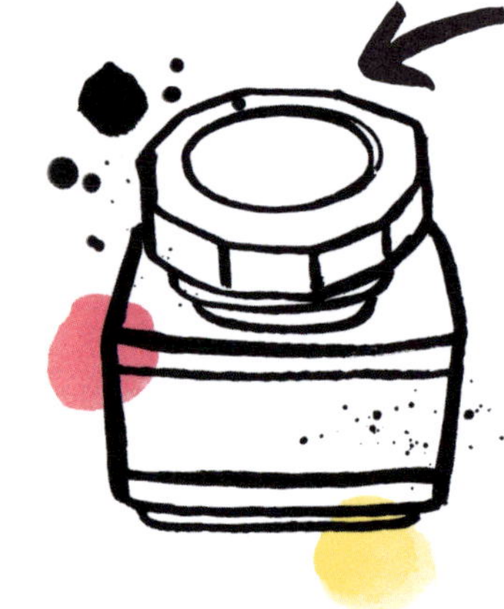

INK

As well as black Indian ink, you can find drawing ink in countless colors, which produce rich and vibrant artwork. Winsor & Newton have a wide selection that is affordable and available in individual colors.

PAINT

Watercolor paint is available in tubes and pans, easy to work with, and is a great choice to start with. It dries quite quickly leaving soft, translucent areas. Gouache is opaque and creates a flatter, matte, solid block of color, but can also be thinned with water for a lighter wash a bit similar to watercolor. Once both have dried, they are perfect for drawing on top of. Acrylic paint can be diluted for a light wash or can be built up into layers. I recommend starting with Winsor & Newton or Liquitex brands, which are inexpensive.

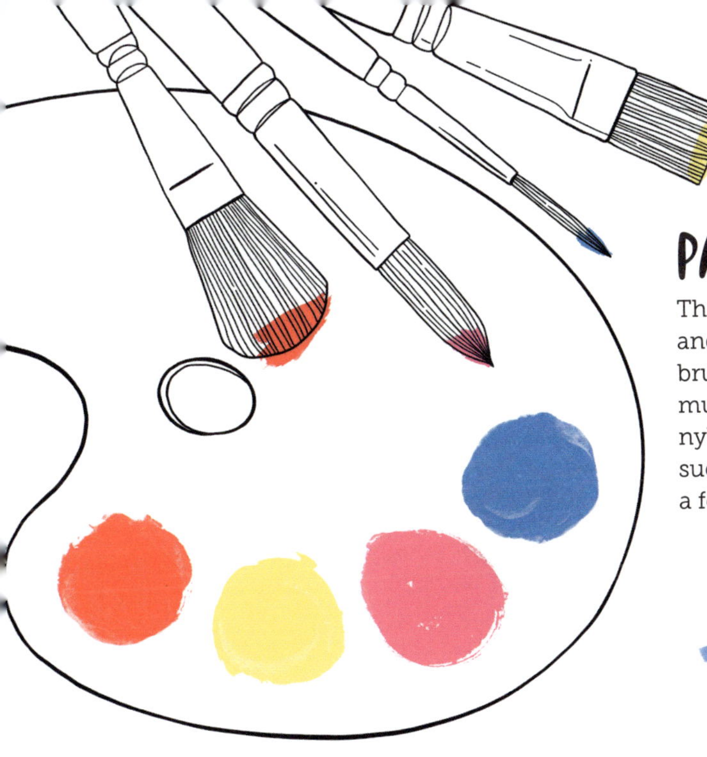

PAINTBRUSHES

There are two types of paintbrushes: natural and synthetic. The best quality is the natural hair brushes, also called sable. Synthetic brushes are much more affordable as they are made from nylon or polyester. There are many brush types, such as round, flat, filbert, and stippler to name a few; each one is for a specific paint and effect.

PALETTES

There are plastic, wooden, porcelain, and tear-off paper palette pads available, although an old china plate is just as good and reusable plastic containers are also very handy. If you have paint left over, just pop the lid back on and keep it for another day!

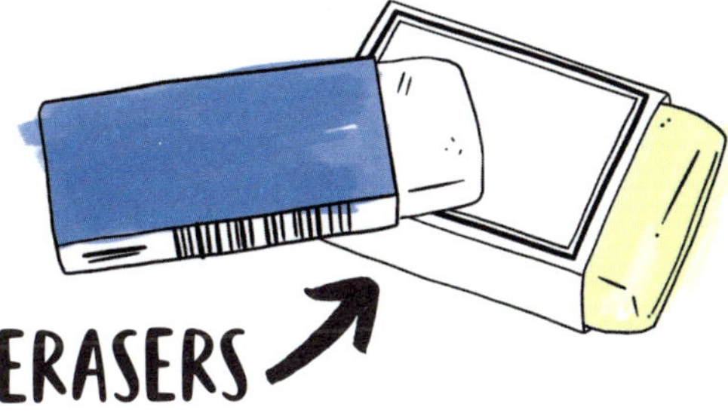

ERASERS

There are two basic erasers: the common eraser made from rubber, gum, or plastic that will crumble and is good at removing your sketch marks. The putty rubber is kneadable and great at making highlights in materials like charcoal.

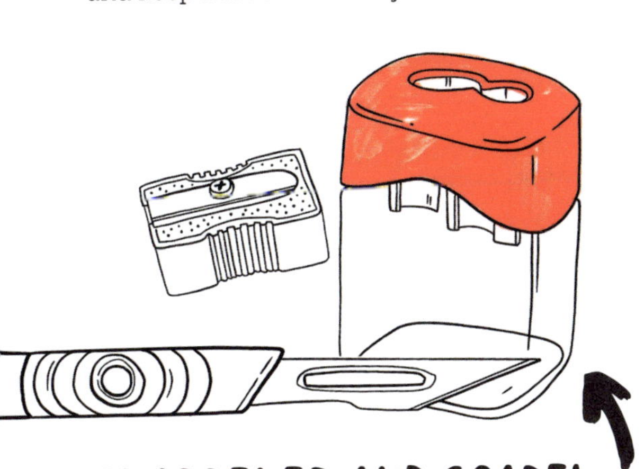

FIXATIVE

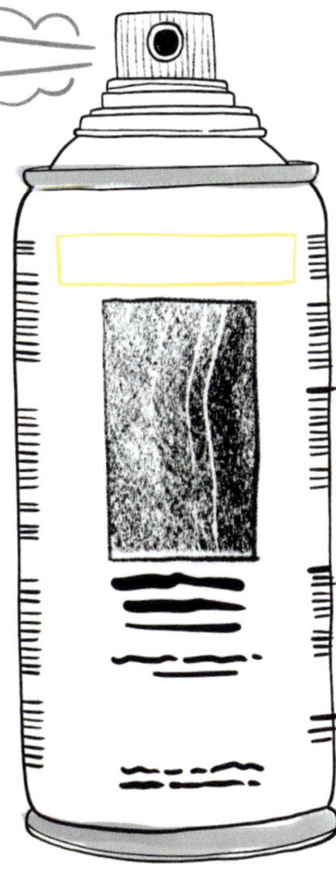

A colorless spray that seals materials like charcoal and pastels to prevent your artwork from smudging. A more affordable option is a standard hairspray; not quite as good but still does the job!

SHARPENER AND SCAPEL

Plastic and metal sharpeners are great for a standard pencil but be mindful of what you choose for materials such as pastel pencils where the lead is more fragile. Personally, I always use a scalpel; with a bit of practice you will have more control and can make a finer point with less breakage.

RECORD YOUR DRAWING GOALS

Write down your main goals for this book. Is it to develop your drawing skills, explore your creativity, or to give yourself a break from your phone or screen? Or all of the above?

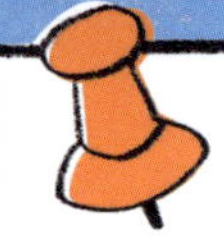

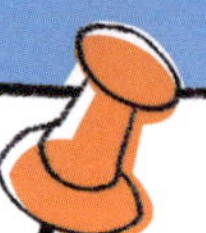

WRITE HERE

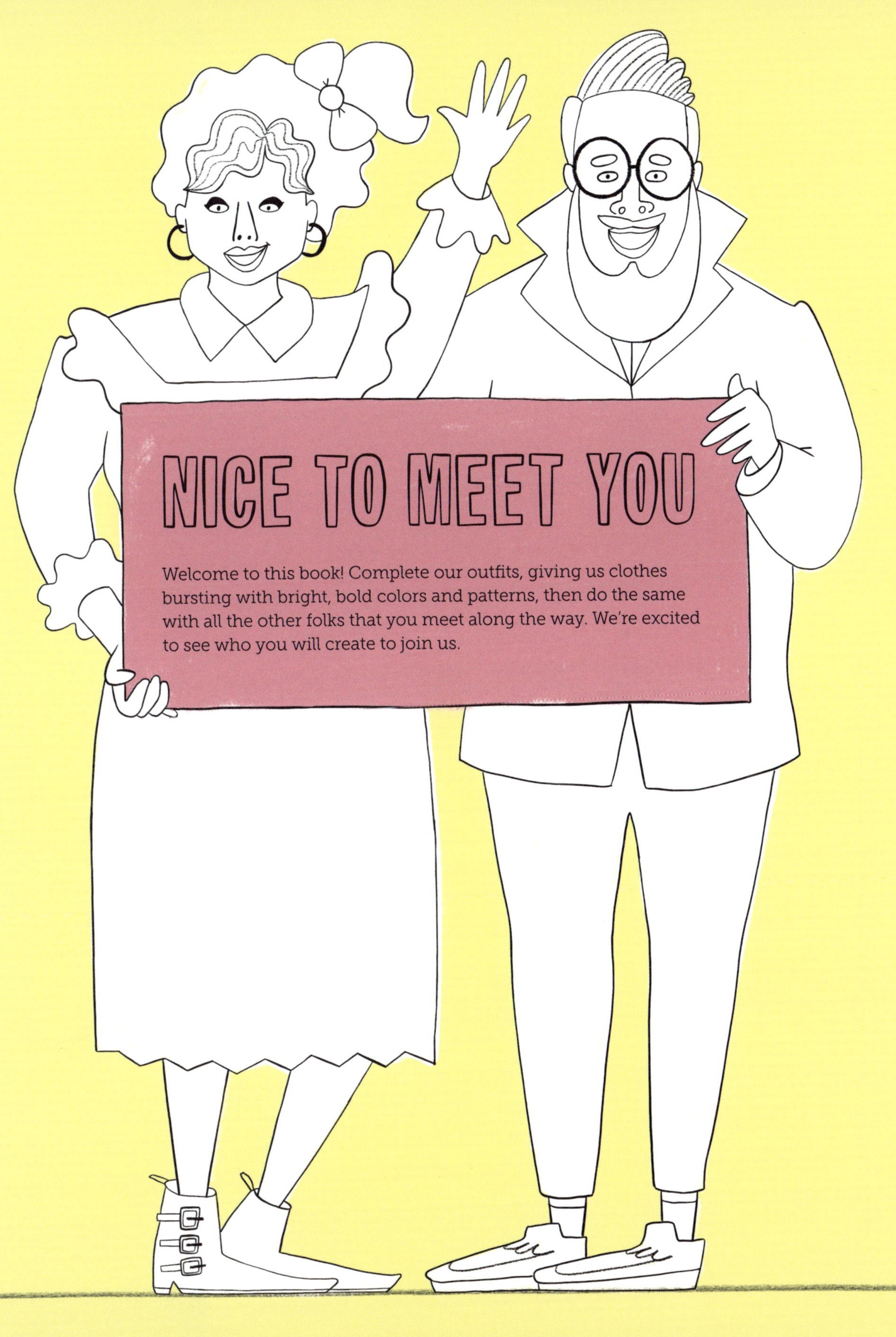

NICE TO MEET YOU
Welcome to this book! Complete our outfits, giving us clothes bursting with bright, bold colors and patterns, then do the same with all the other folks that you meet along the way. We're excited to see who you will create to join us.

FACIAL FEATURES: NOSE

Noses come in all shapes and sizes and can really change a face and make a character. Below are examples of different ways you can draw a nose. Fill in the remaining space with your versions, practicing from various angles. You might find using reference photos or a mirror helpful.

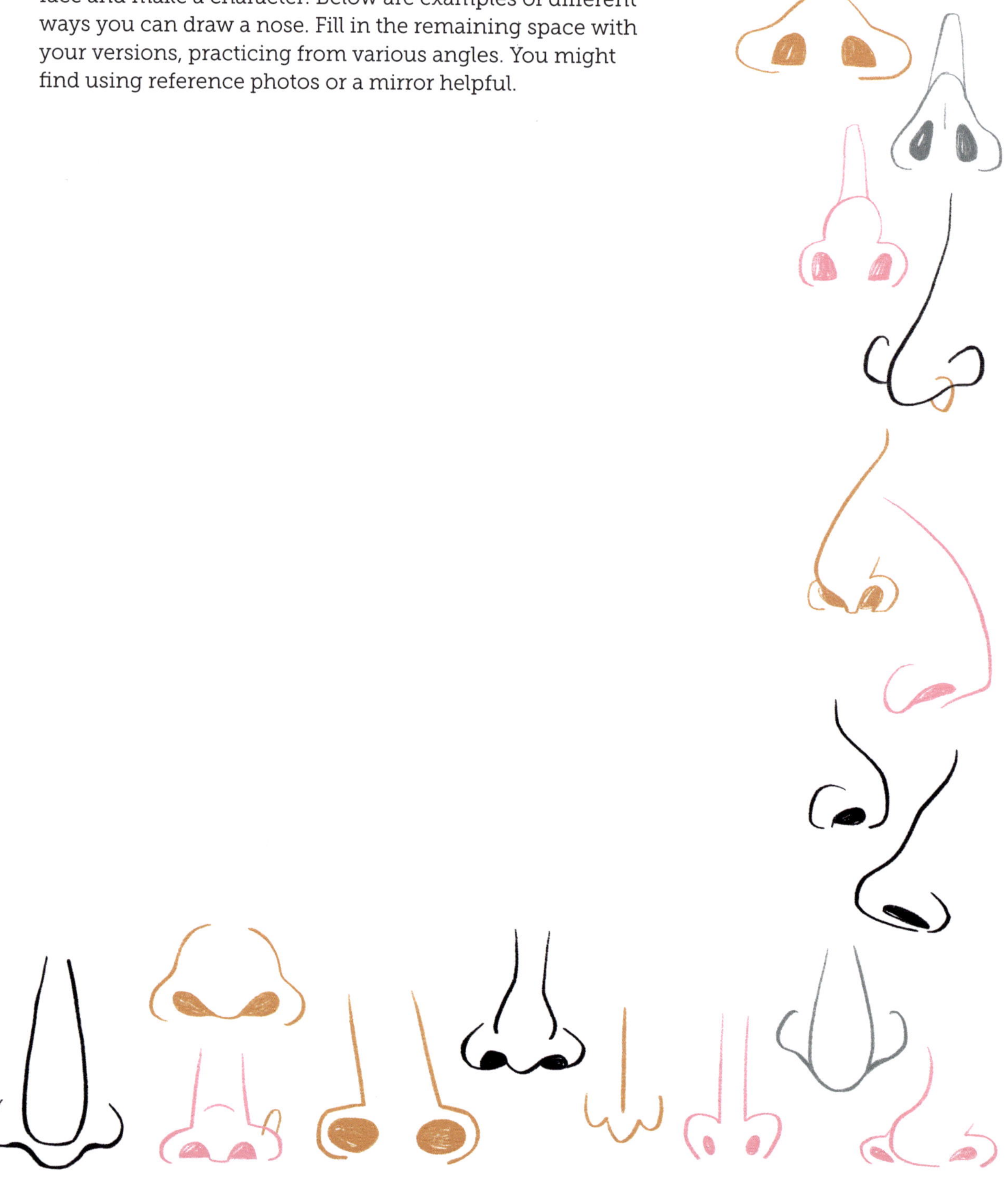

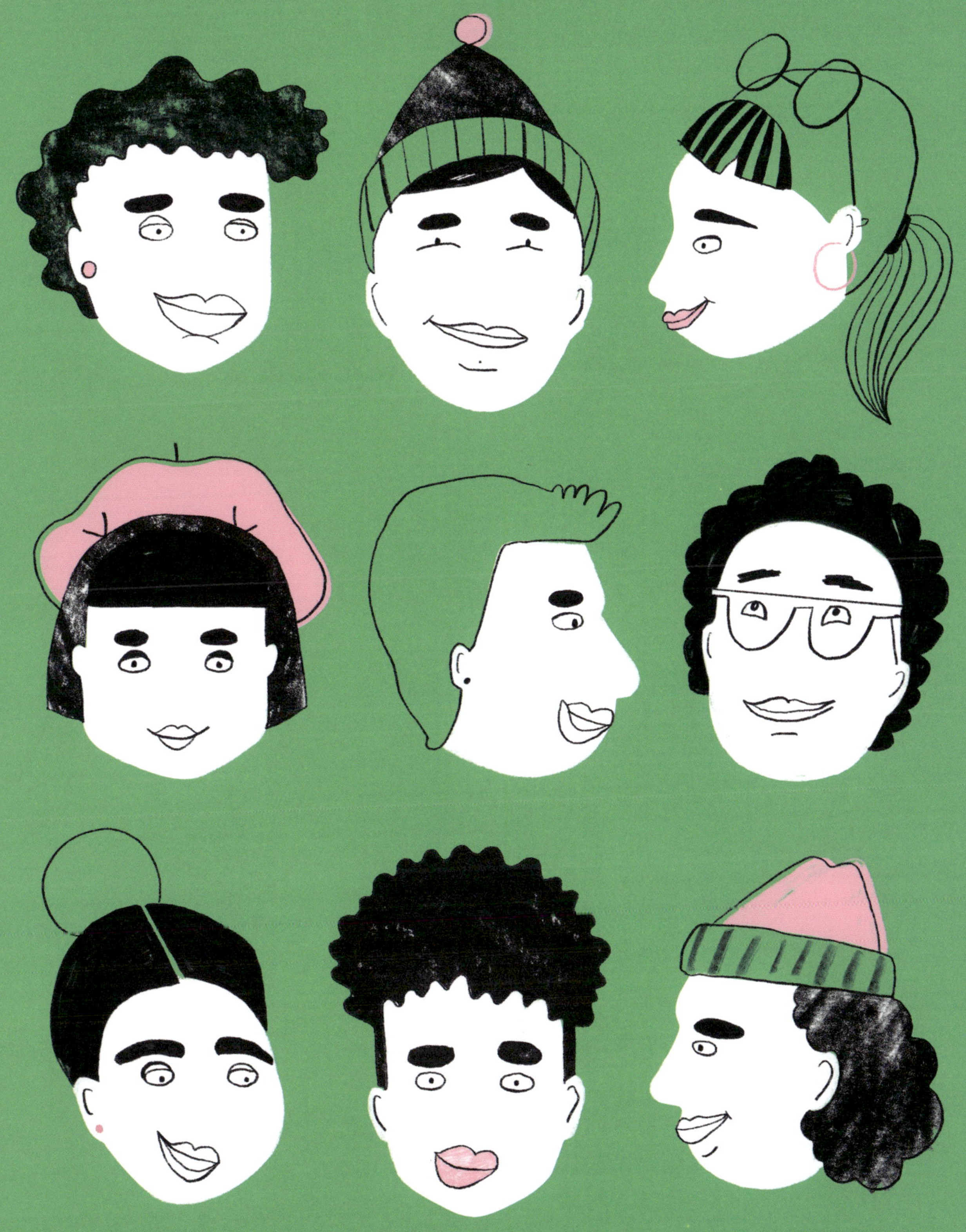

NOW, CHOOSE YOUR FAVORITES AND COMPLETE THESE FACES!

A COLLECTION OF BUSTS

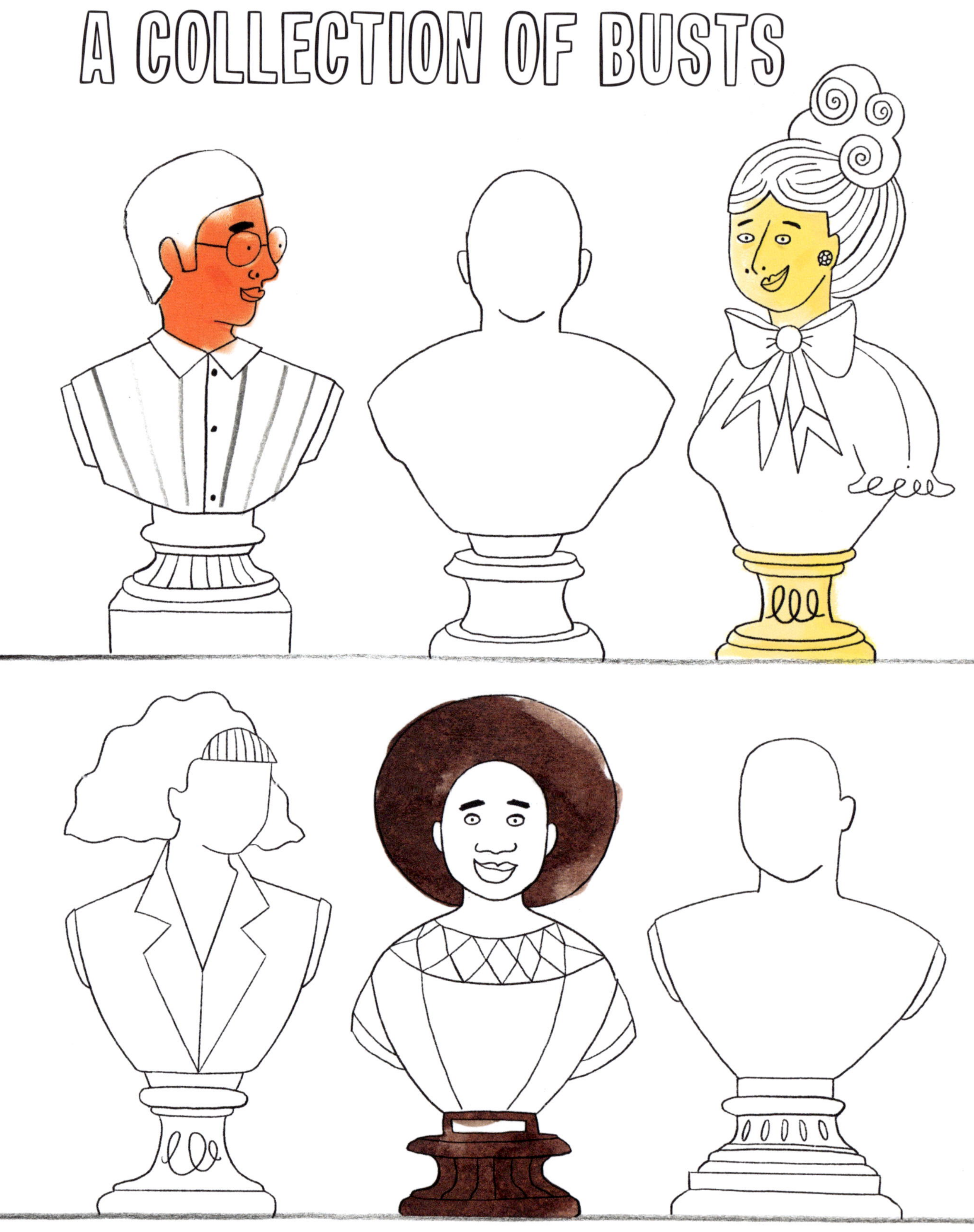

Complete this museum collection of busts by adding the people you would like to display as sculptural portraits. Choose the materials you'll use carefully—select ones that will resemble the quality and texture of traditional sculpture, such as ink for bronze or colored pencils for stone.

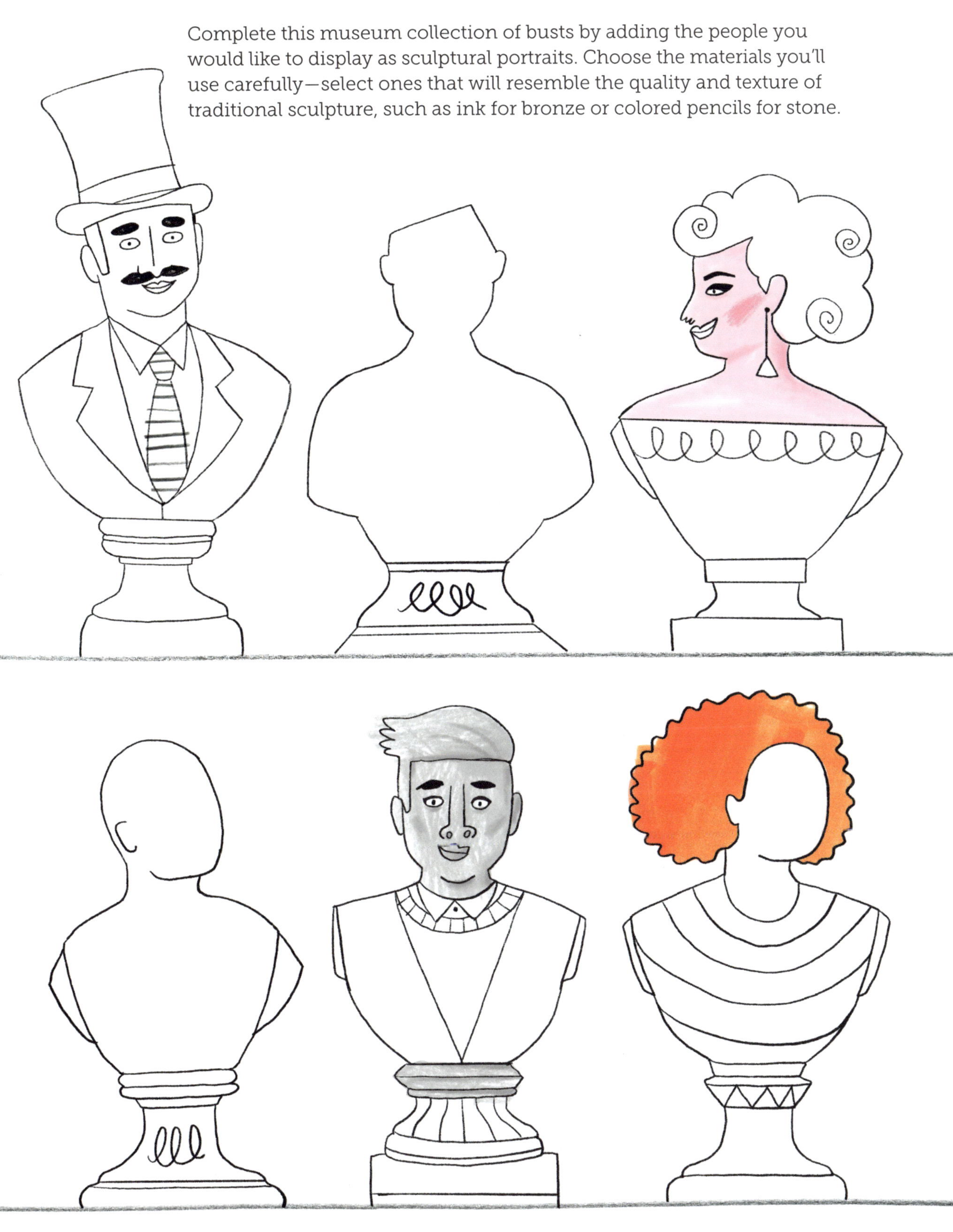

SELF-PORTRAIT

Drawing faces can be a bit intimidating, but this four-step technique can help, along with lots of practice. Before you know it, you will be confident in creating recognizable facial features and emotions.

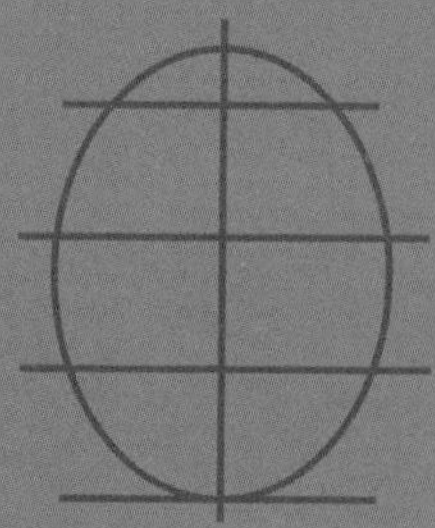

1 Draw an oval shape for the face with four evenly spaced lines across and one down the center of the face.

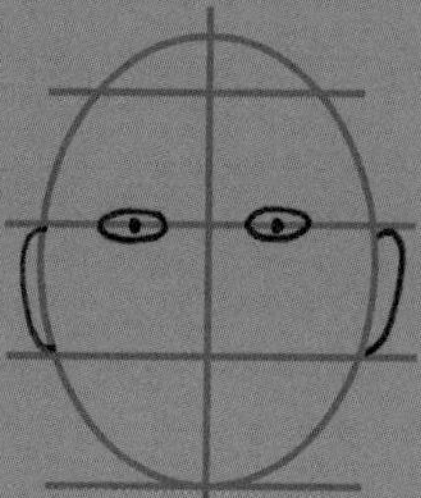

2 The eyes and ears sit on the second line, then place the ears between the second and third lines.

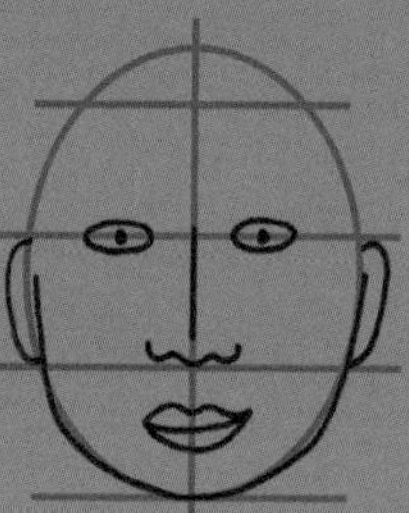

3 The end of the nose sits on the third line. The mouth is central between the nose and chin.

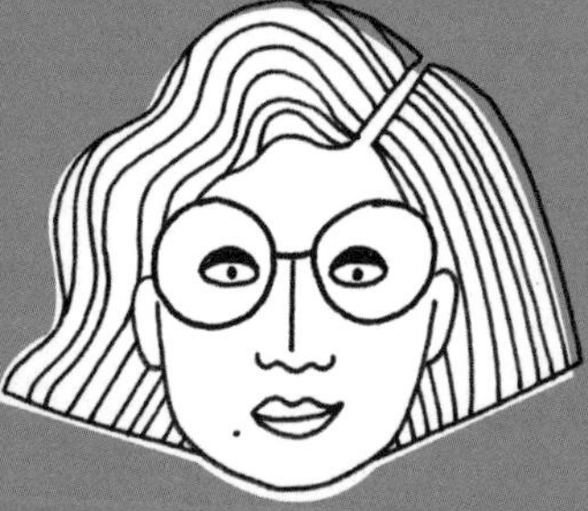

4 Add more details to bring your character to life! Then, rub out your pencil marks.

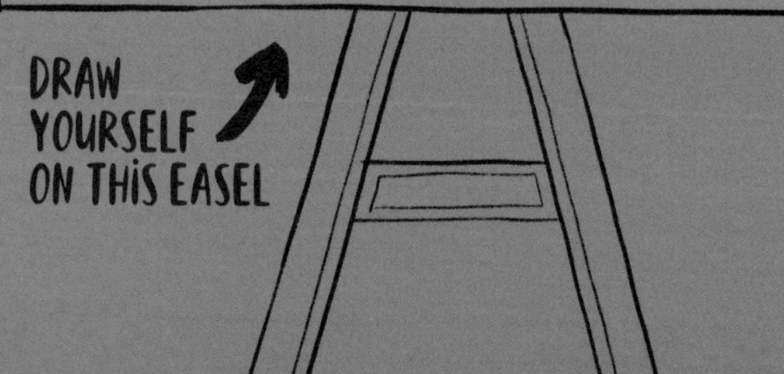

EXPLORING TONE

Practice how to make faces appear three-dimensional by adding tone (the range of light and shadow). Draw your own face in the box below with a graphite pencil. Use a bright light that will give you strong tone. Start with gentle marks, then gradually build up pressure and the pencil weight for stronger shadows.

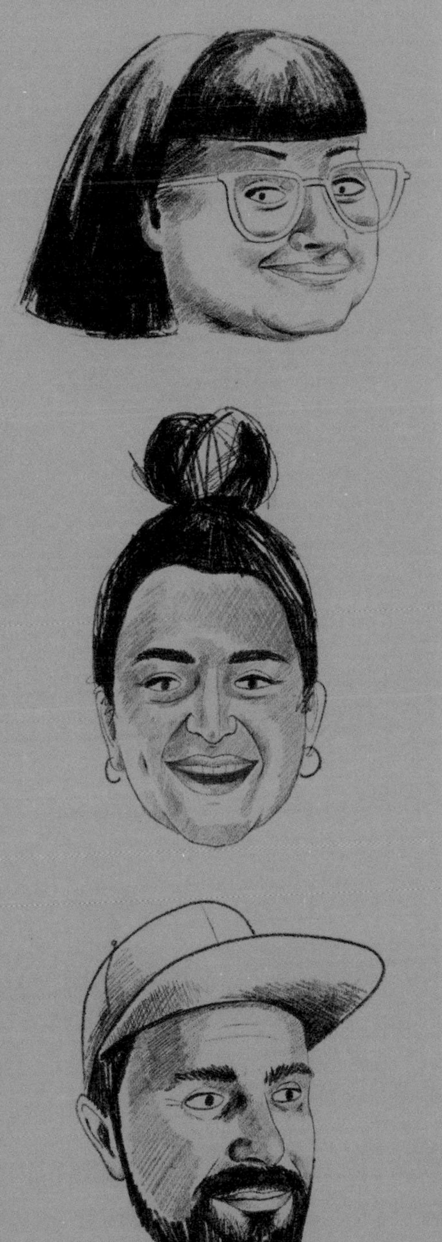

SQUINTING YOUR EYES CAN HELP YOU PICK OUT AREAS OF LIGHT AND DARK MORE EASILY

FACIAL FEATURES: EARS

The shape of ears vary immensely from tiny, tucked back ones to narrow and pointy. They are also a fun way to express style and personality with jewelry! Using reference material or your imagination, fill in the remaining space below with as many different types of ears as you can fit in.

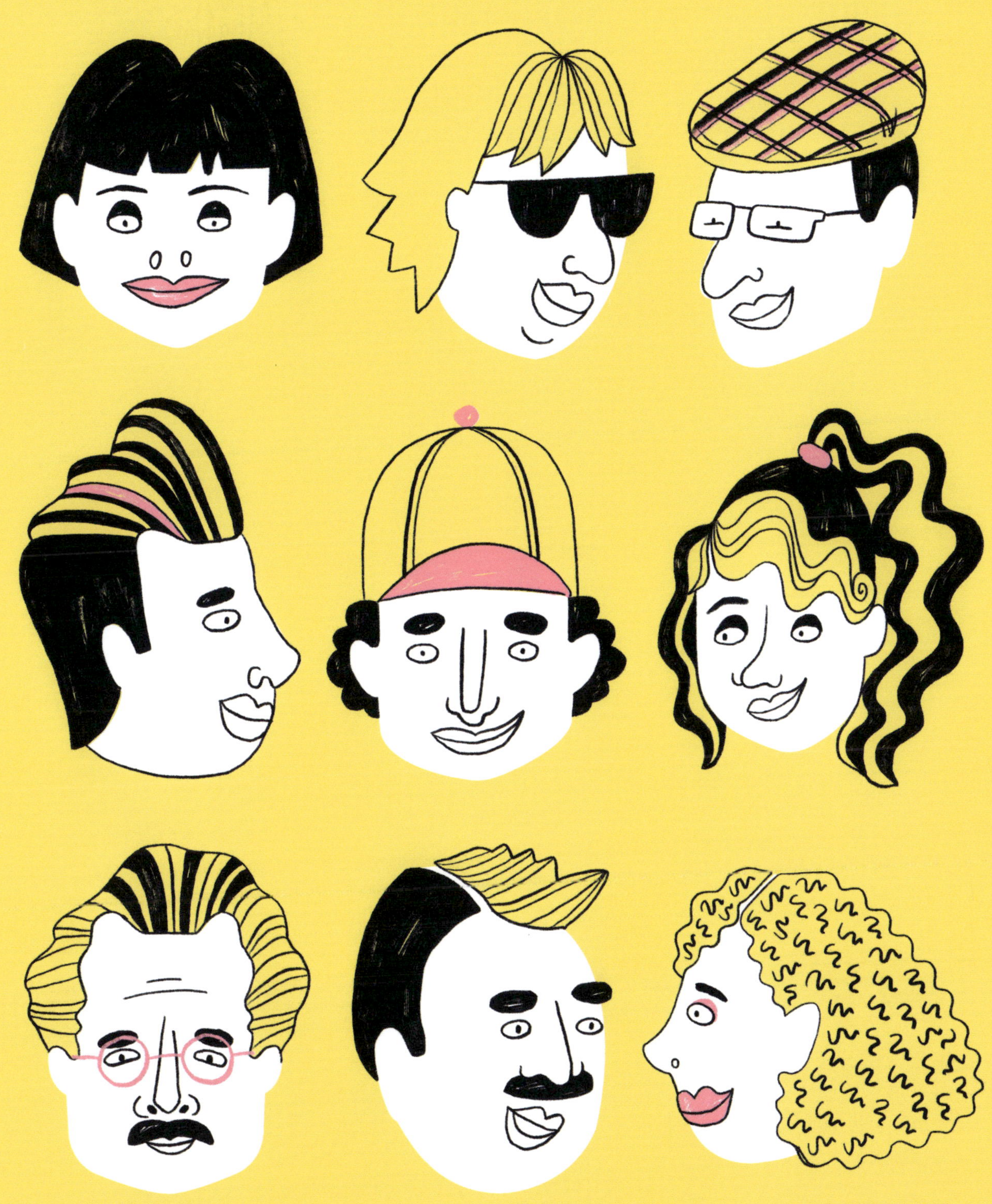

NOW, CHOOSE YOUR FAVORITES AND COMPLETE THESE FACES!

HOW TO DRAW FEET

This is a simple way of drawing a stylized foot by dividing it into a series of shapes. It is also a good place for beginners to start. The foot has 26 bones, so don't aim for a perfect anatomical drawing. Use your own feet or a photo as reference when practicing.

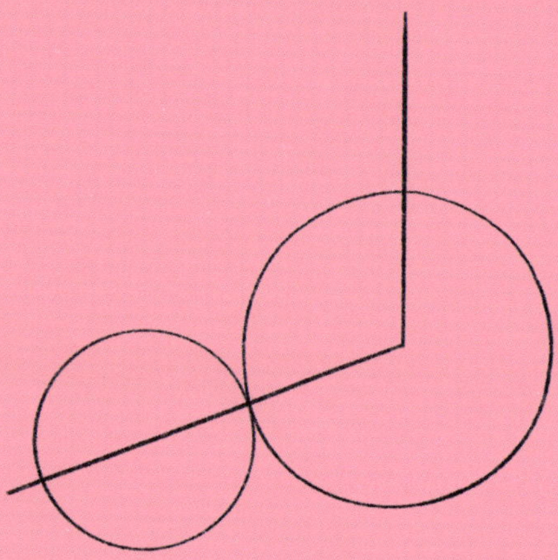 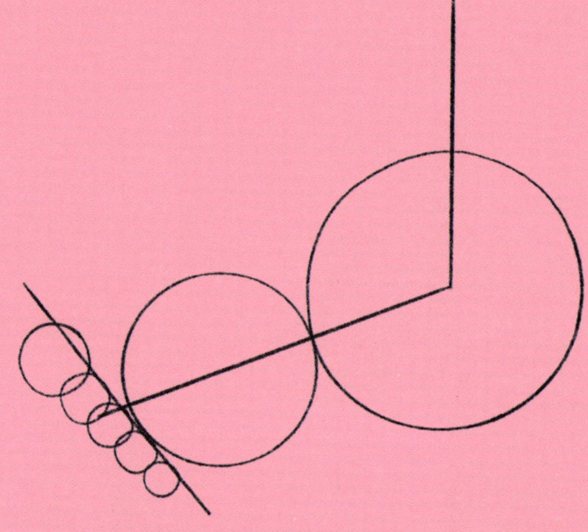

1 Draw two lines pointing at 8 o'clock. Draw a large circle at the center point of the lines for the base of the foot and a smaller circle for the bridge of the foot.

2 Draw a vertical line at a 45-degree angle and five connecting circles getting progressively smaller in size for the toes.

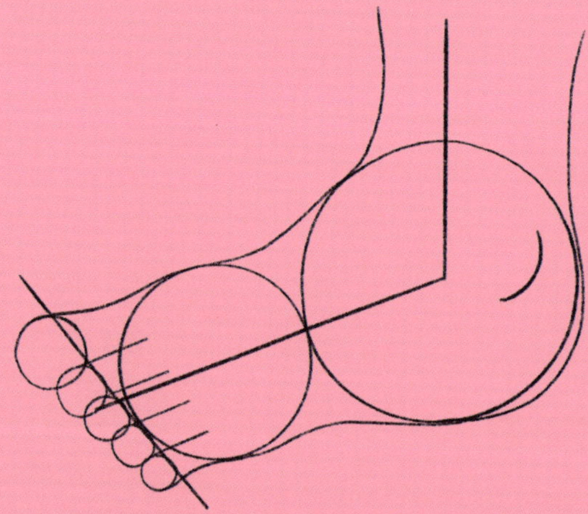 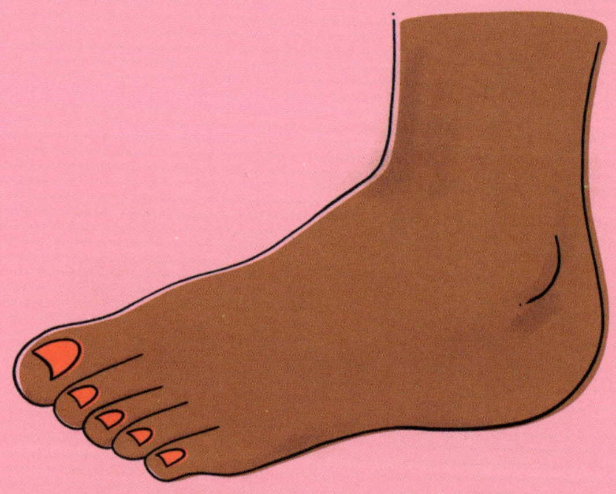

3 Connect the circles with lines following the natural curve of the foot. Add lines that lead off each circle for the toes and mark the position of the ankle.

4 With a fineliner, draw over your pencil work, refining the lines and adding in the toenails. Finish by rubbing out your pencil lines.

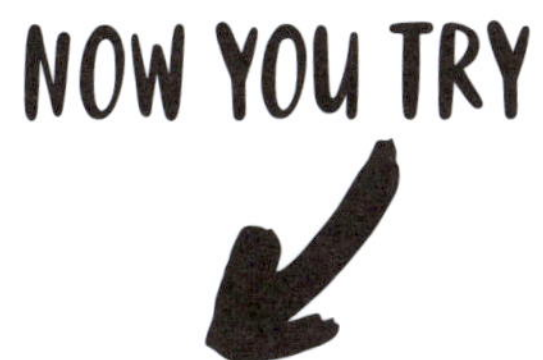
NOW YOU TRY

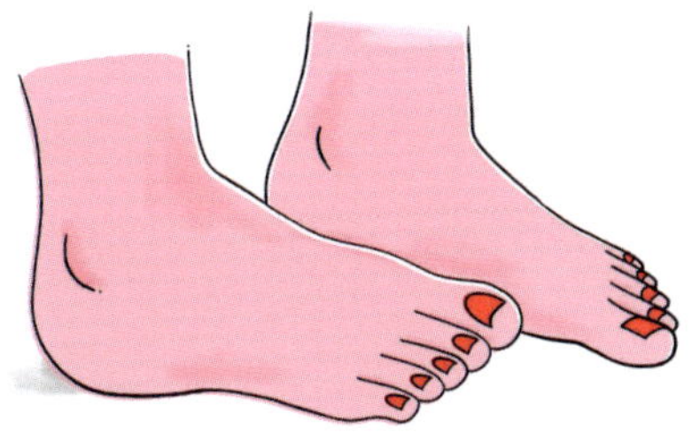

FACIAL FEATURES: EYES

Eyes come in many different shapes, such as almond, downturned, or upturned. They also change shape depending on what emotion that person is expressing. Fill in the remaining space with examples of different eyes, using a mirror or reference material to help.

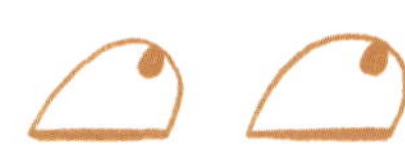
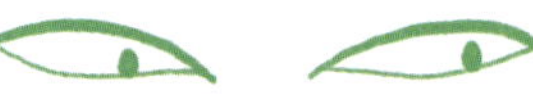
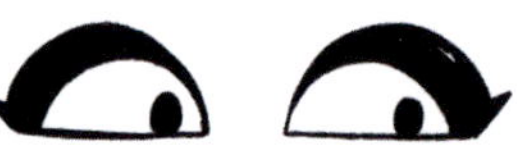
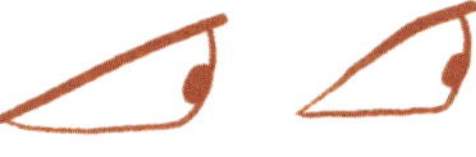
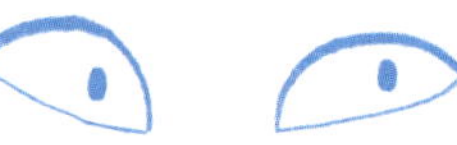
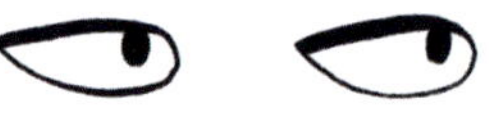
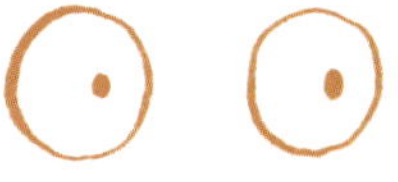
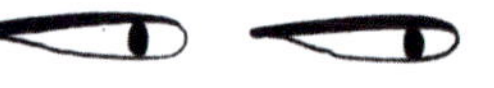
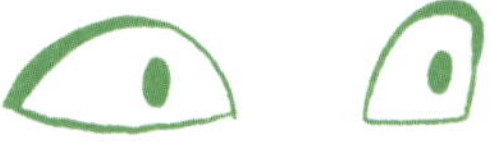
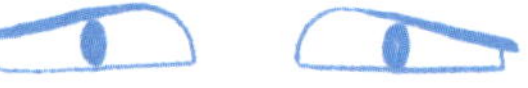
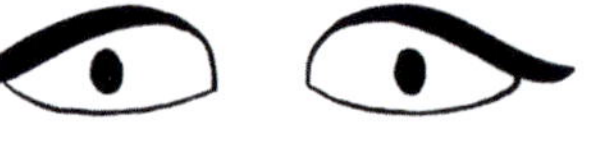
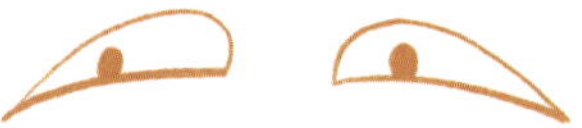
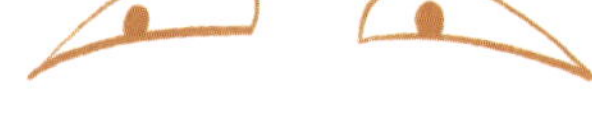

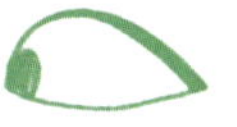
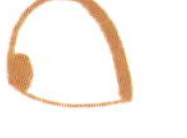
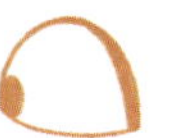
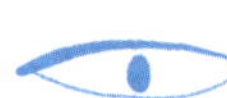

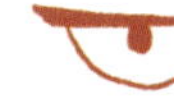
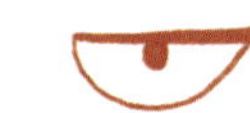

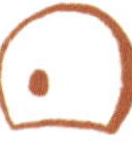
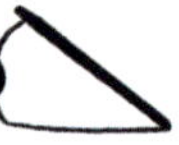
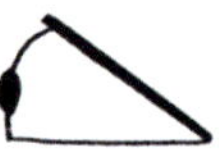

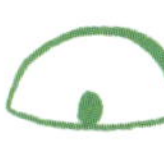
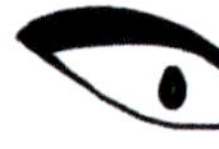
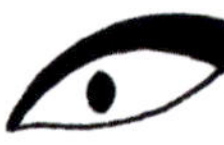

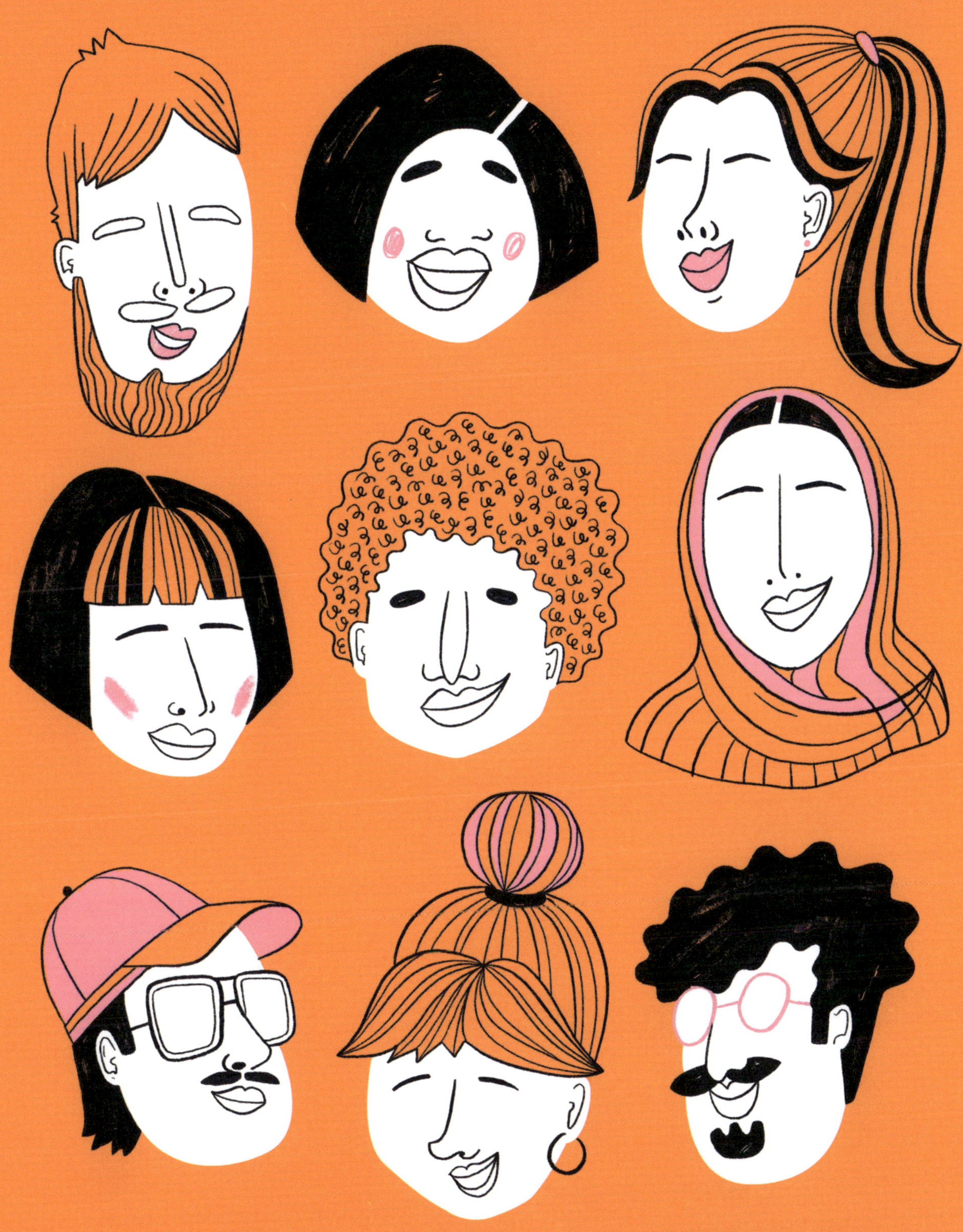

NOW, CHOOSE YOUR FAVORITES AND COMPLETE THESE FACES!

WHO'S THERE?

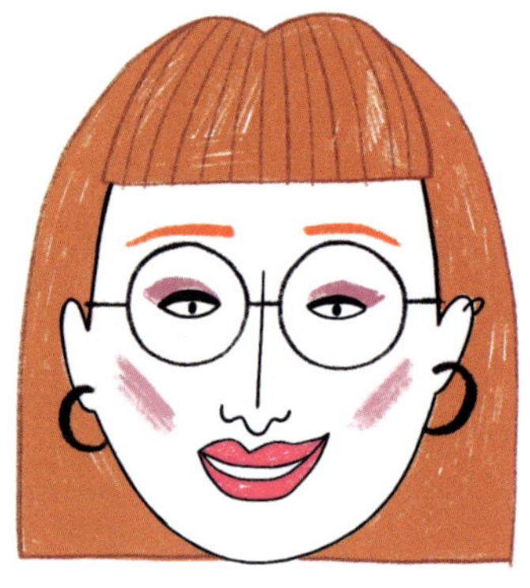

GINGER HAIR WITH ROUND GLASSES

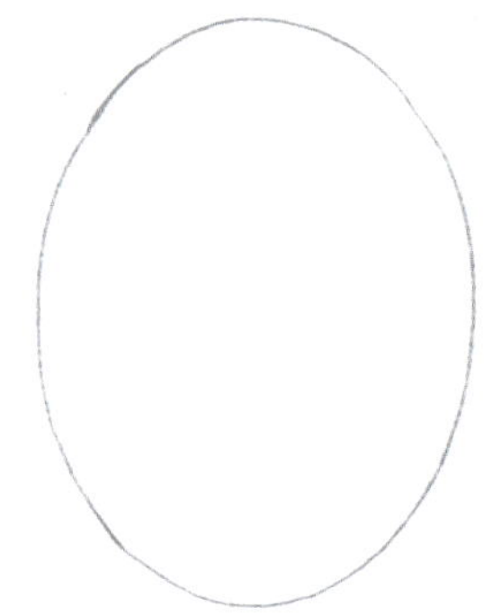

MOUSTACHE, LAUGHING, EYES CLOSED

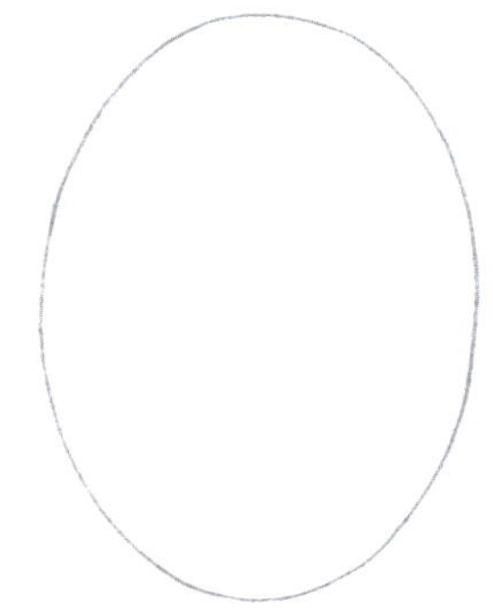

MOHAWK WITH A FACE TATTOO

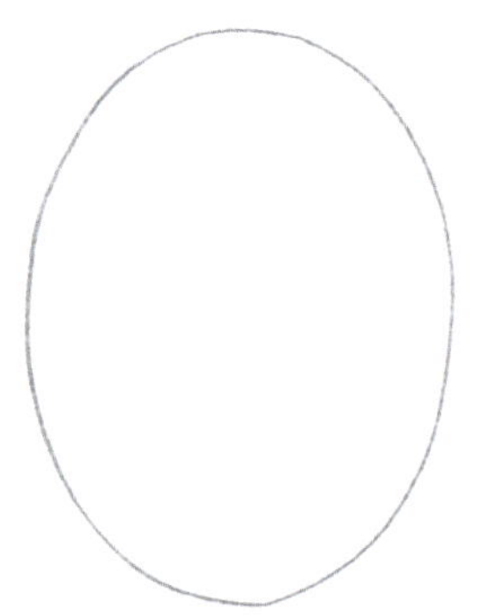

HUGE SMILE AND BIG, BOLD EARRINGS

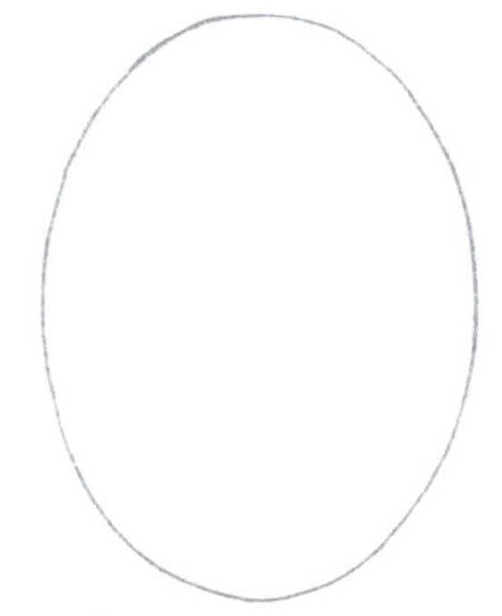

BALD HEAD AND SQUARE GLASSES

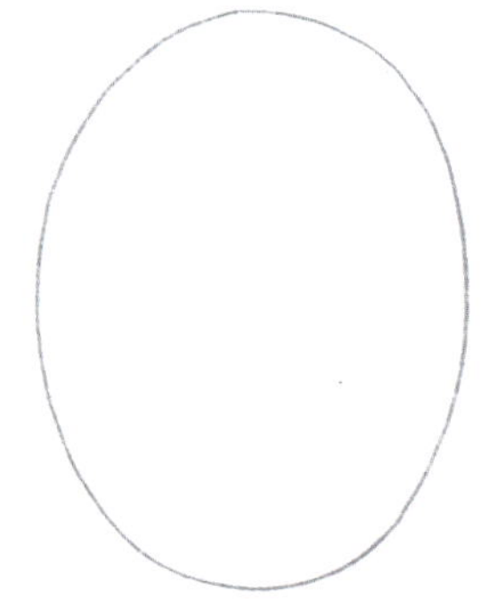

BIG SIDE BURNS AND WAVY HAIR

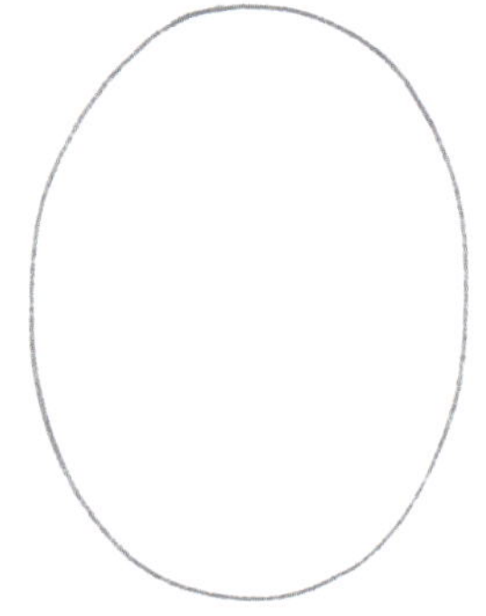

PINK FRIZZY HAIR AND FRECKLES

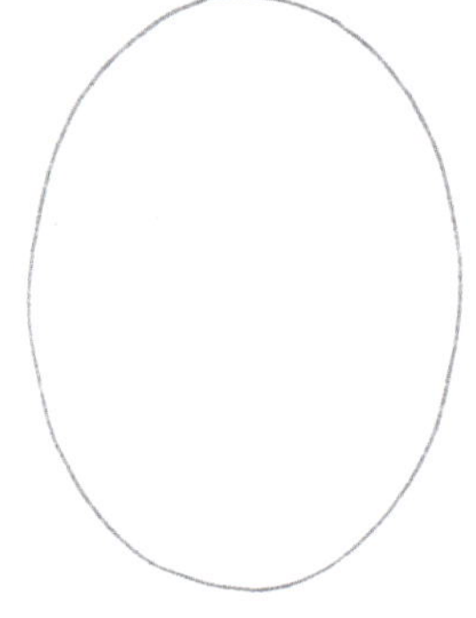

BRUNETTE WITH SHORT BANGS

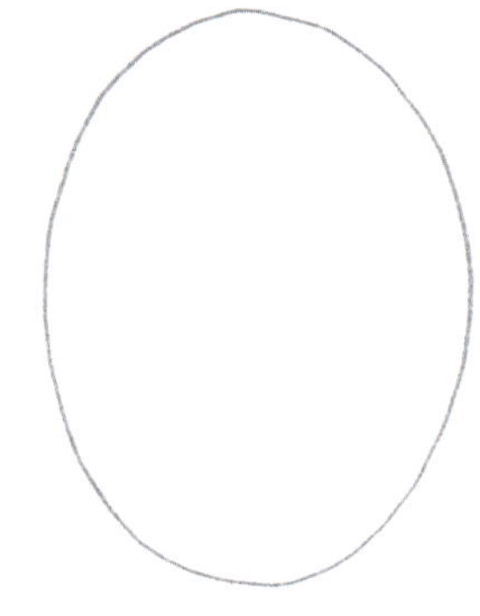

ELDERLY WITH A GRAY BEARD

Use these prompts as inspiration to design your own characters. Fill the page with individuals of all ages to create a diverse mix of people. Who will you and your pencils discover?

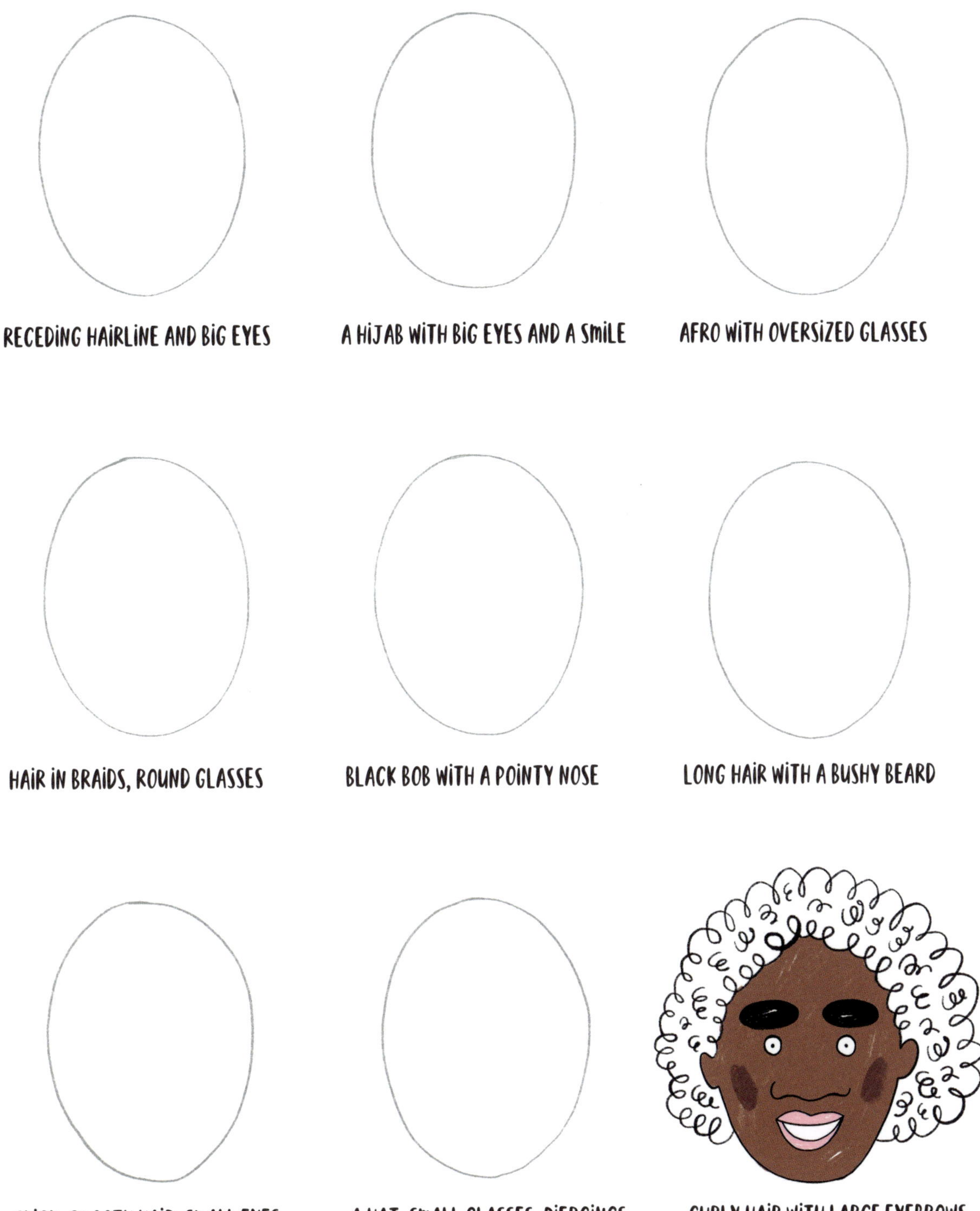

HOW TO DRAW HANDS

Drawing hands can feel daunting and a challenge to master, but if you break them down into their basic anatomical form you can see them as just a series of shapes and lines. Use your non-drawing hand as reference and remember, try to be patient—it just takes practice!

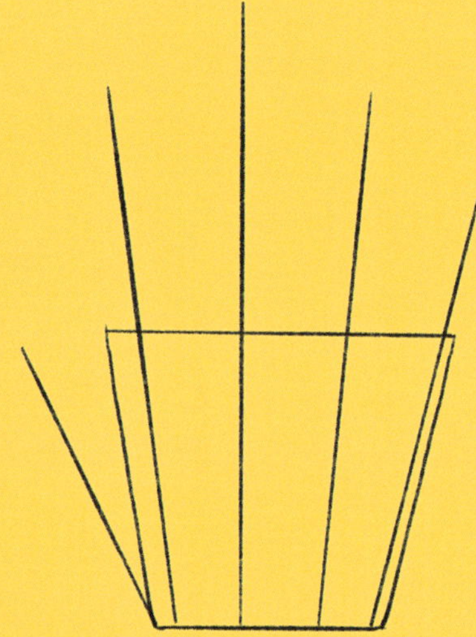

1 In pencil, begin by drawing the palm as a box shape that widens at the top. Then, add five lines extending upward for the fingers.

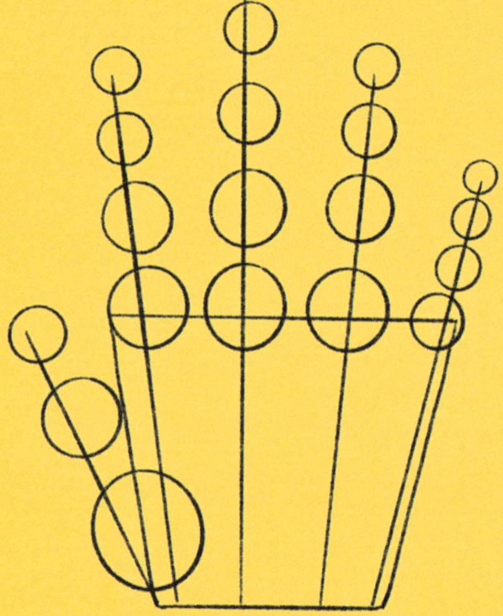

2 Add three circles to each line for the knuckles and a final one for the fingertips. Make each one smaller as they get closer to the fingertip.

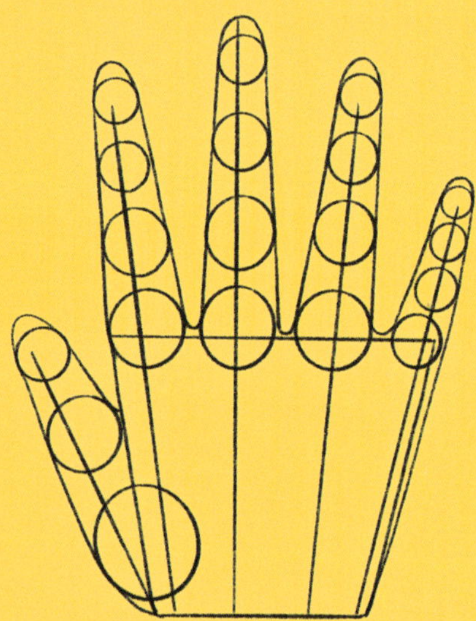

3 Next, connect the circles with lines to form the shape of the fingers. Keep the lines rounded to follow the natural shape of a finger.

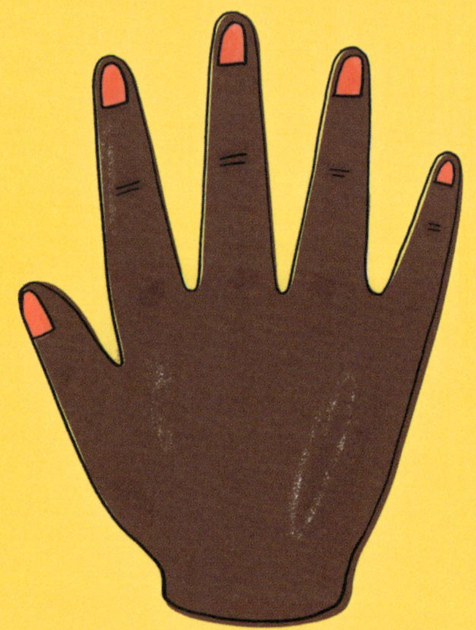

4 With a fineliner, draw over your pencil work, refining the lines and adding in the fingernails, then rub out your pencil lines.

NOW YOU TRY

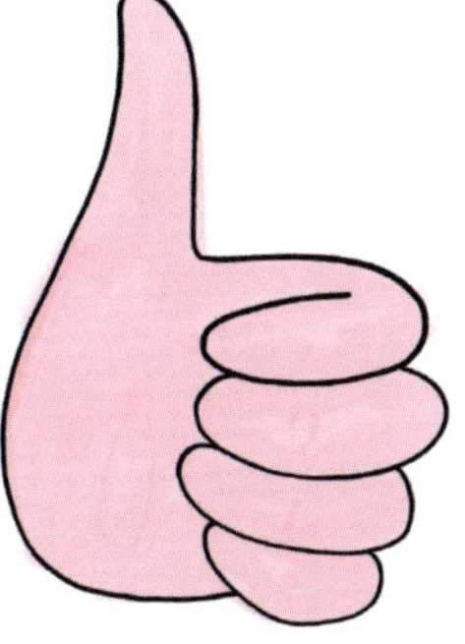

DRAW A FEMALE FIGURE

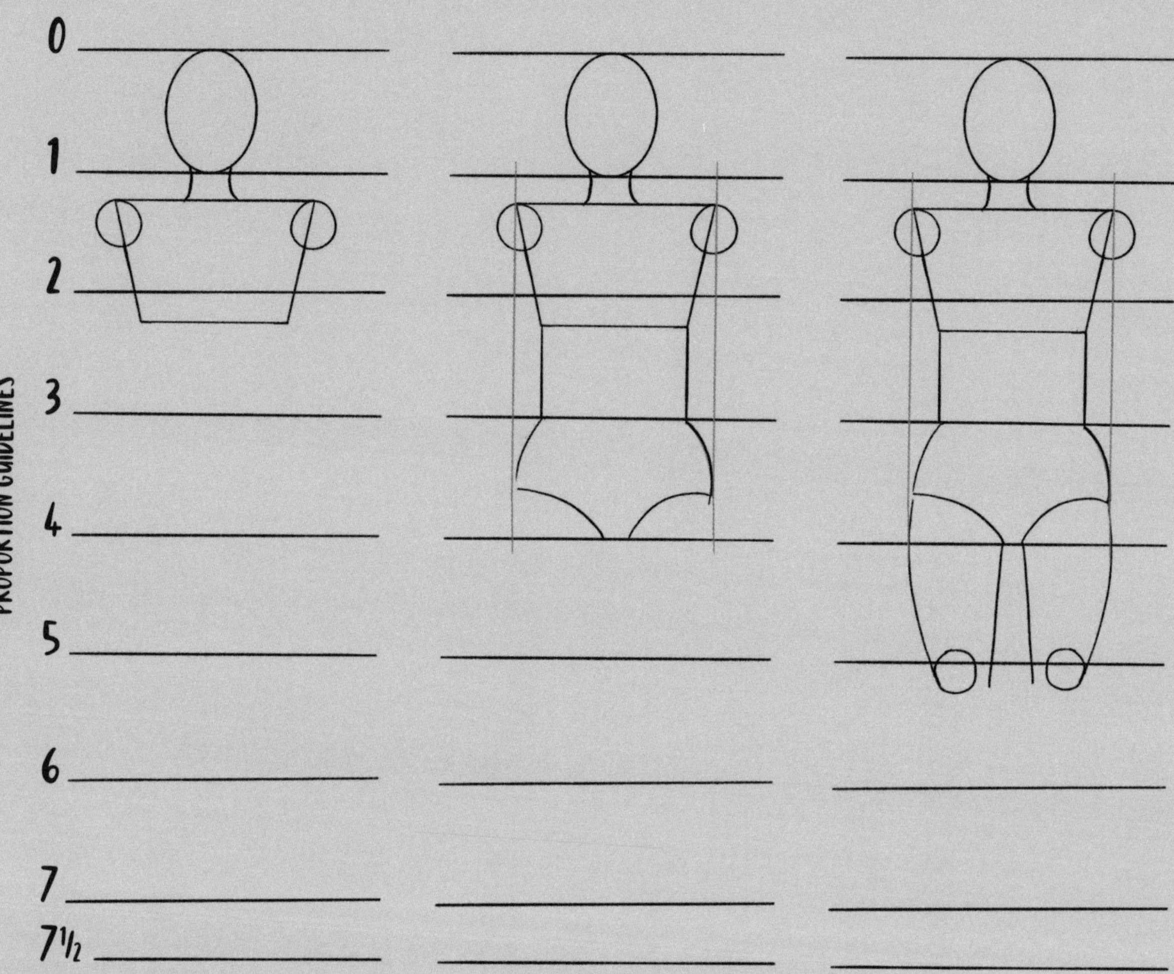

1 In pencil, sketch your character's head. Draw the neck about one-third its length. Then, sketch a square for the chest with the top edges tilting outward. Next, add two circles for the shoulders.

2 Draw a rectangle for the torso. Then, draw the hips, simplifying them as if you were drawing that character's underwear. When drawing the female form, the widest point should line up with the edges of the shoulders.

3 Next, are the thighs. Draw these as rectangles that curve slightly at the outer edges, as shown. Then, add two circles for the knees.

Practice the basics of drawing the human figure with this step-by-step tutorial. Here, we are looking at the female form. The average human body is about seven and a half heads tall, so use this as a guide to help you create a balanced figure proportionally. Align your drawings at the same points on the proportion guidelines, as illustrated below.

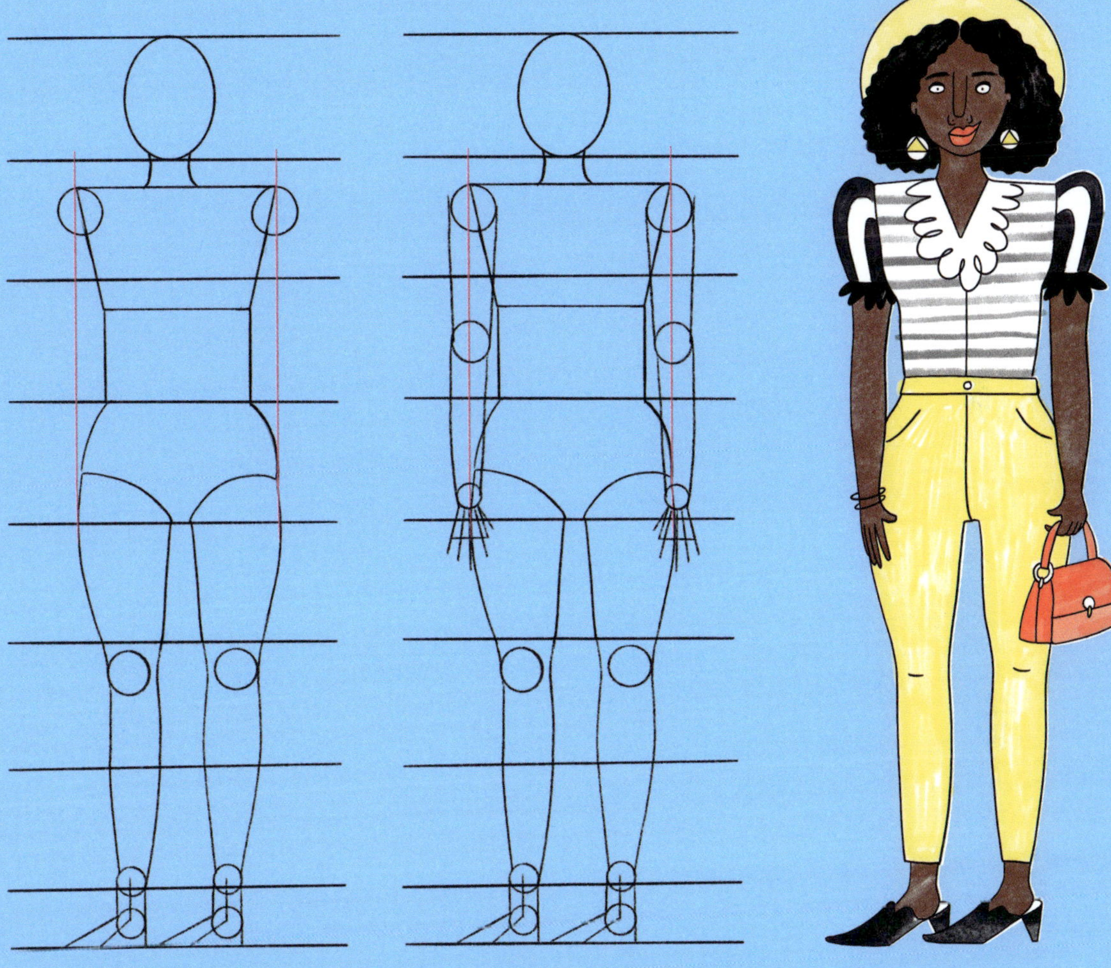

4 For the calves, draw another pair of thinner rectangles that narrow toward the bottom at the ankle. Add circles for ankle joints, then draw the feet.

5 For the upper arms, draw two more rectangles, with circles for the elbows. Add a set of rectangles for the forearms, and circles for the wrists, then draw the hands and fingers.

6 With a fineliner, draw over your pencil work. Have fun adding in the character's details and style. Once the pen has dried, finish by rubbing out your pencil lines.

TURN OVER TO PRACTICE →

PRACTICE WITH THE PROPORTION
GUIDELINES TO START

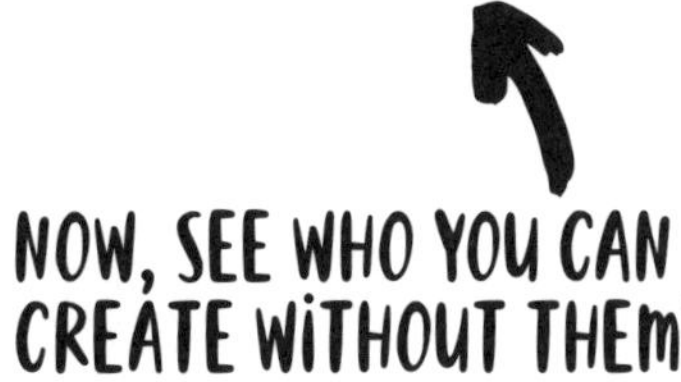
NOW, SEE WHO YOU CAN
CREATE WITHOUT THEM!

SUBCULTURES: PUNK

Fill the remainder of this page with your own punk characters. Dress them in the iconic mohawk hairstyle, tartan and ripped pants, leather jackets, and heavy chains.

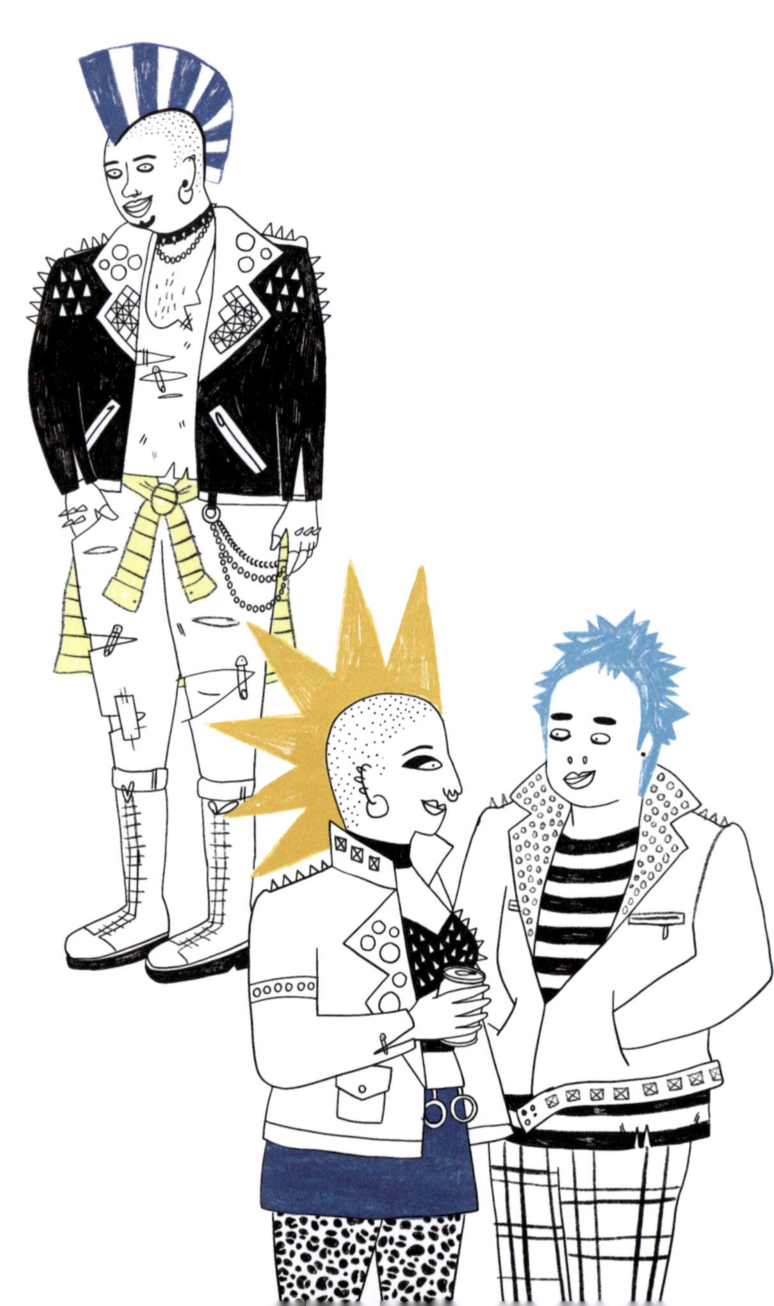

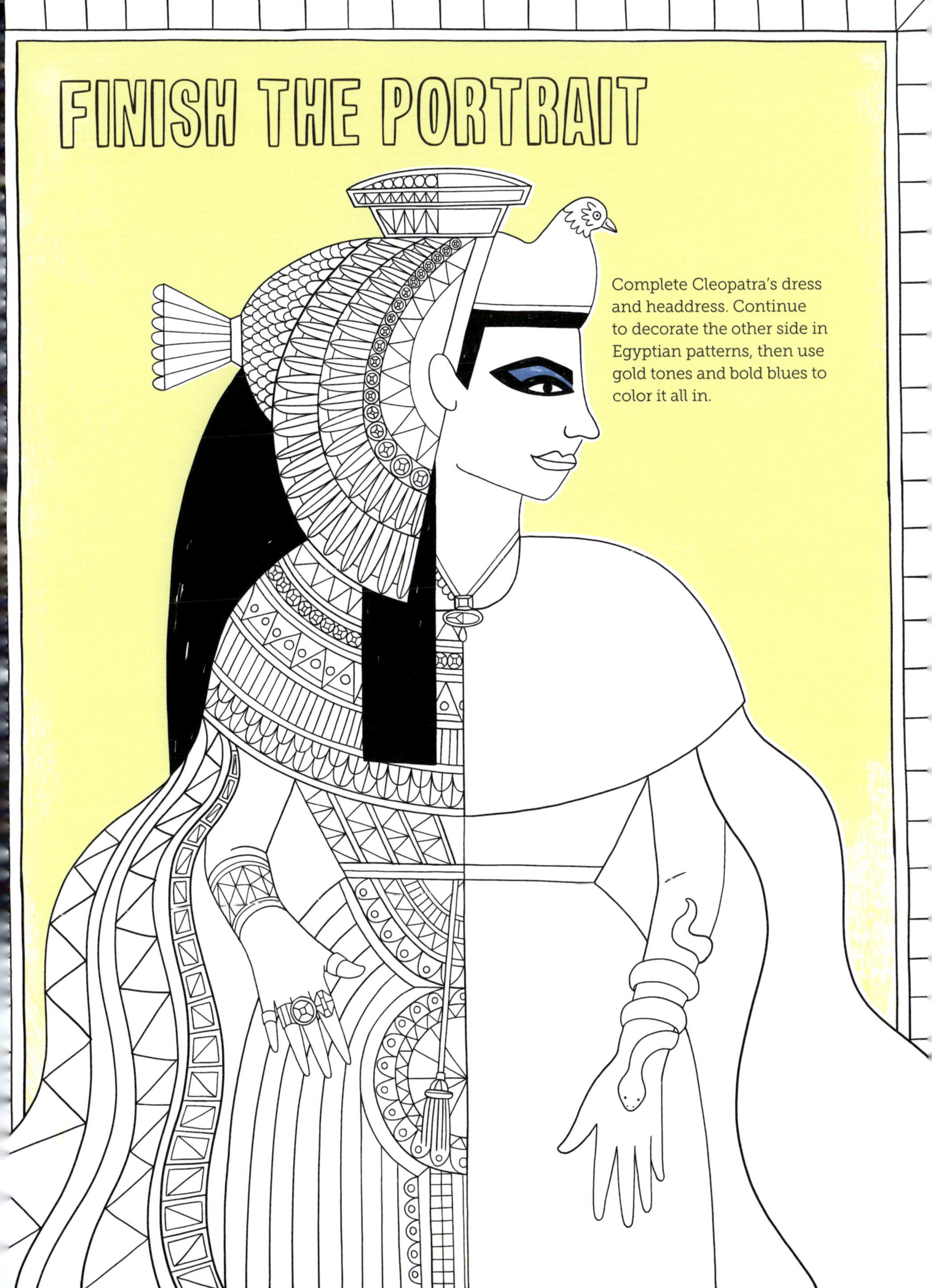
FINISH THE PORTRAIT
Complete Cleopatra's dress and headdress. Continue to decorate the other side in Egyptian patterns, then use gold tones and bold blues to color it all in.

FACIAL FEATURES: MOUTH

The mouth is not only the way we communicate, we also show how we are feeling by its shape and if it's open or closed. Here are some examples of various ways to draw a mouth displaying a happy emotion. Sit next to a mirror and mimic that emotion, then fill in the remaining space below.

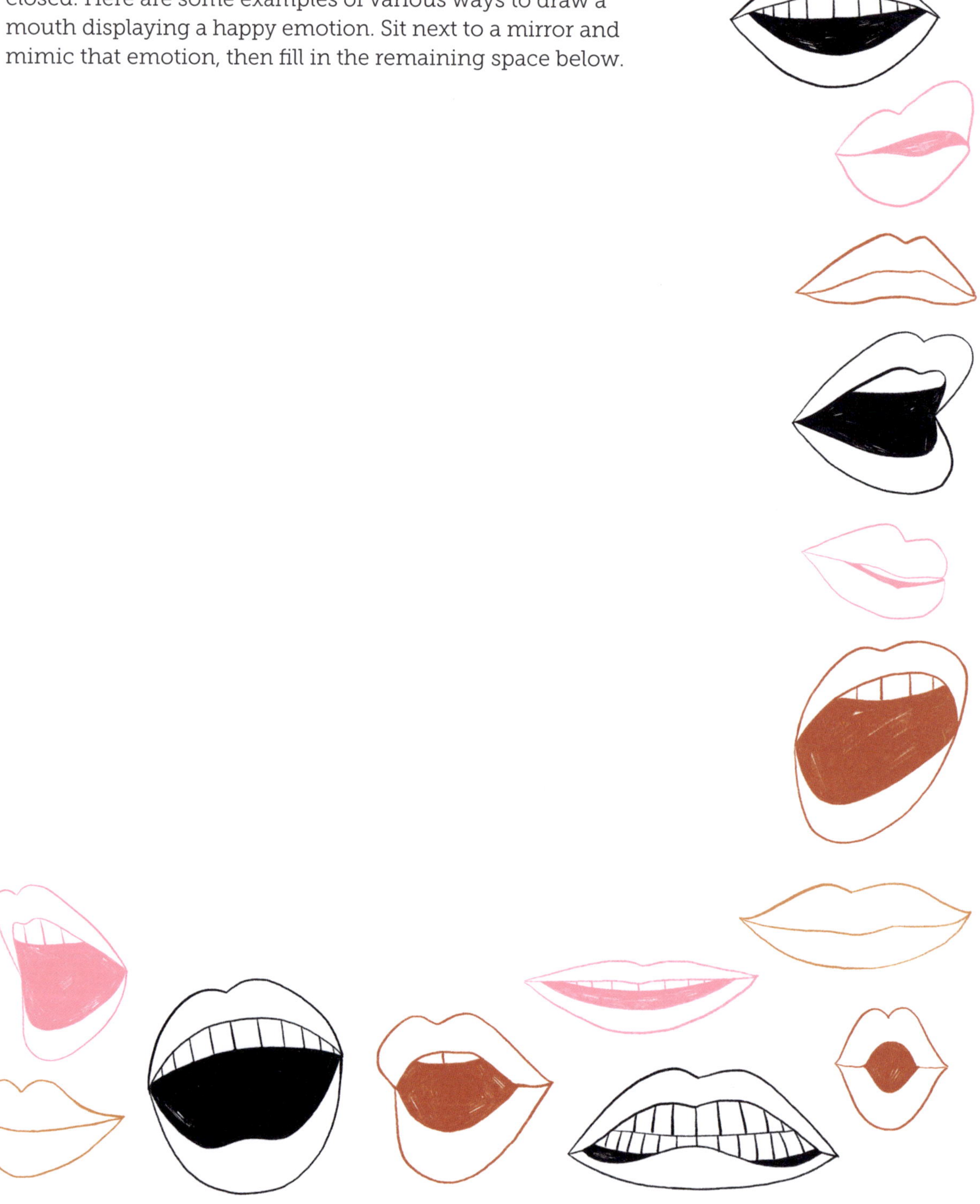

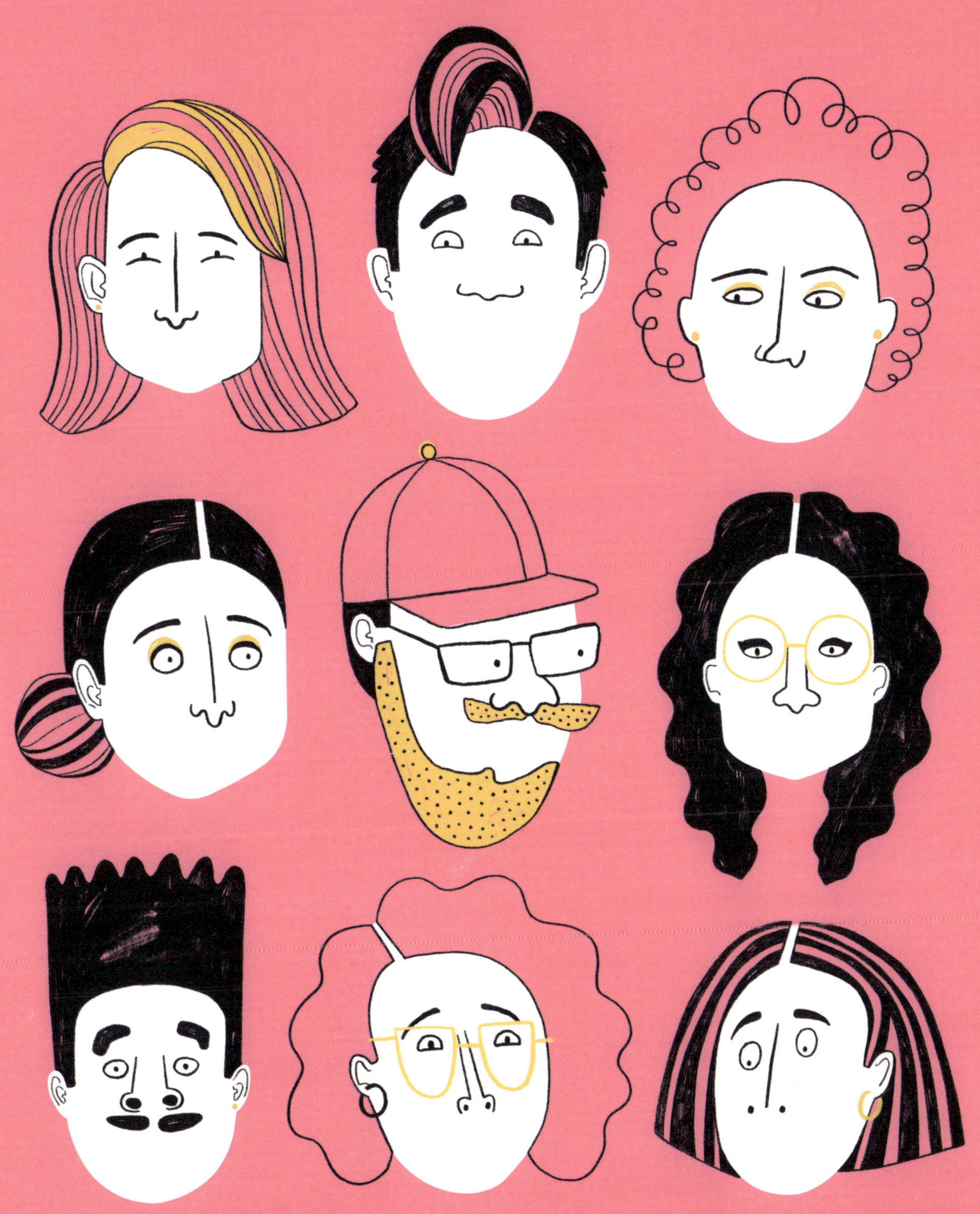

NOW, CHOOSE YOUR FAVORITES AND COMPLETE THESE FACES!

FUN ON THE FERRIS WHEEL

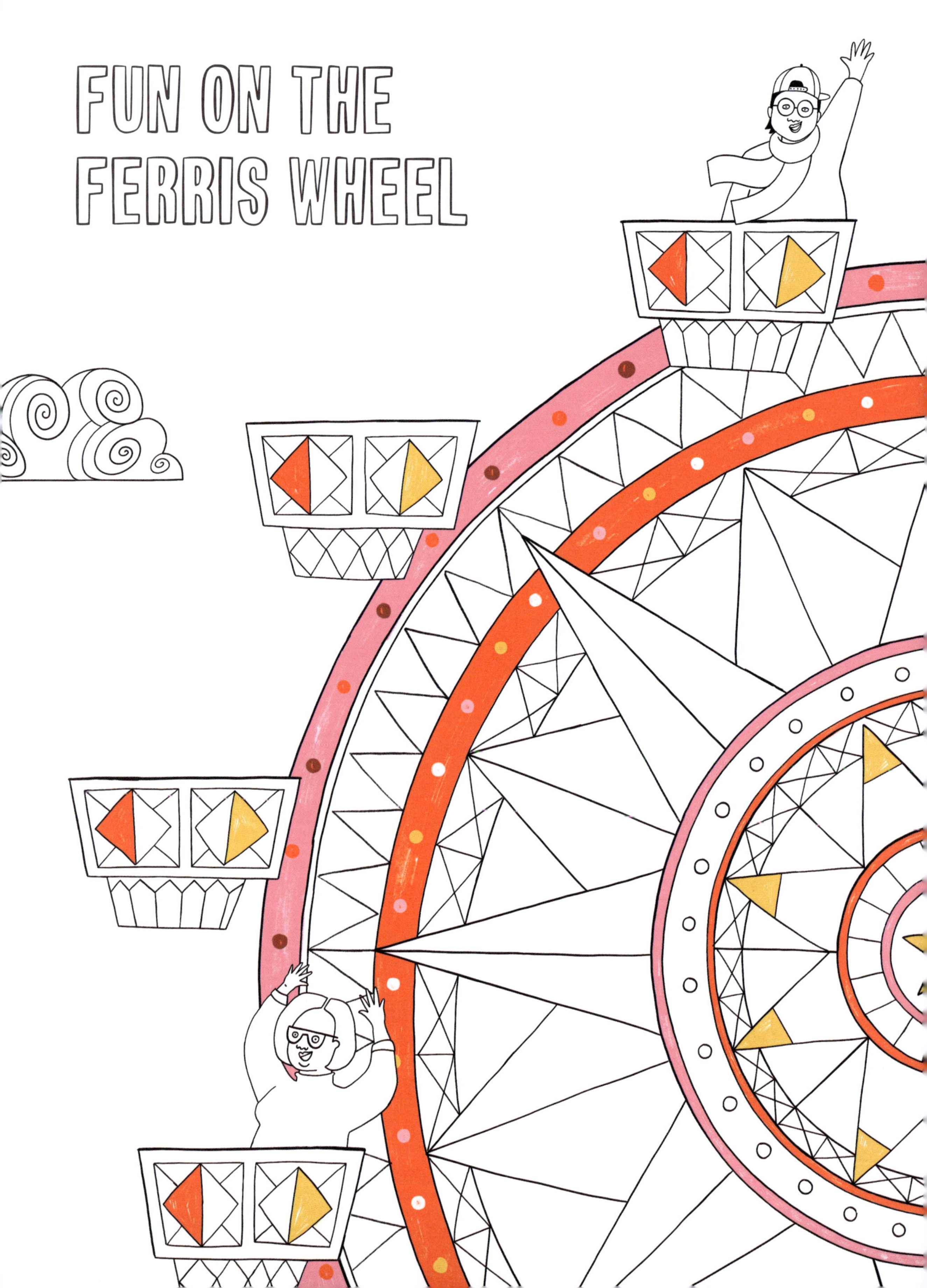

Fill these ferris wheel carts with people having fun at the fairground. Will you add characters on their first date, families on a fun day out, or people there to enjoy the view?

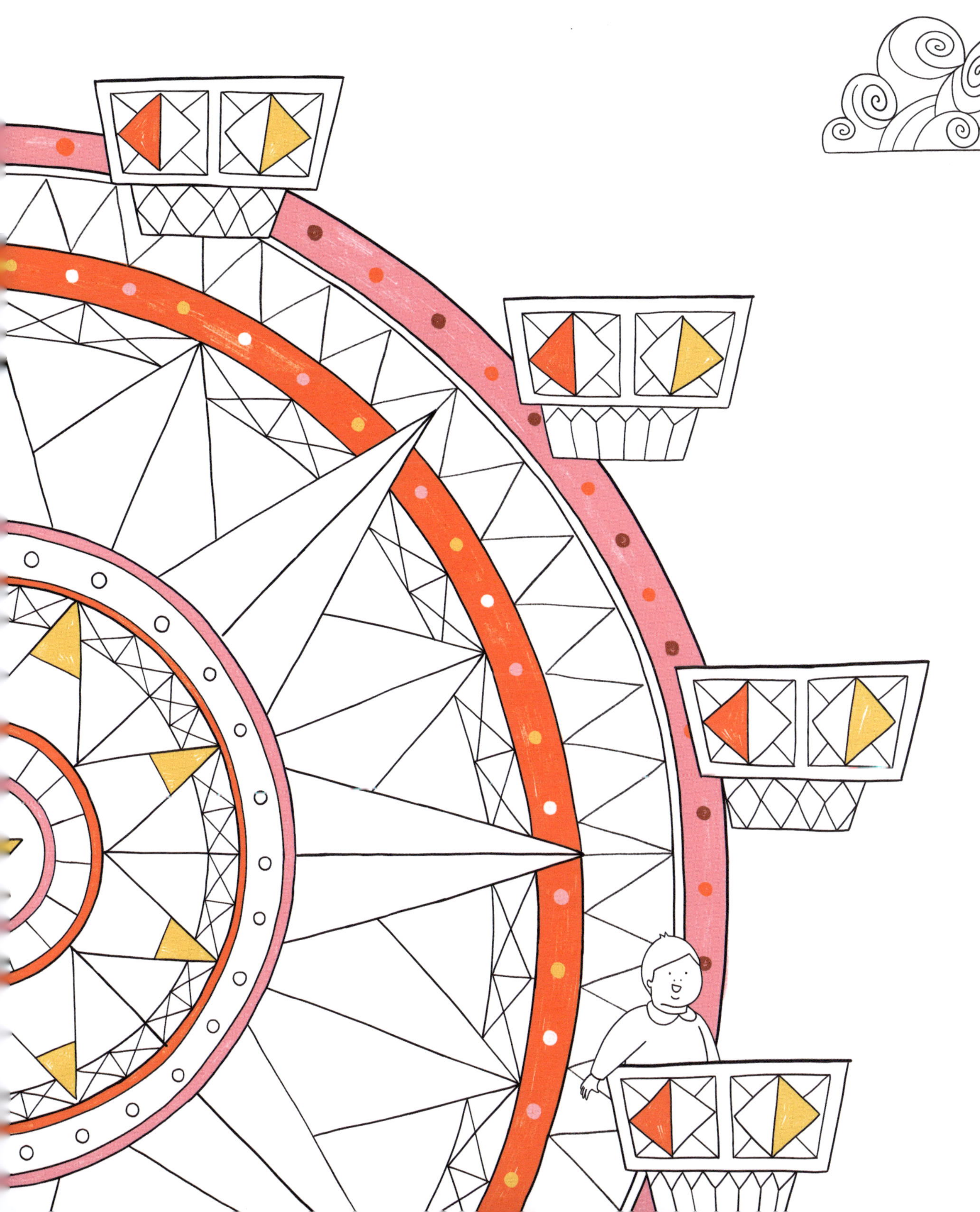

THE SEVEN FACE SHAPES

Fill these boxes with character drawings of the seven main face shapes listed below. Read the descriptions and add these details to your drawings.

OVAL
Curved edges, longer than wide

ROUND
Fuller symmetrical shape

TRIANGLE
Wide jawline and narrow forehead

SQUARE
Wide jawline, symmetrical

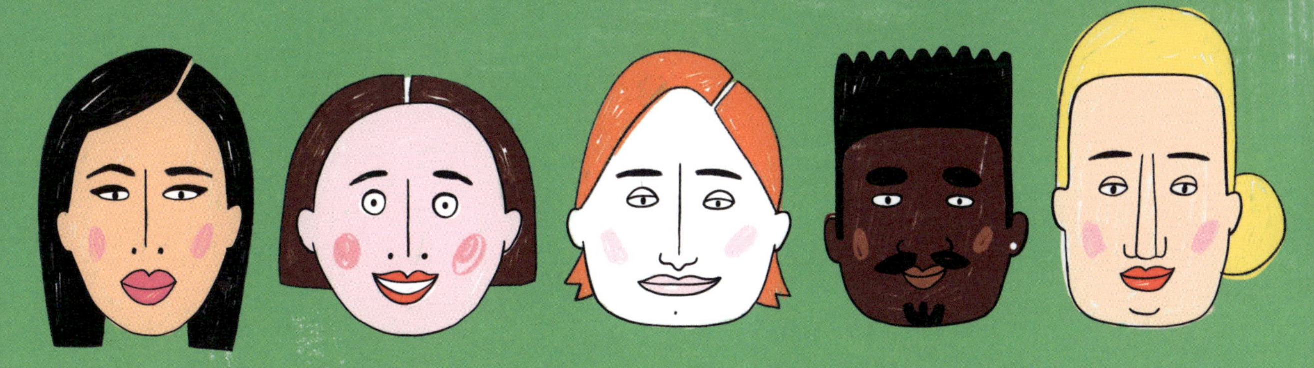

HEART

Narrow chin and a wider forehead

RECTANGLE

Longer face

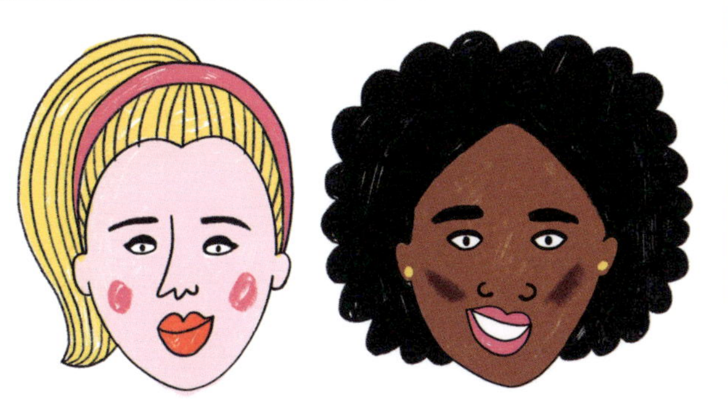

DIAMOND

Narrow chin and forehead, wider at the eyes

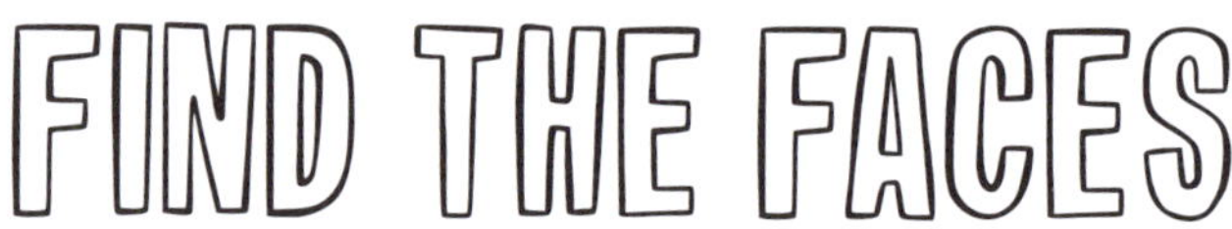

FIND THE FACES

Use your imagination to create different characters from these ink, pastel, and watercolor shapes. Fill the page with a diverse and colorful collection of people!

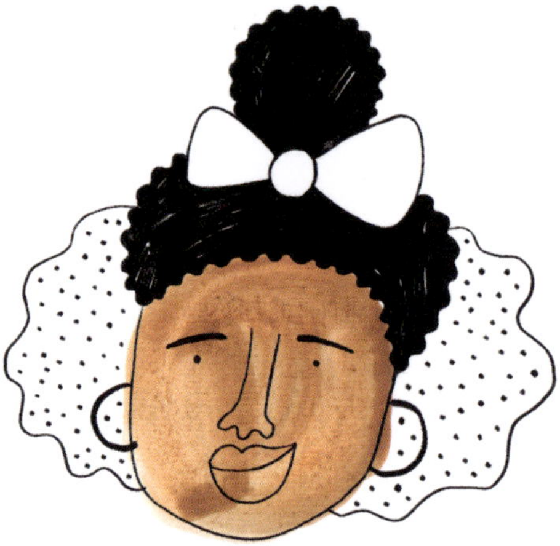

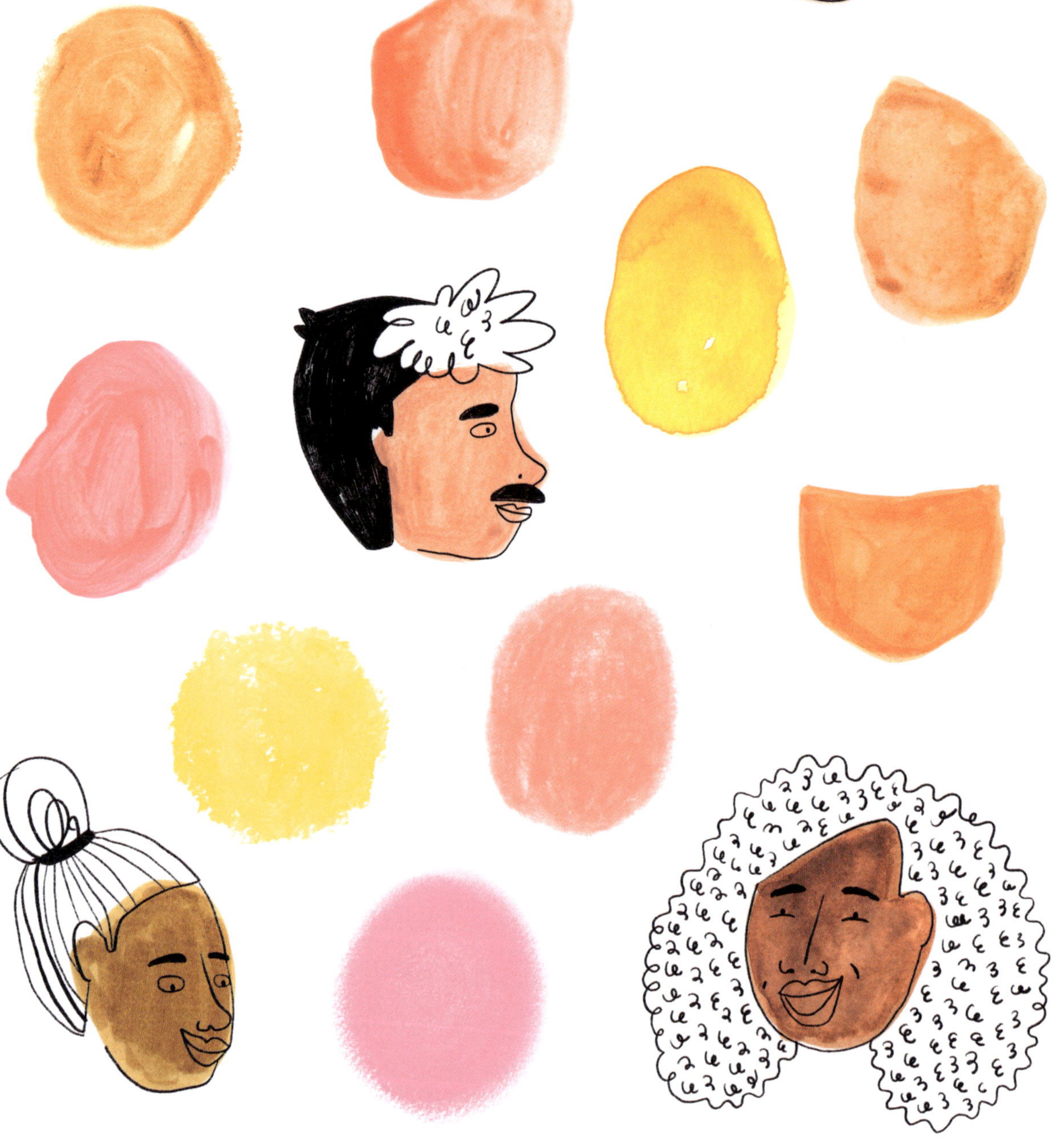

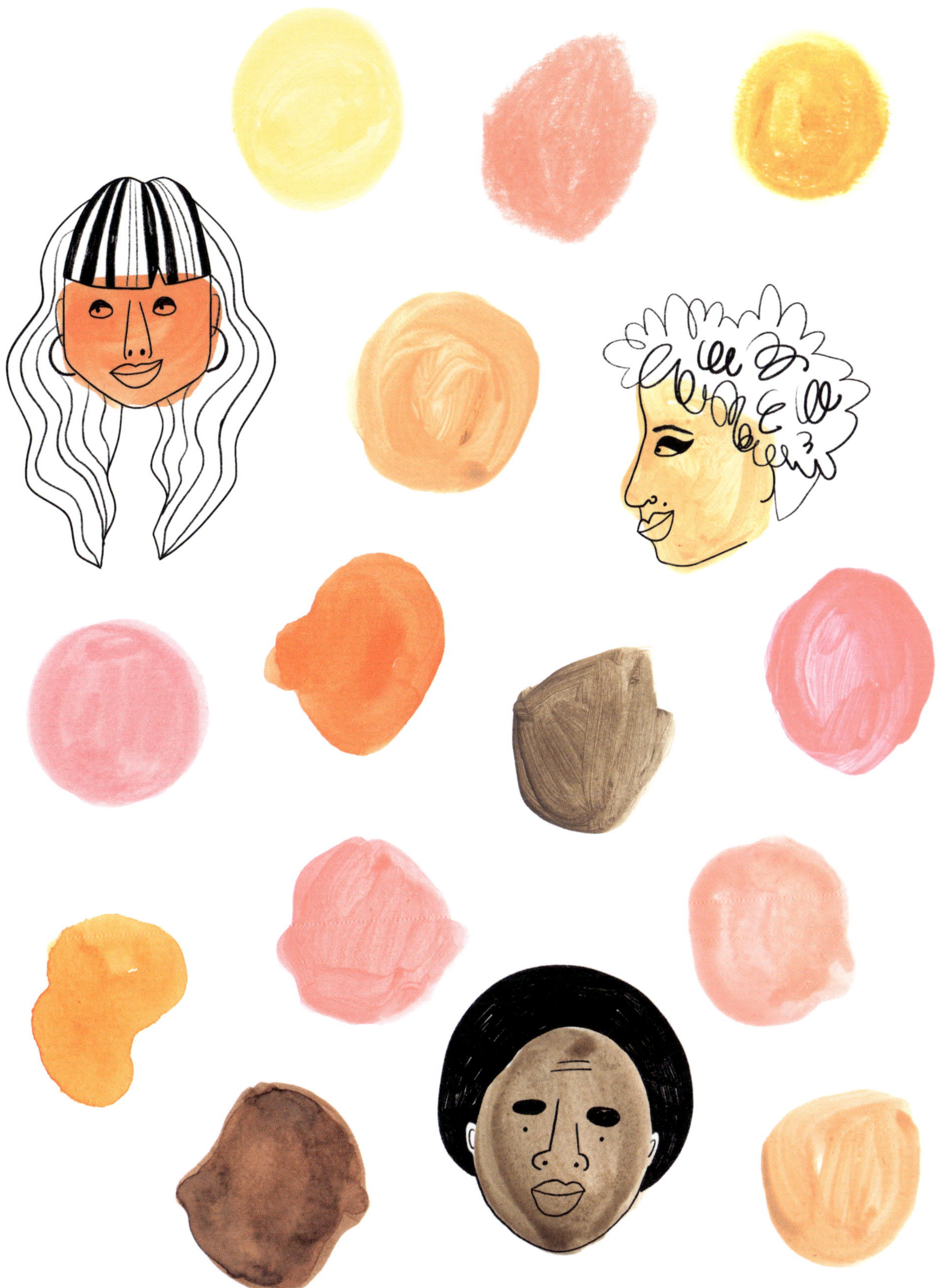

HAT STYLES

Here are a series of prompts for some well-known styles of hats, from the celebratory to the fabulous and the functional. Draw a hat in each corresponding box and a character to go with it. What personality suits which hat?

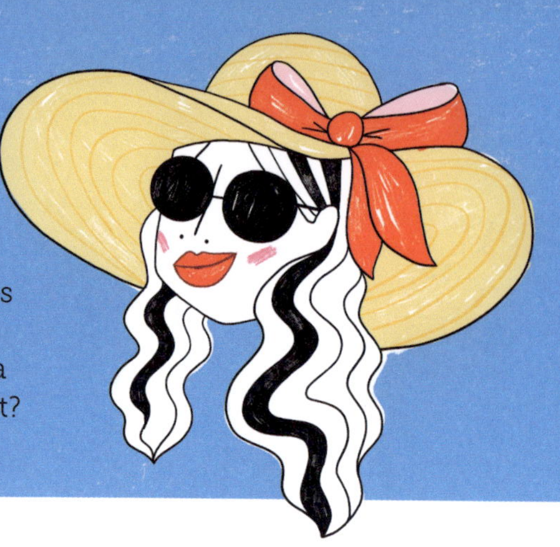

BERET

SUN HAT

FLAT CAP

MORTARBOARD

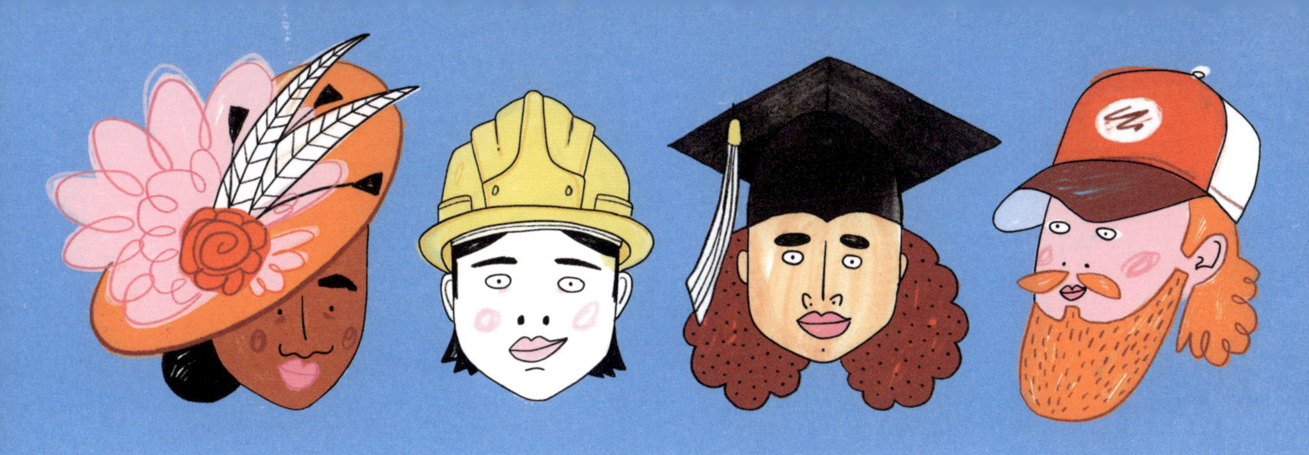

FASCINATOR

TRUCKER

HARD HAT

BOATER

WAITING FOR THE BUS

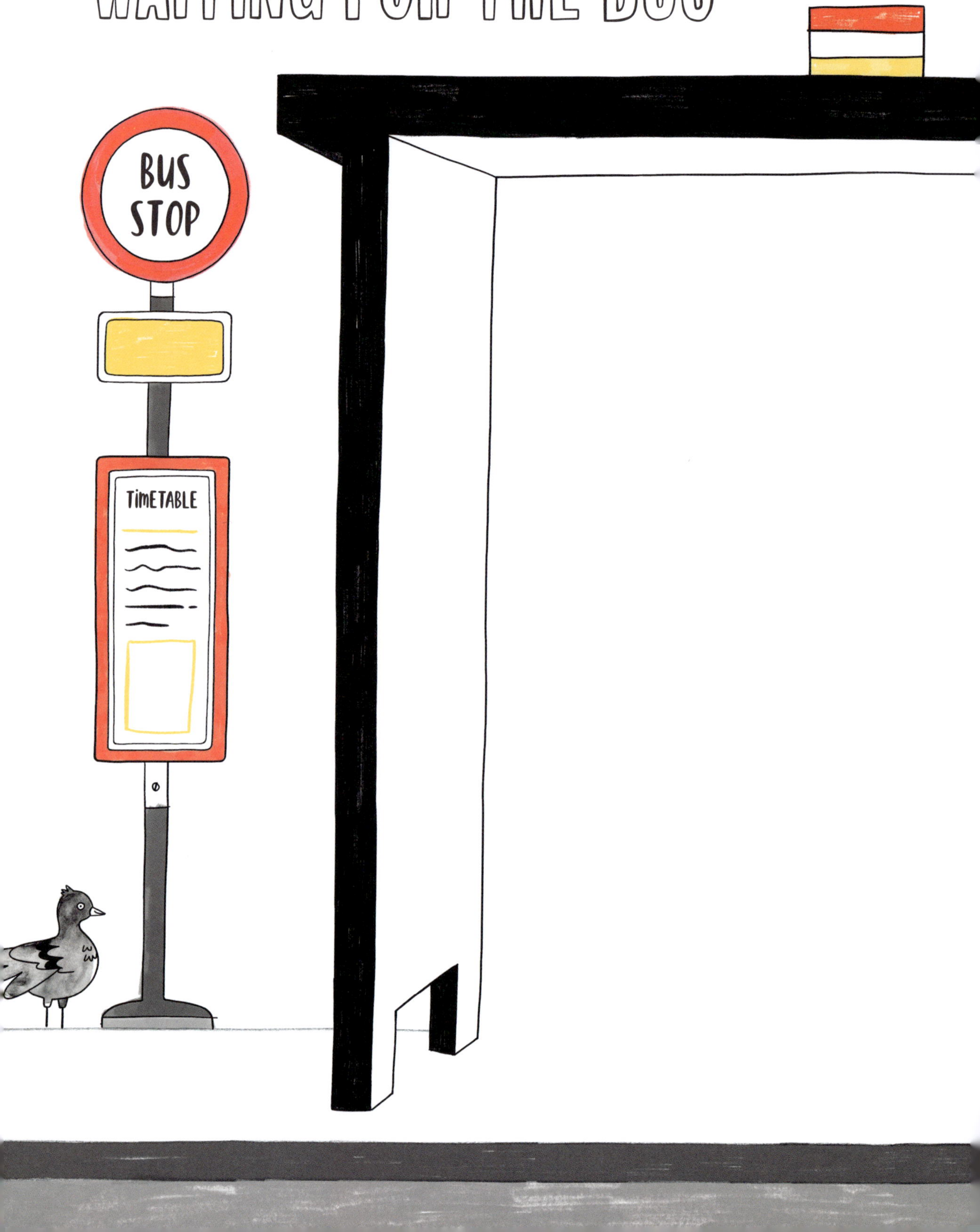

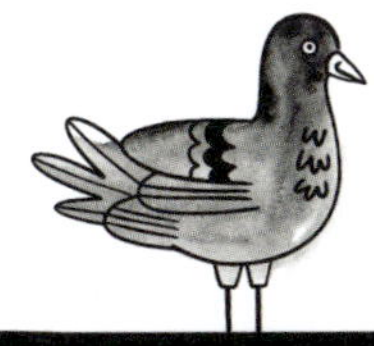

People are waiting at this bus stop for their bus to arrive. Draw more characters. Who do you want to include and where are they going? Have they been shopping or are they on their way to work?

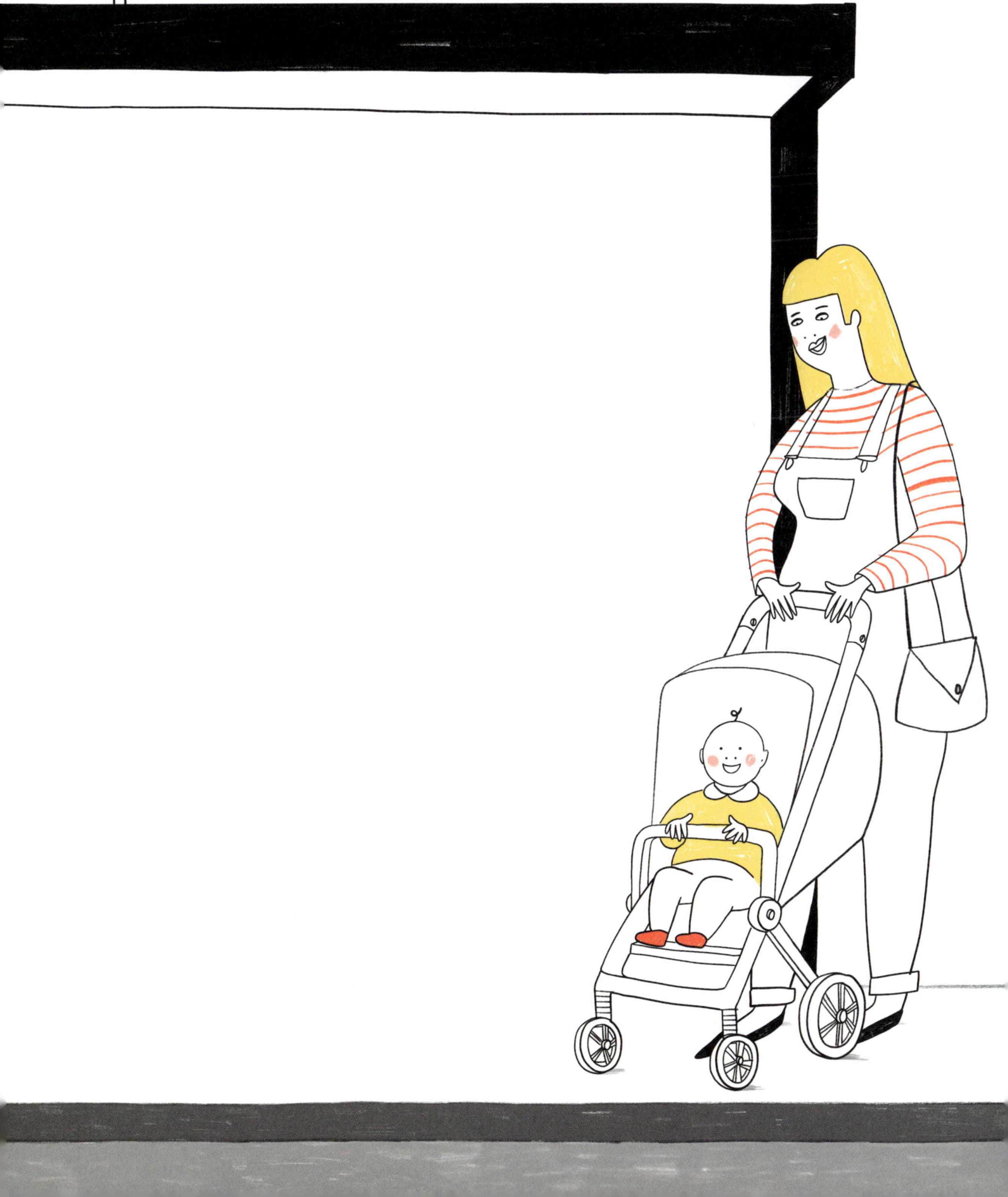

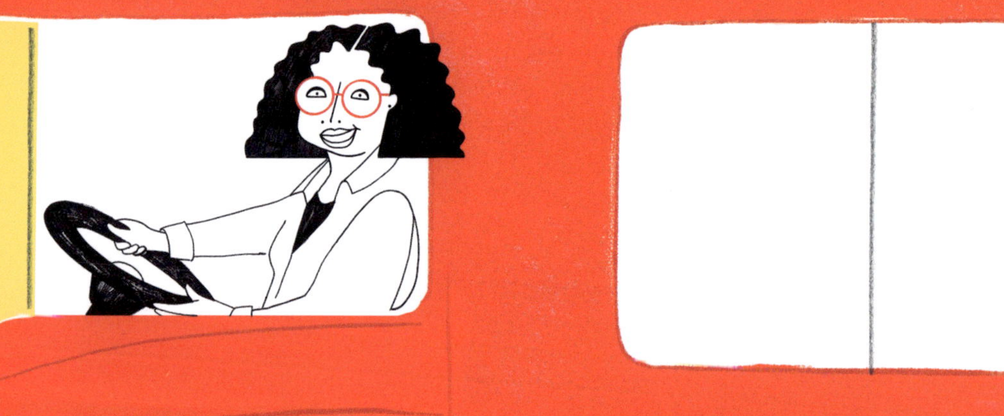

ALL ABOARD!

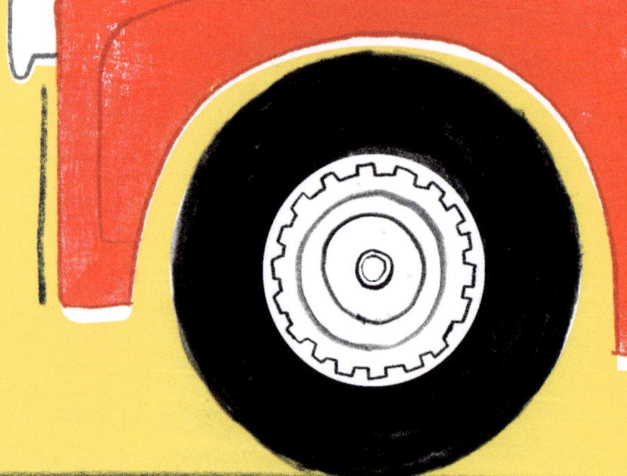

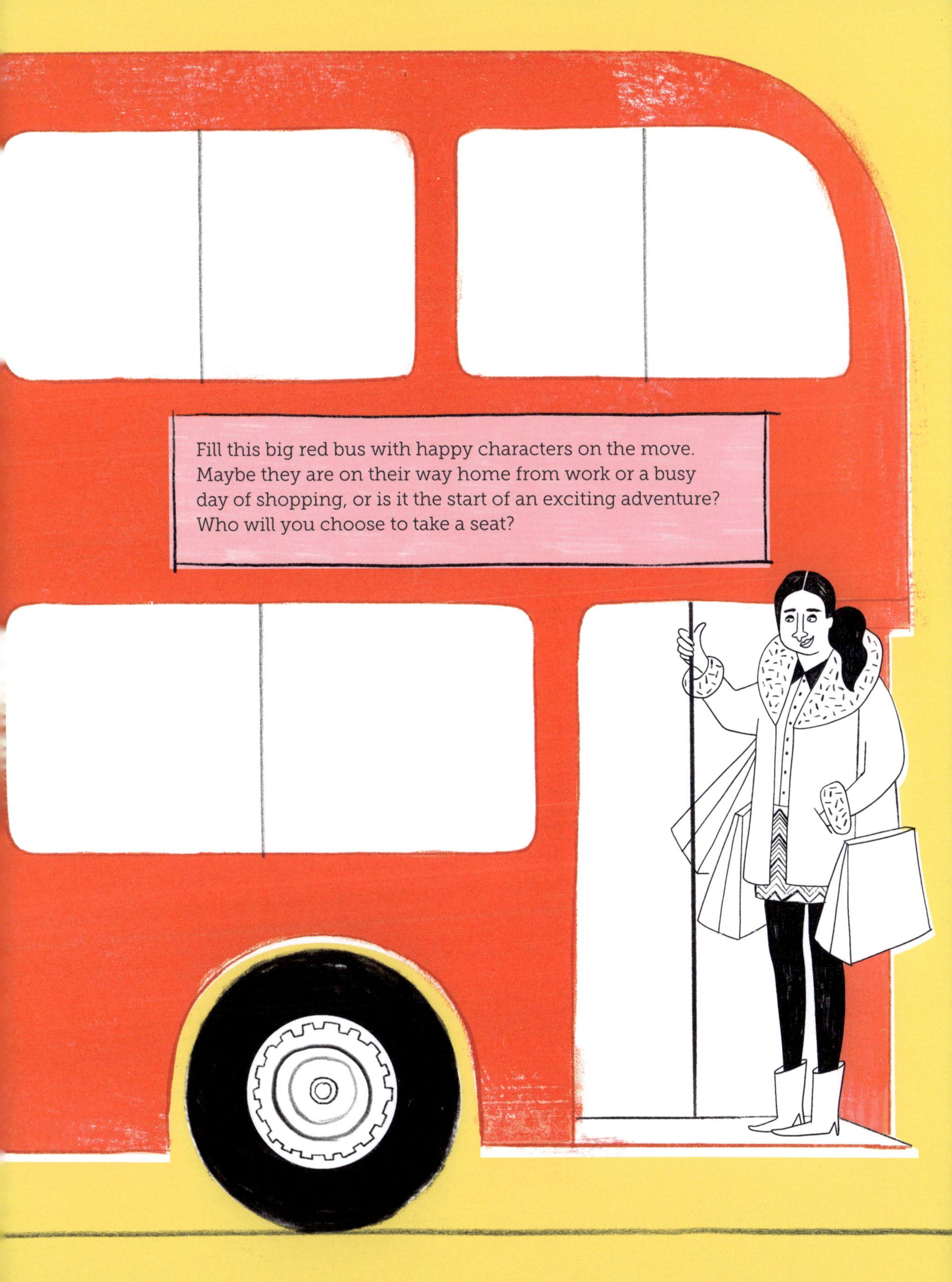

Fill this big red bus with happy characters on the move.
Maybe they are on their way home from work or a busy
day of shopping, or is it the start of an exciting adventure?
Who will you choose to take a seat?

DRAW A MALE FIGURE

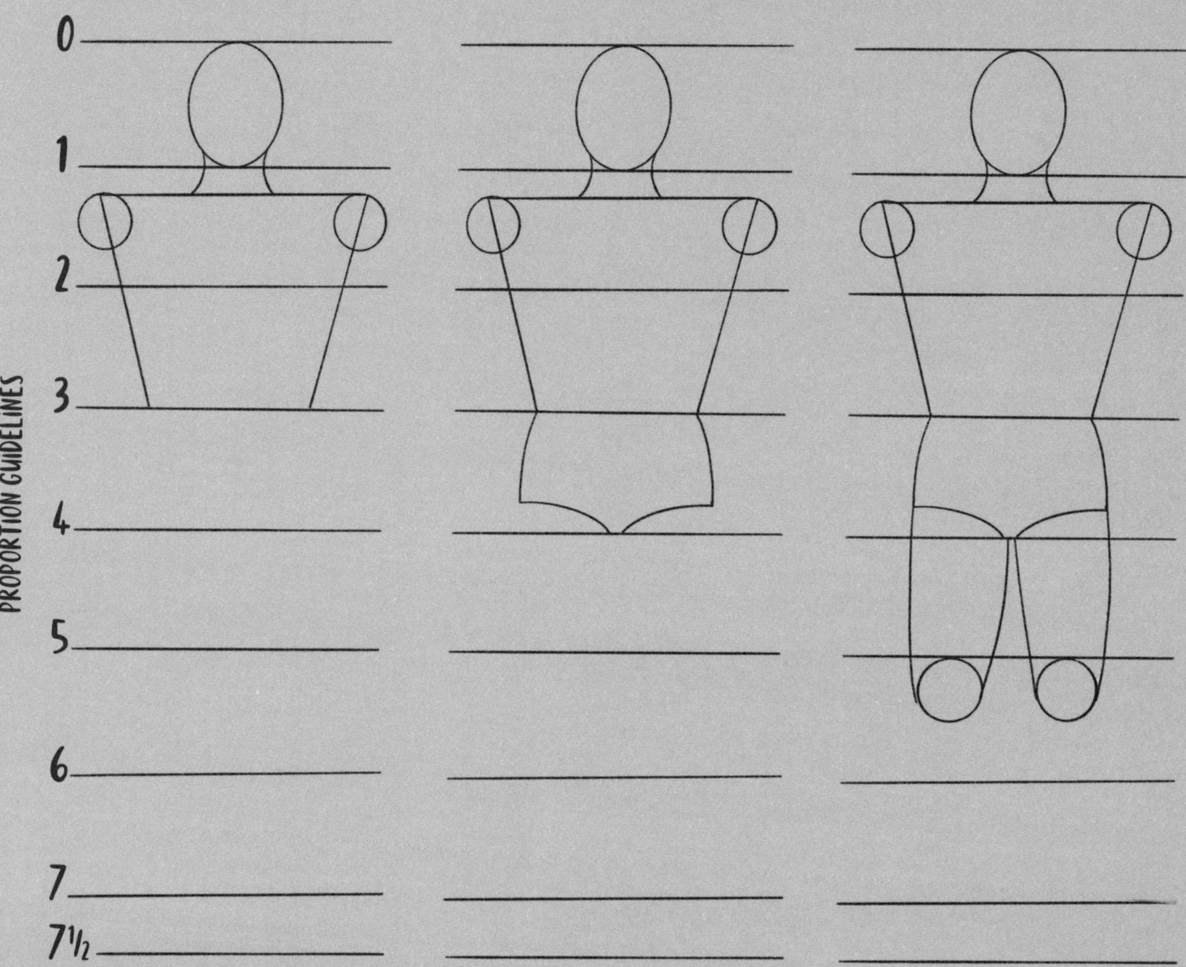

1 In pencil, sketch your character's head and neck. Then, draw a trapezium for the chest and shoulders. The more the top edges tilt outward the broader the shoulders. Add two circles for the shoulder joints.

2 Draw the hips, simplifying the shape as if you were drawing underwear. When drawing the male form, the hips are narrower than when drawing a female body.

3 Next are the thighs. Draw these as rectangles that curve slightly at the outer edges, as shown. Then, add two circles for the knee joints.

Here you will learn the basics of drawing the male form in this step-by-step tutorial. It's similar to drawing the female form, except men's proportions are different, noticeably the shoulder-and-hip width ratio.

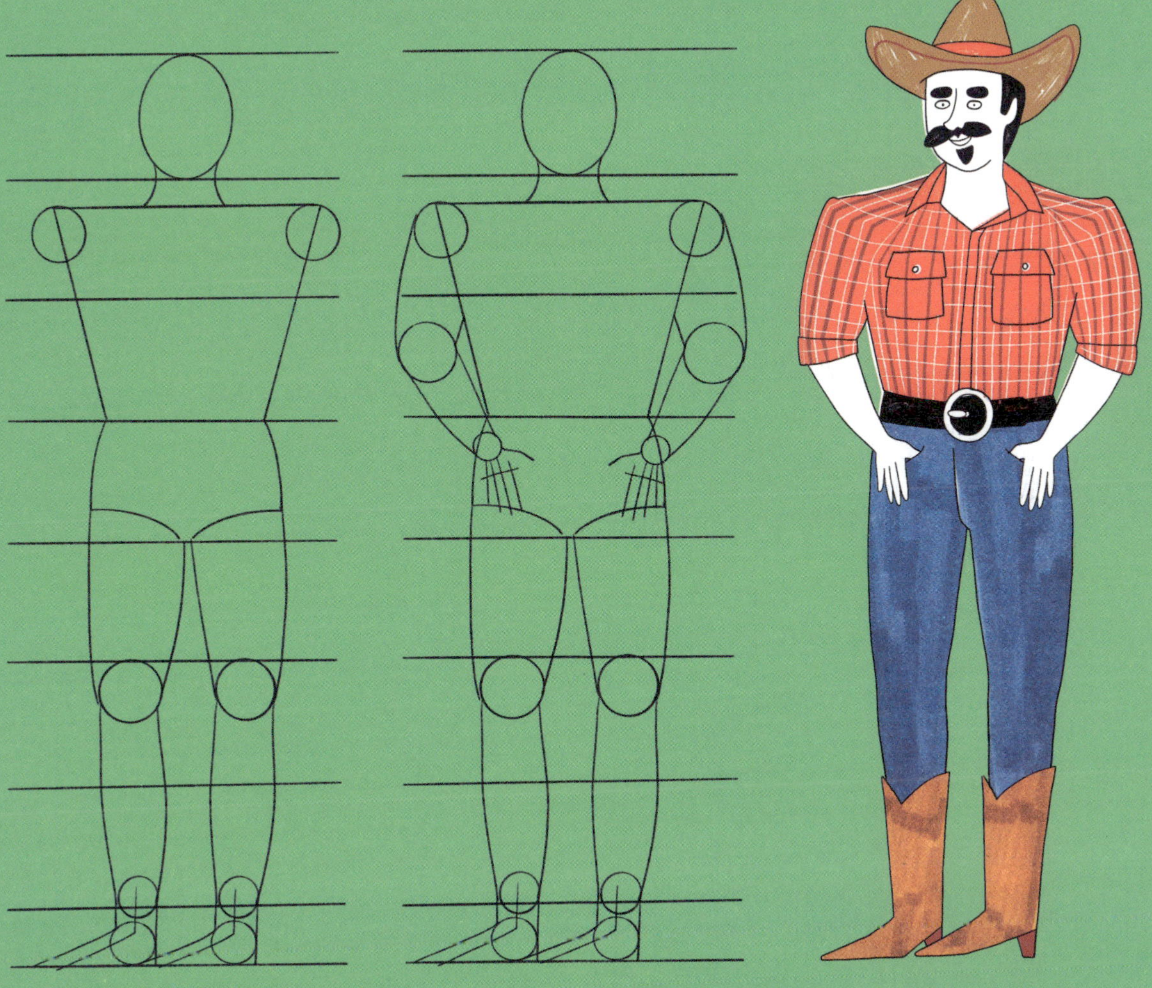

4 For the calves, draw another pair of thinner rectangles that narrow toward the bottom at the ankle. Add circles for ankle joints, then draw the feet. (Refer to the tutorial on how to draw feet if needed.)

5 For the upper arms, draw two more rectangles with circles for the elbows. Add another set of rectangles for the forearms, and circles for the wrists, then draw the hands and fingers.

6 With a fineliner, draw over your pencil work. Have fun adding in the character's details and style. Once the pen has dried, finish by rubbing out your pencil lines and color in!

TURN OVER TO PRACTICE →

PRACTICE WITH THE PROPORTION
GUIDELINES TO START

NOW, SEE WHO YOU CAN
CREATE WITHOUT THEM!

WHO'S HOME?

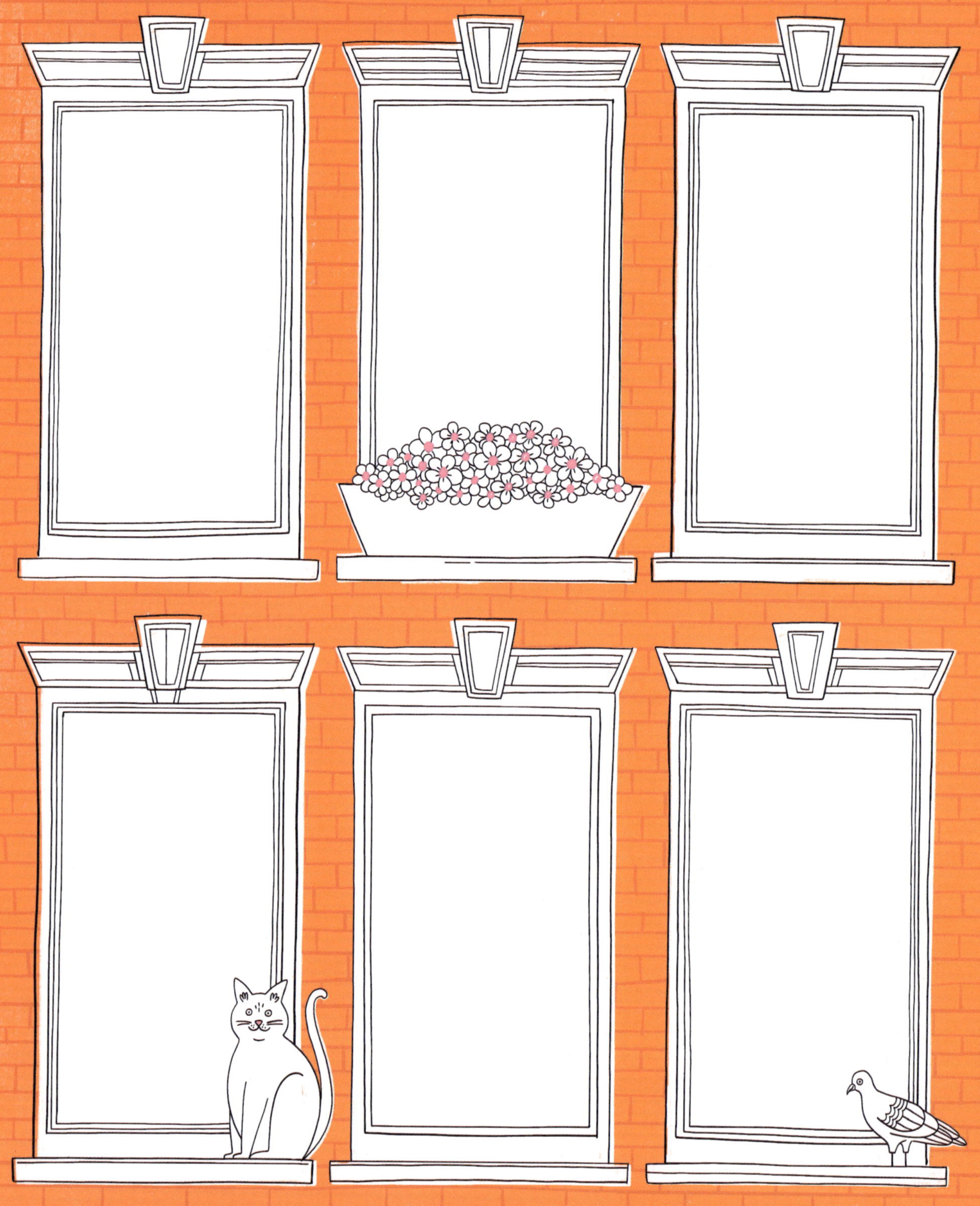

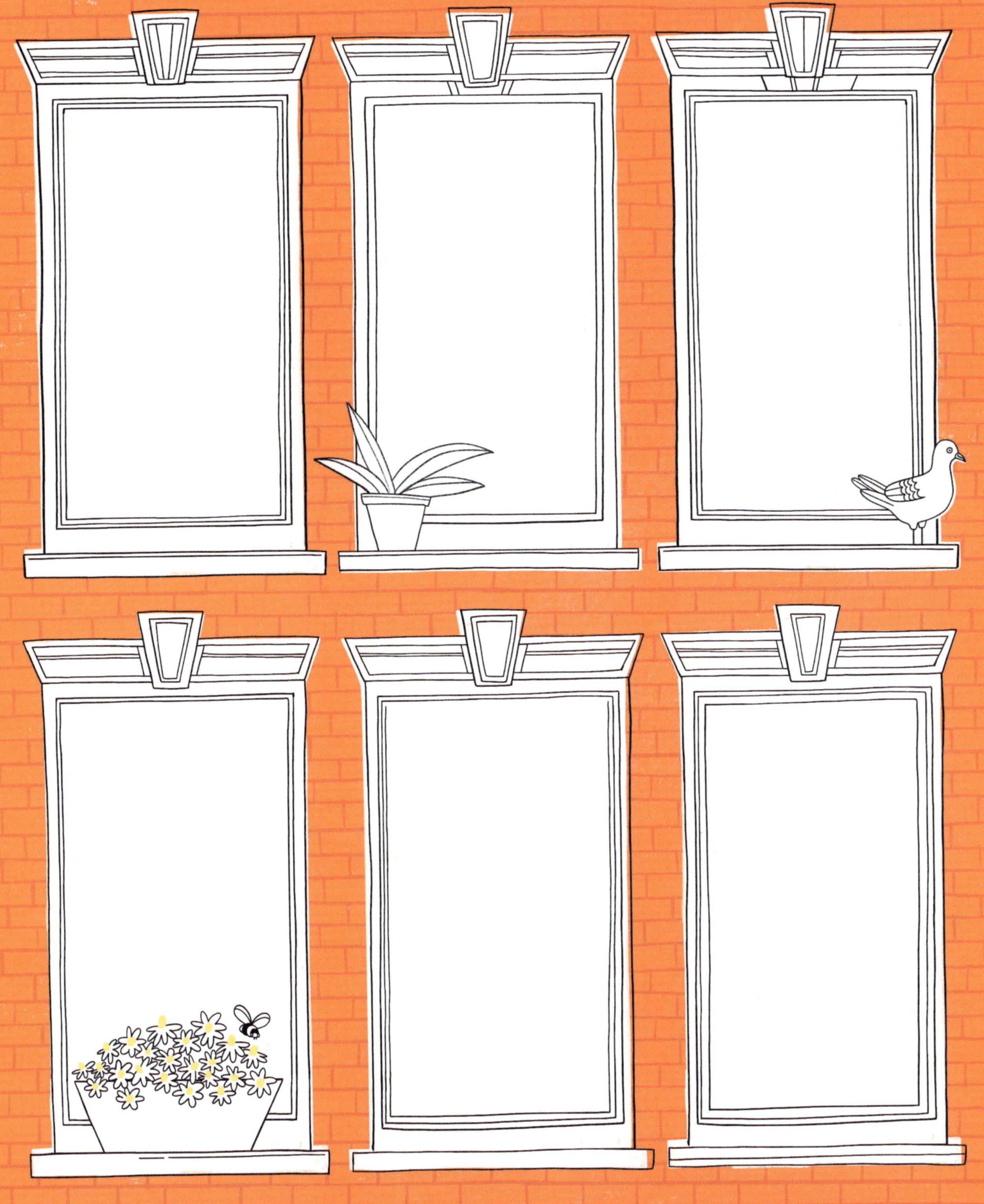

Fill these apartment windows with people in their homes. Are they in the kitchen cooking or in the lounge watching TV? Maybe they're watering their window boxes? Who will be home, and what will they be doing?

FASHION FOR ALL SIZES

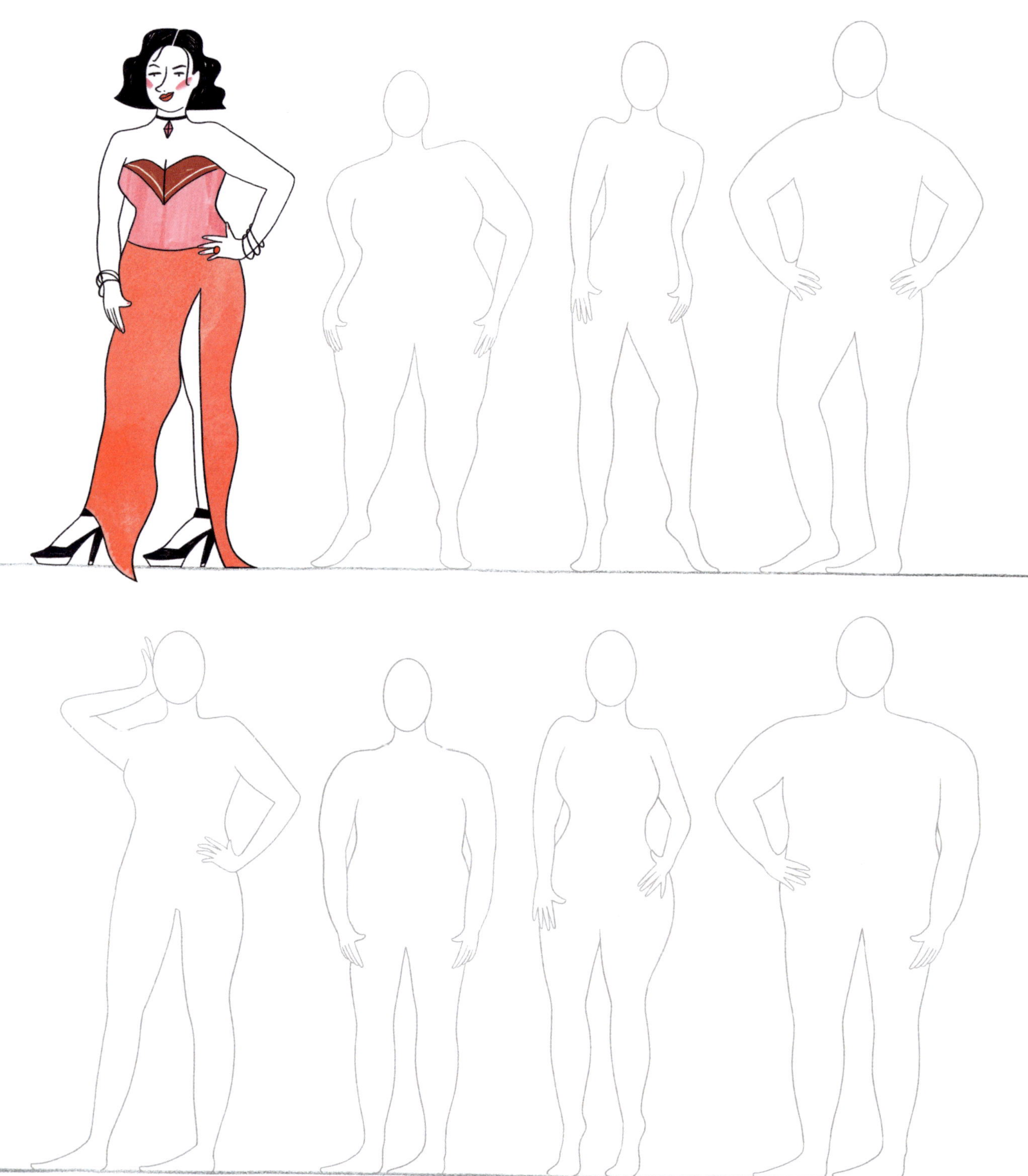

Bodies come in all shapes and sizes. Using these outlines, create characters and dress them in clothes to suit their shape. You can play with tone to show how the fabric falls or explore textures, such as using pastels for wool.

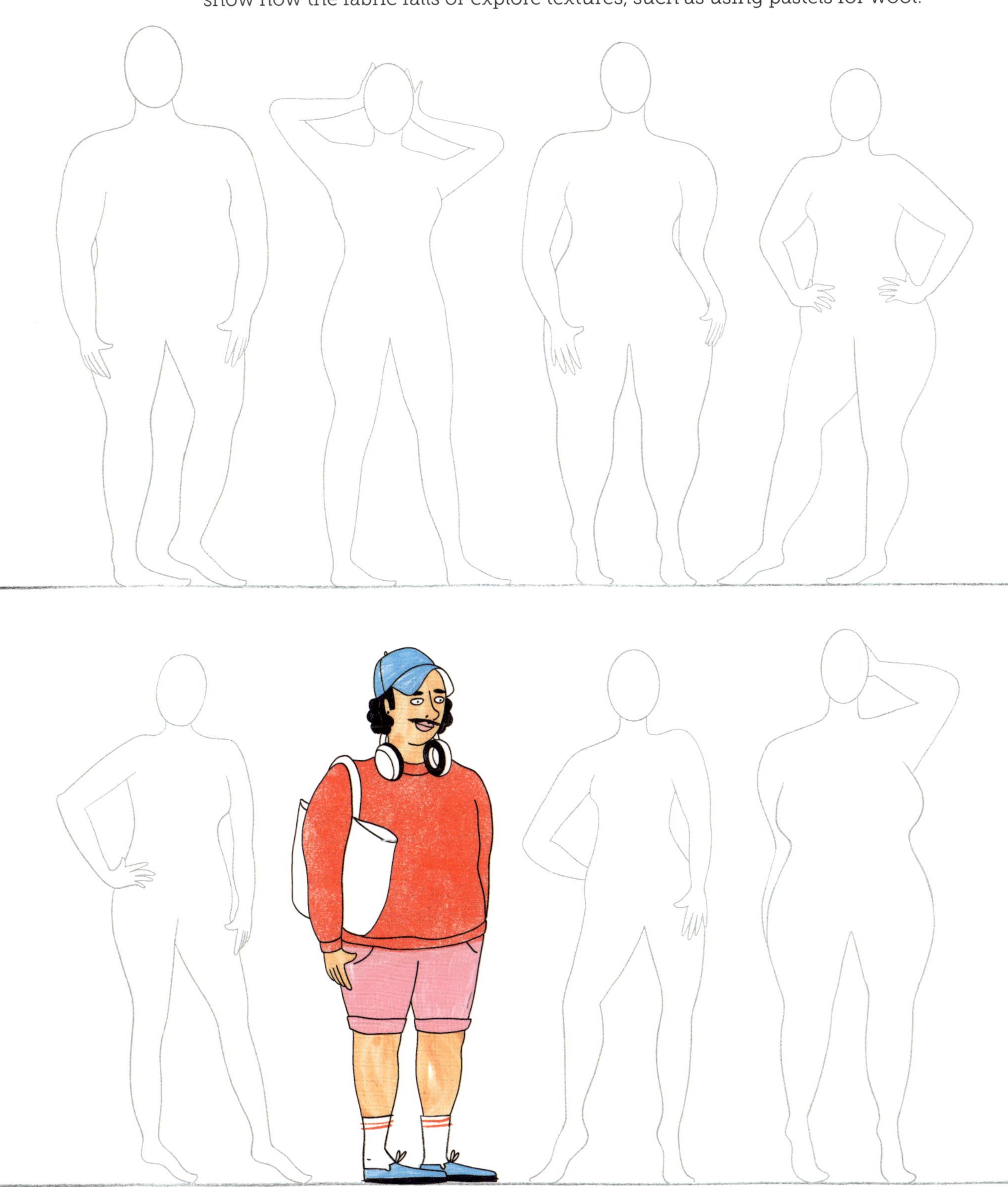

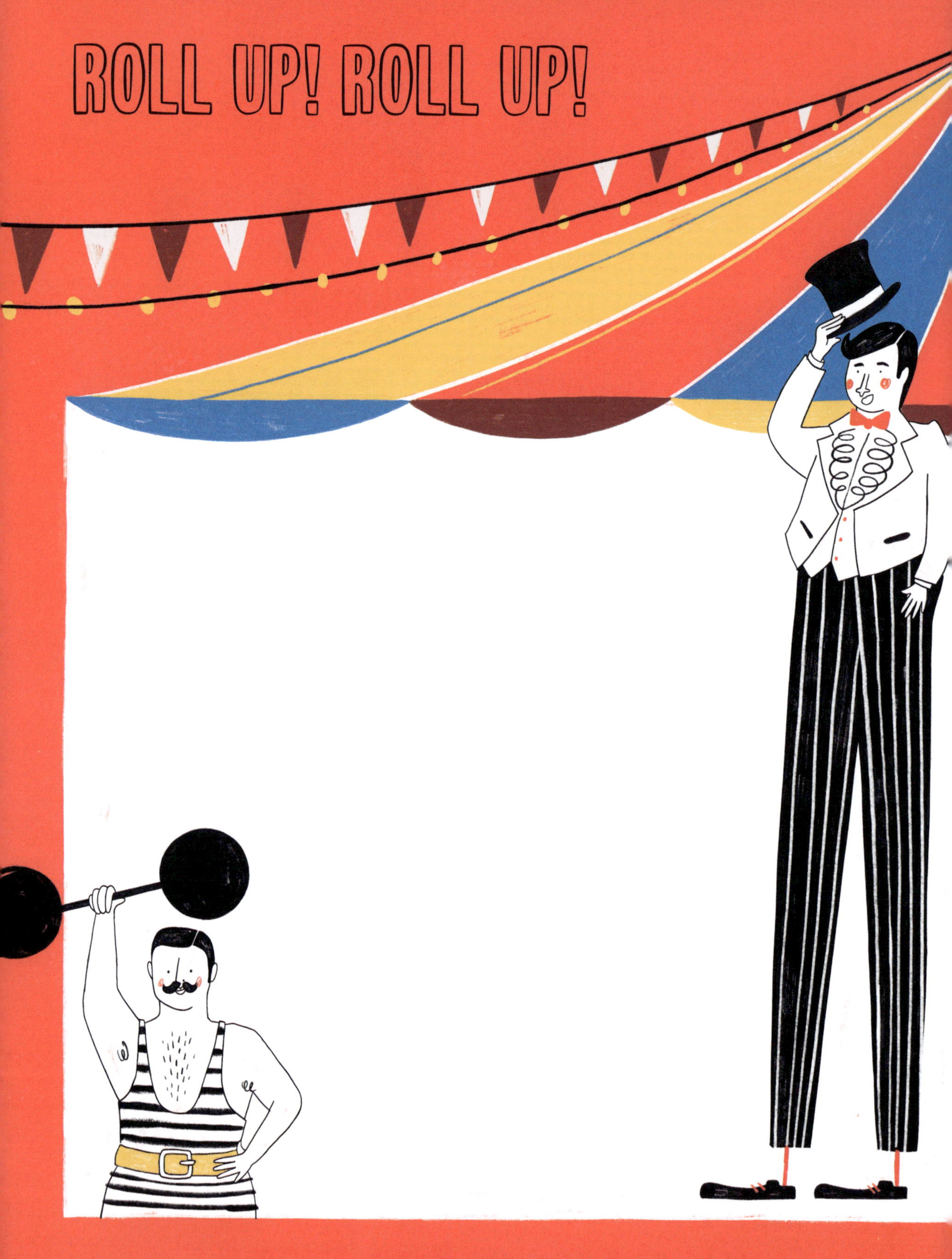
ROLL UP! ROLL UP!

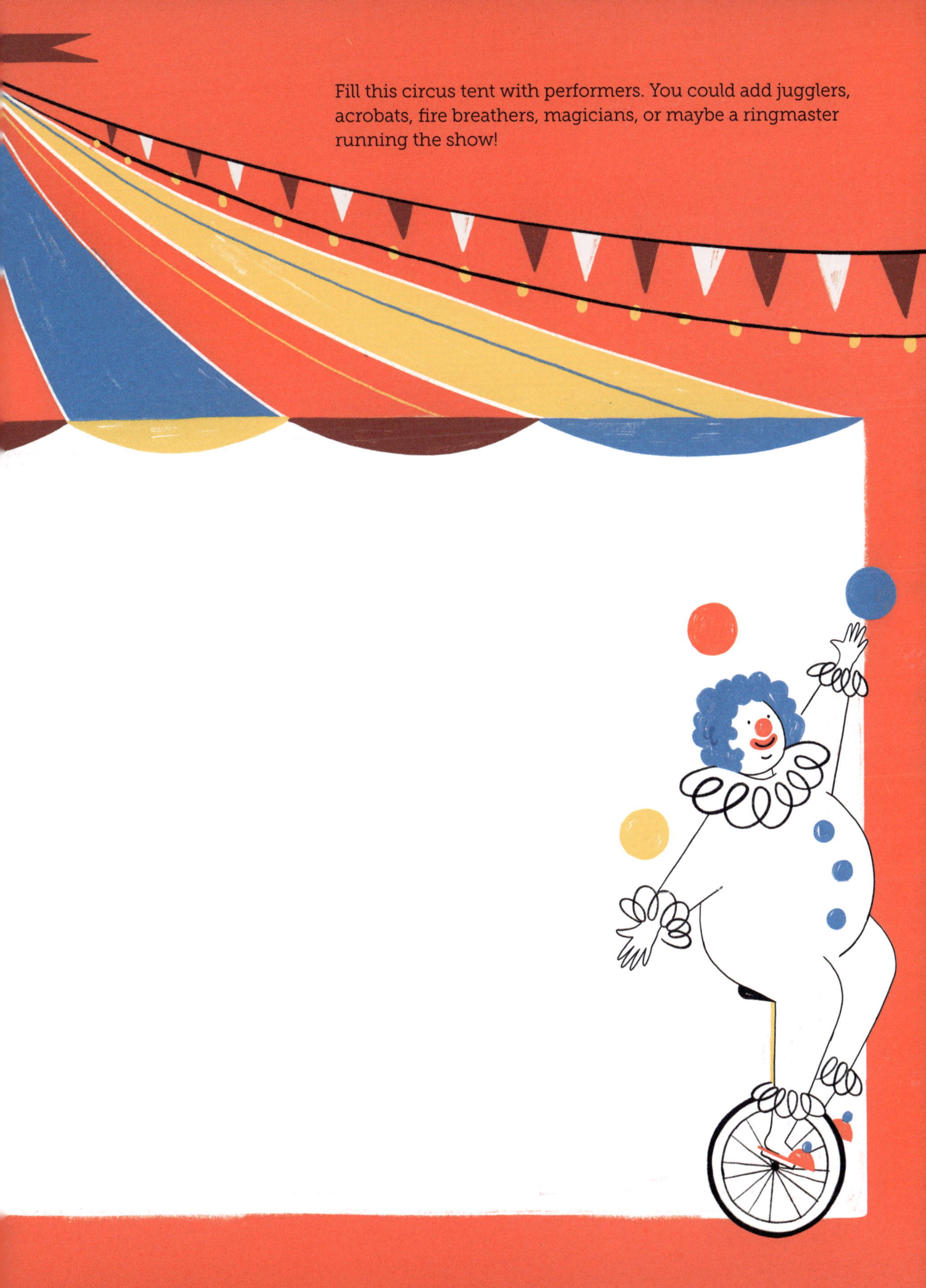

Fill this circus tent with performers. You could add jugglers, acrobats, fire breathers, magicians, or maybe a ringmaster running the show!

SUBCULTURES: MODS

Add more characters to this mod crew gathered around their iconic scooter. Popular in 1960s Britain, they were known for wearing slim-fitting tailormade suits, parka jackets, and short straight dresses with Mary Jane shoes.

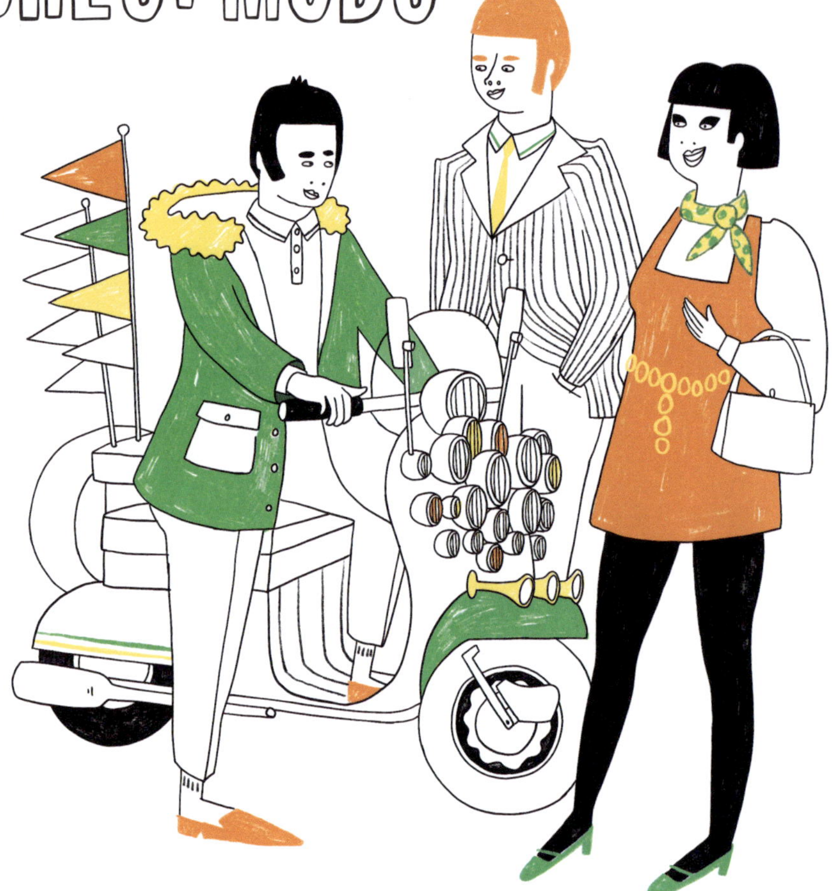

FINISH THE PORTRAIT

Complete Leonardo da Vinci's outfit by adding patterns to his tunic and fur trim. Then finish illustrating the details of his long, flowing beard.

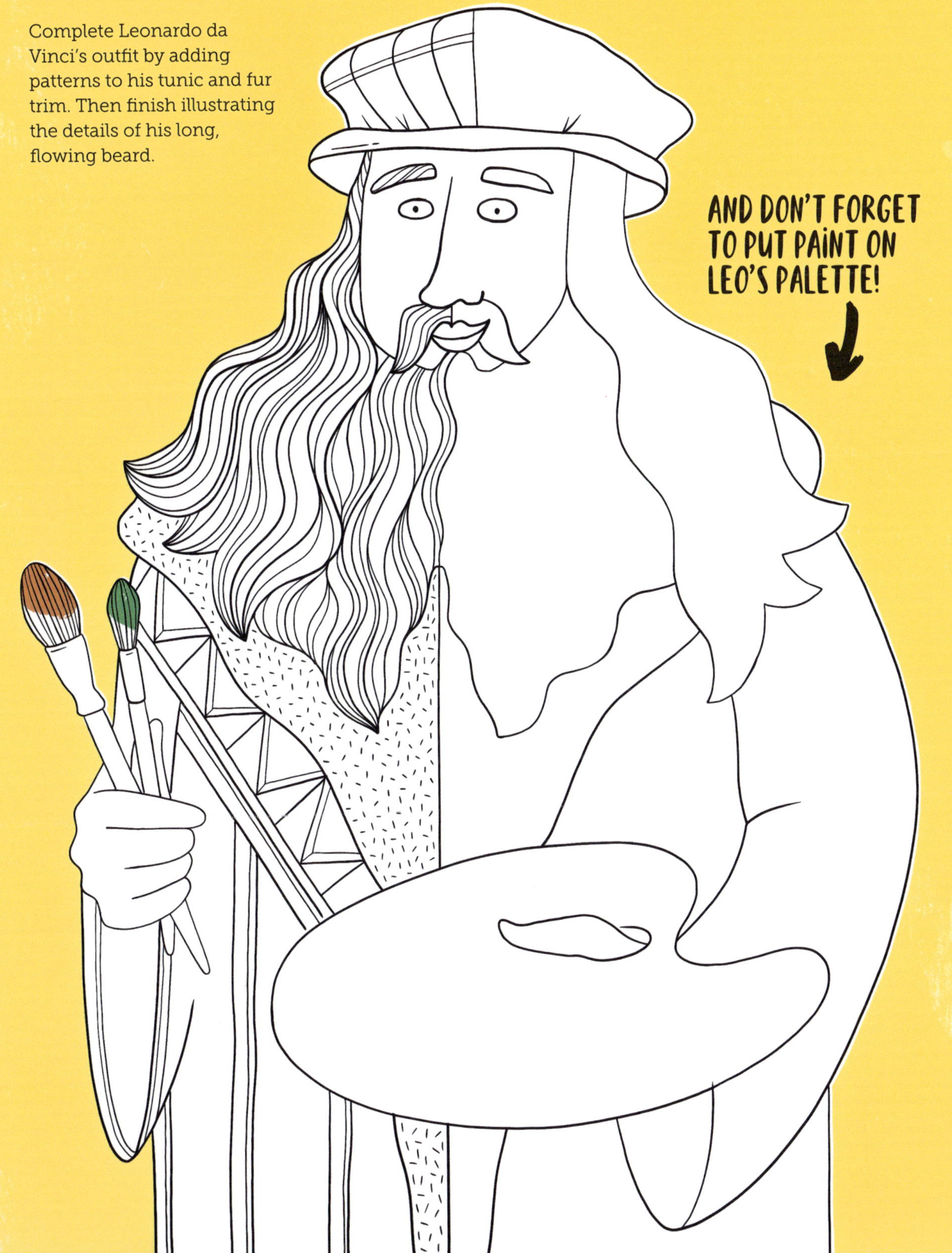

DRAW A PERSON DANCING

Here, you will learn the basics on how to draw a person in motion, using dancing as an example. Once you break the task down into simple shapes and see how each limb moves with another, you will find it a lot easier. Then you can start placing the limbs at different angles to change the dance moves your character makes.

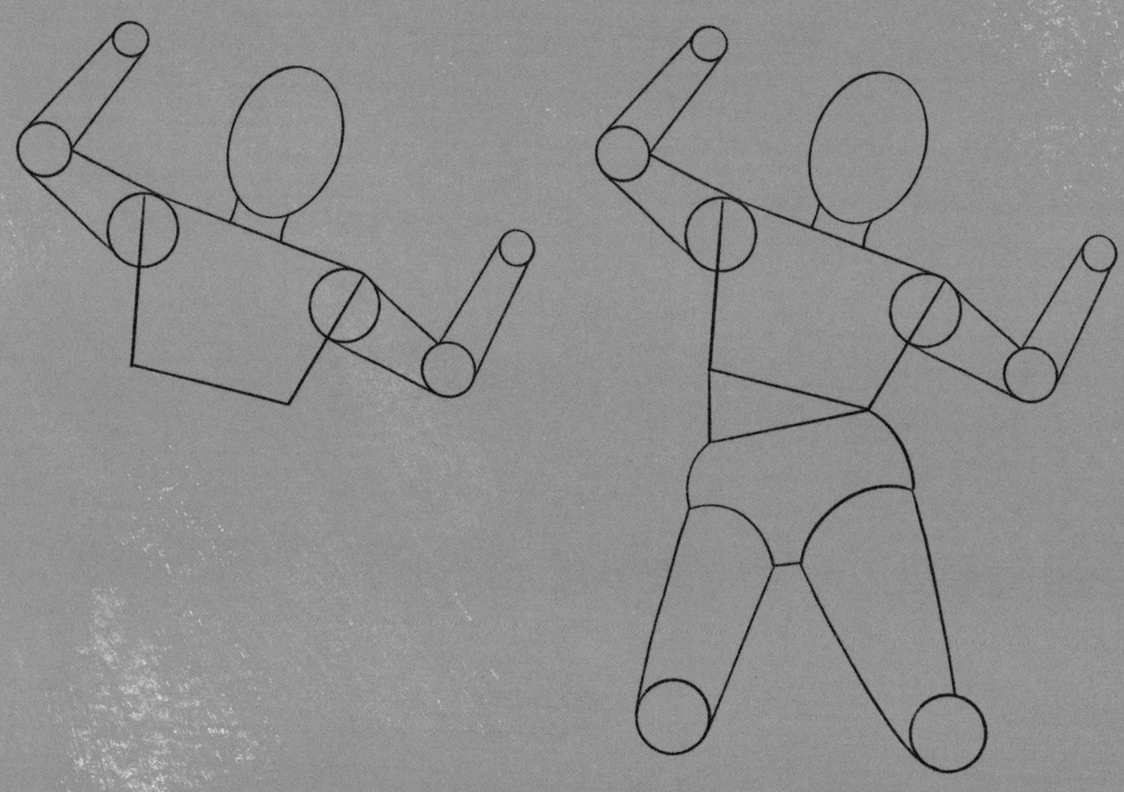

1 First, sketch the head and neck tilting to the right. For the chest, make a square with the top edges slanting outward. Add two circles for the shoulders as shown. Draw rectangles for the upper arms and forearms with the latter bending up at the joint. Then add circles for the elbows and wrists.

2 Add a triangle for the torso and draw the hips as shown, wider on the right to show the hip position. Sketch two rectangles for the upper legs and draw circles for the knees, making the outer right leg meet the middle of the right knee circle.

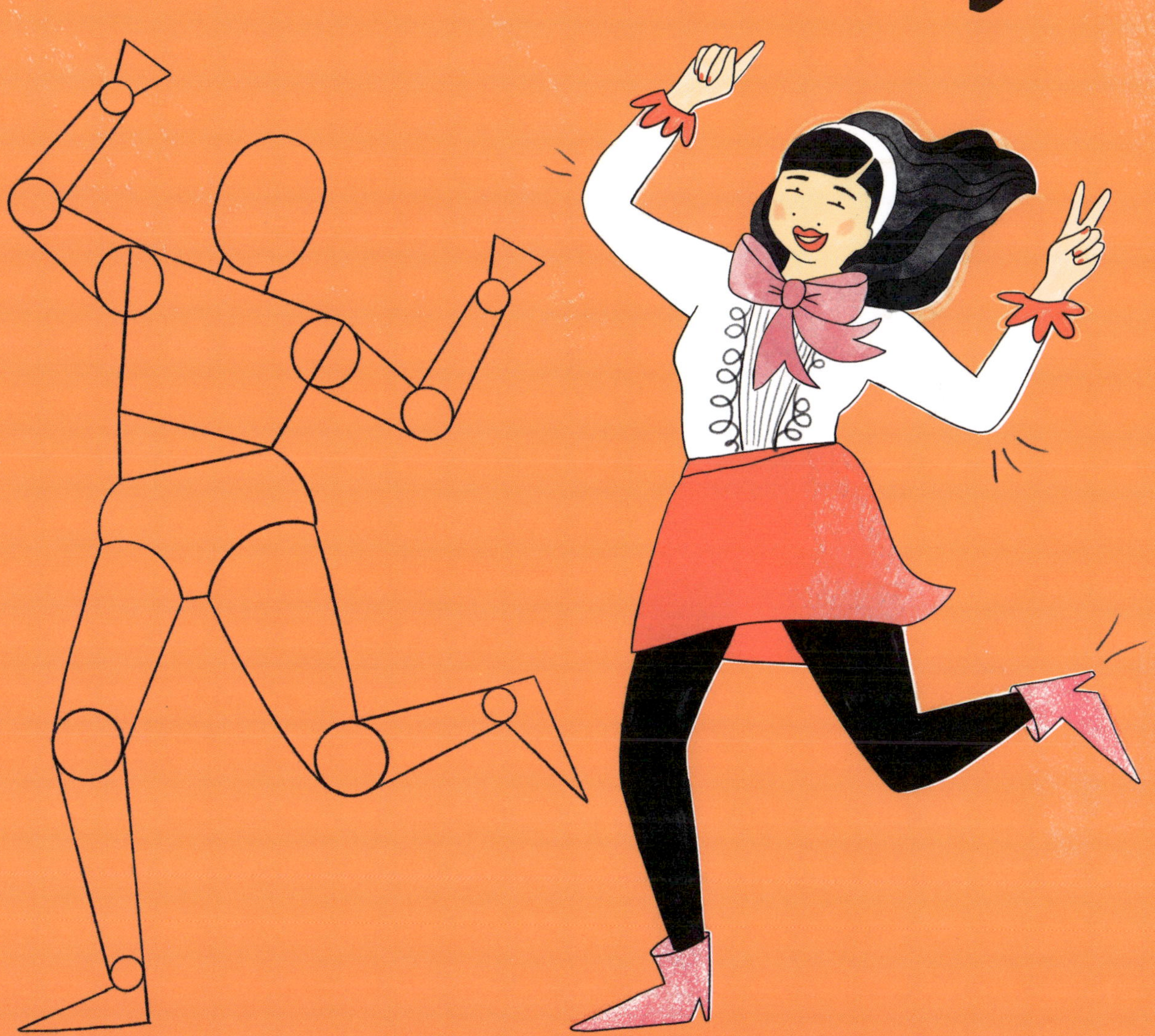

3 For the calves, draw another set of rectangles tapering toward the bottom and narrowing at the ankles. Add a circle for the ankle, and then draw the feet. Sketch in the shape of the palm.

4 Now, for the best bit! With a fineliner, draw over your sketch adding in the character's details and style. Finish by rubbing out your pencil marks; make sure the pen is dry first!

TURN OVER TO PRACTICE →

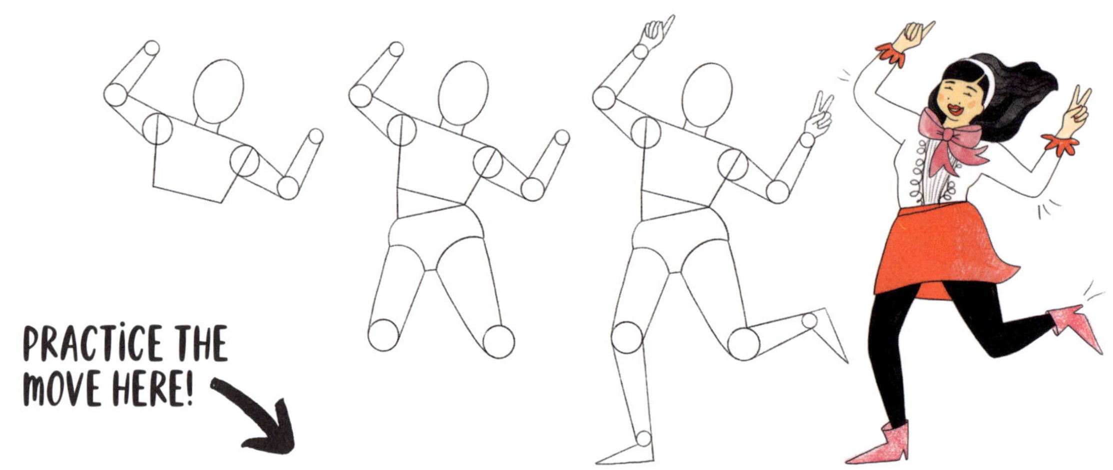

PRACTICE THE
MOVE HERE!

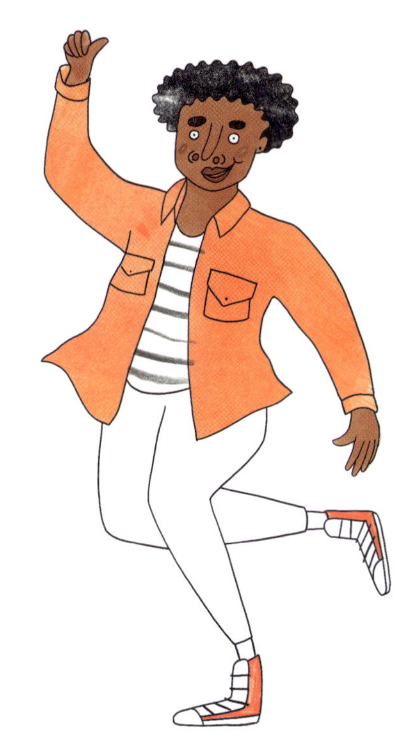

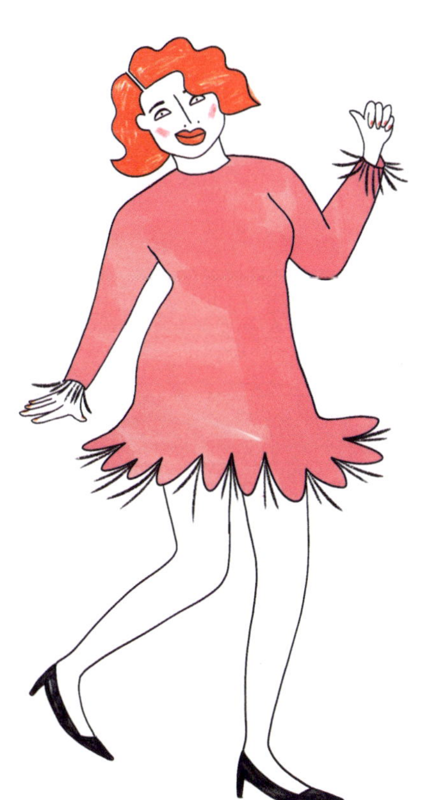

NOW, SEE WHAT OTHER POSES YOU CAN CREATE!

ATHLETIC APPAREL

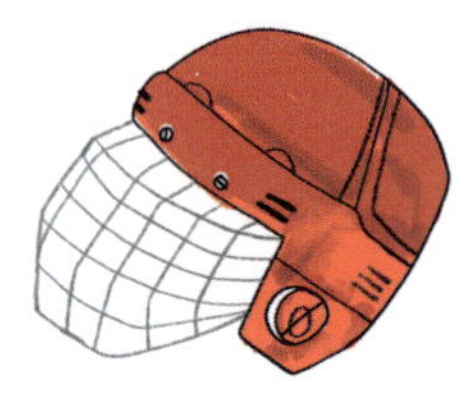

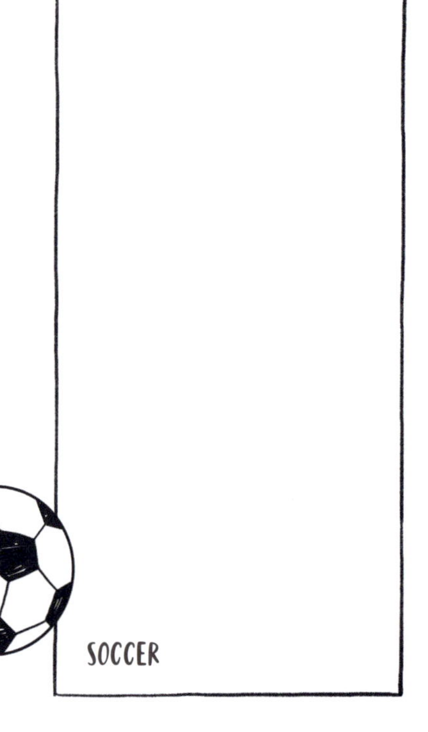

SOCCER

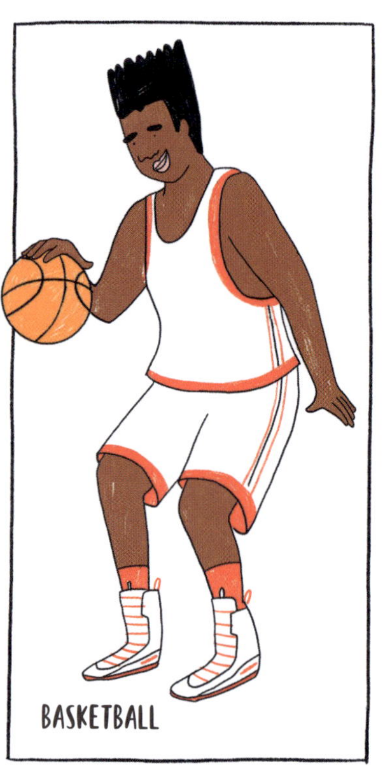

BASKETBALL

ICE HOCKEY

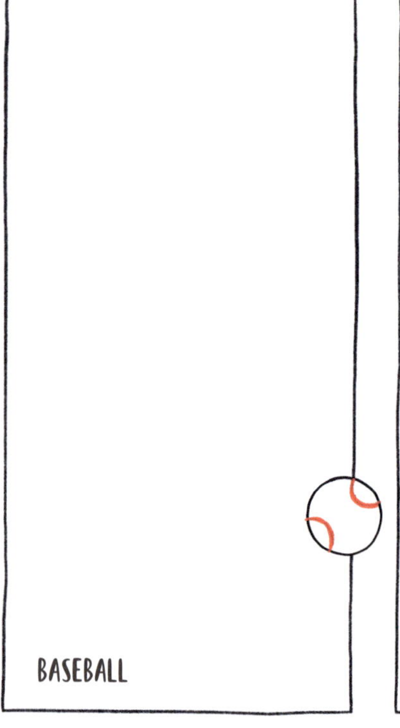

BASEBALL

FENCING

AMERICAN FOOTBALL

Draw the athletes in their sportswear next to the corresponding sport. You could draw them stationary, posing with their equipment, or in an action shot. Are there any sports you would like to try? Draw yourself in that box.

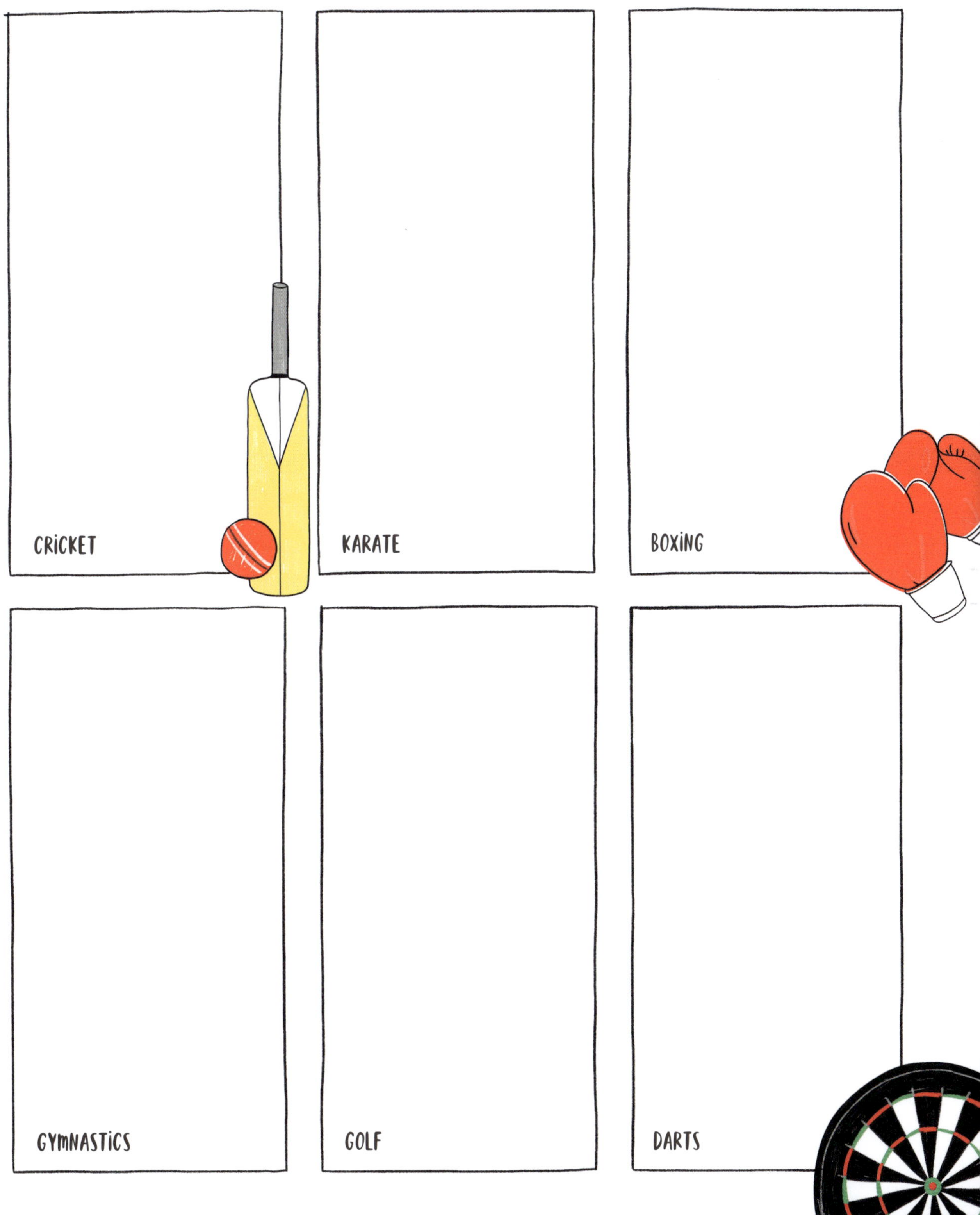

FACES AT AN ANGLE

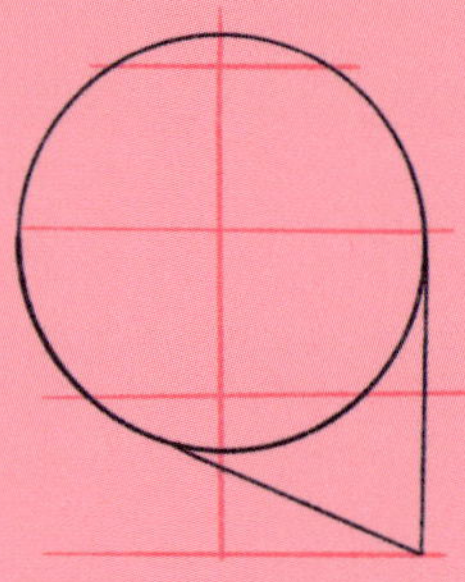 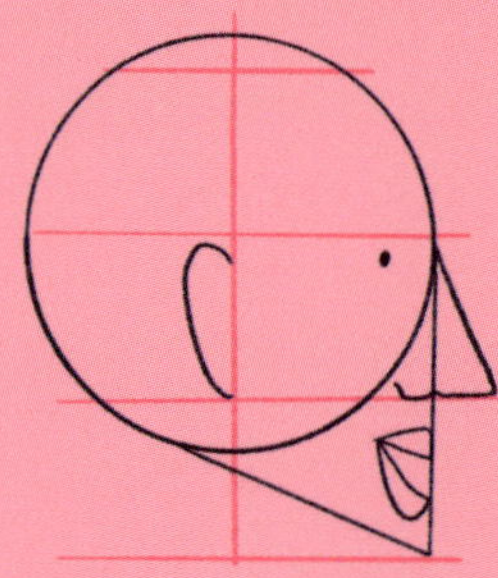 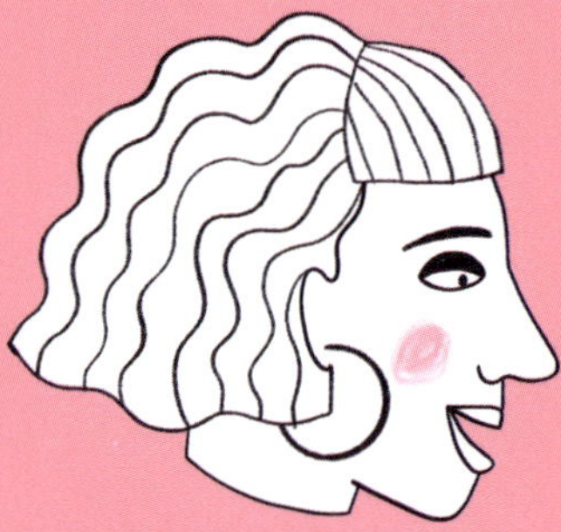

1 Draw a circle with a line down the center and four evenly spaced lines across. Add the shape for the chin.

2 The ear sits on the central line; the nose sits on the third line. The eye aligns with the top of the ear. The mouth is central between the nose and chin.

3 Next, add the fun details to develop your character. Finish by rubbing out your pencil marks.

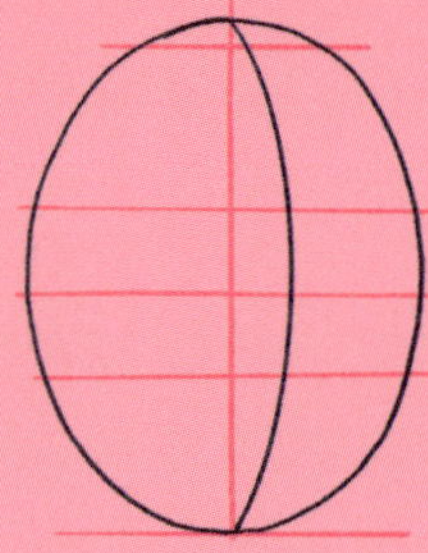 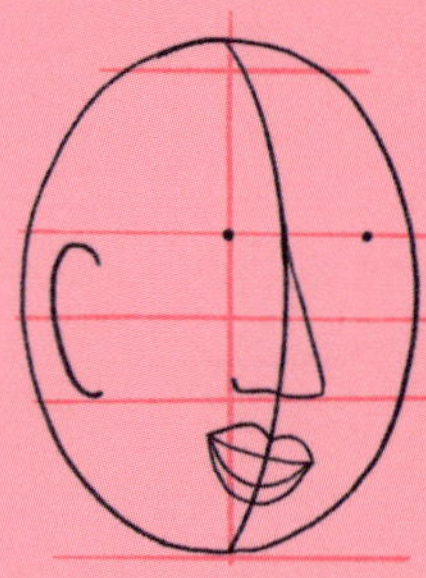 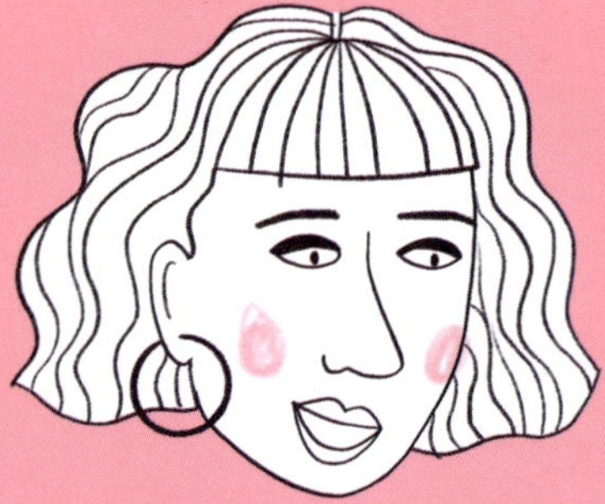

1 Draw an oval with a central line and four evenly spaced lines across. Then, add an extra line in between the third and fourth. Draw a curved line from the top to the bottom line.

2 The nose sits on the fourth line starting from the curved line. The ear is centered on the third line. The eyes sit on the second line, with the mouth centered to the curved line.

3 Draw over your pencil marks to create your character. Finish by rubbing out your pencil marks.

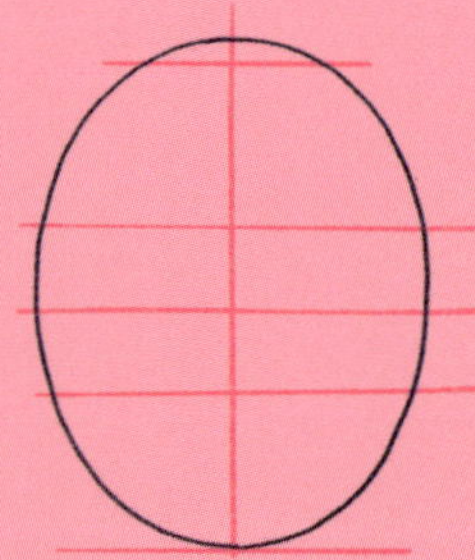 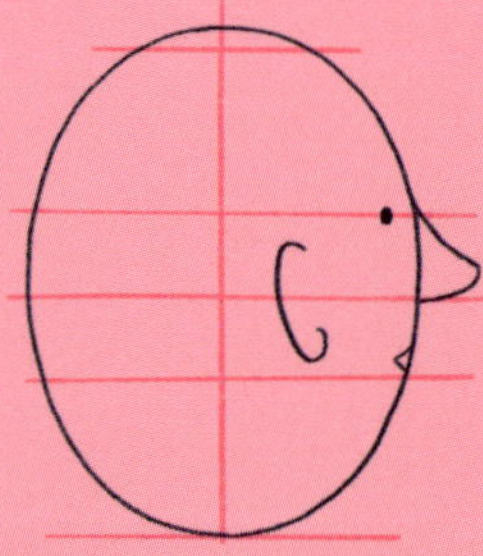 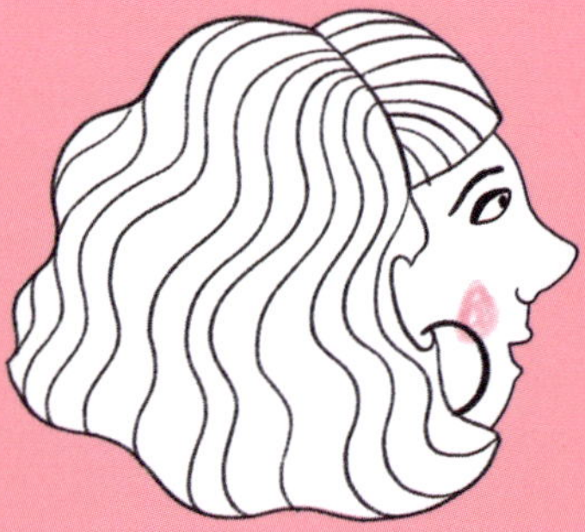

1 Draw an oval shape with a line down the center and four evenly spaced lines across. Add an extra line in between the second and third.

2 The nose sits on the third line; the ear is centered on it, slightly closer to the midline. The eyes sit on the second and the mouth on the fourth line.

3 Next, add your details. Use the direction of the hair to emphasize the angle. Finish by rubbing out your pencil marks.

Learn to draw faces from three different angles in these simple step-by-step tutorials. Use the space below to practice. Try drawing the same character for each pose as an extra challenge!

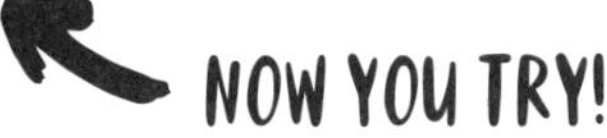

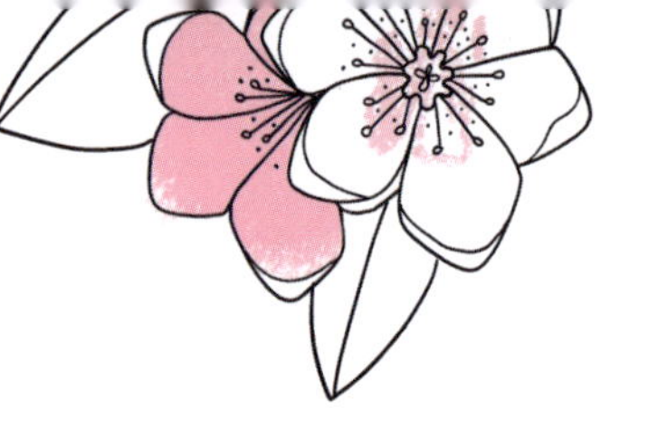

SEASONS: SPRING

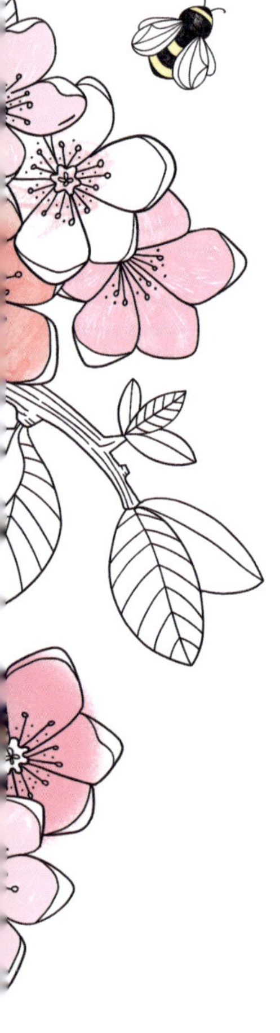

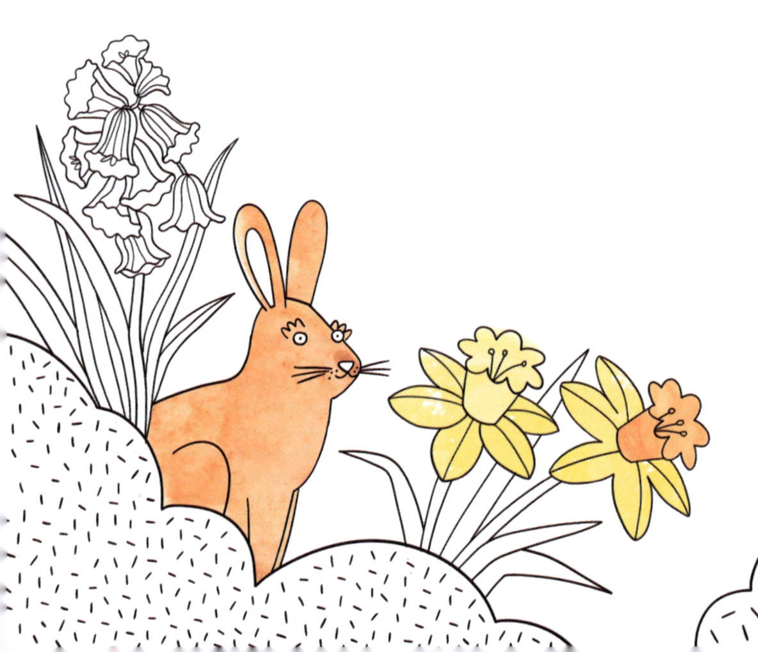

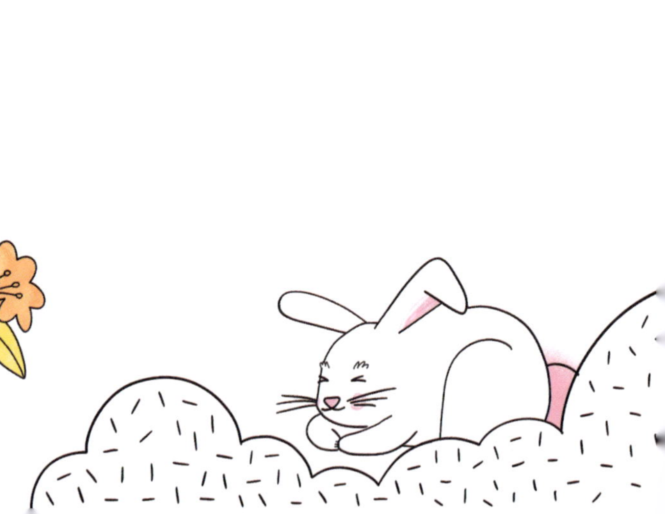

Springtime brings a sense of renewal with warmer days and blossom appearing on trees. Using a soft pastel color palette, draw people enjoying a sunny spring day out, dressing them in florals, light coats, and cardigans.

LET'S LINE DANCE

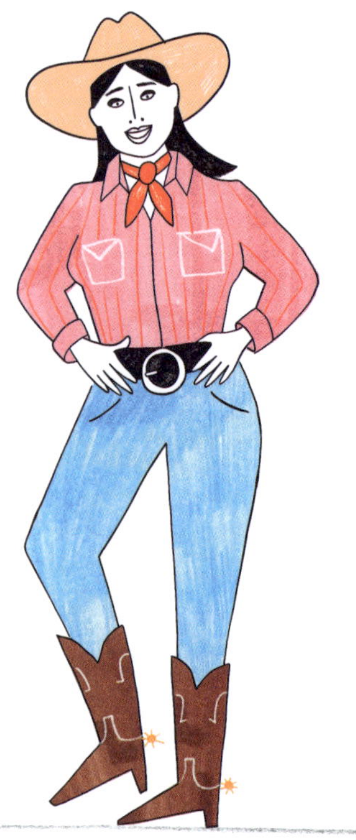

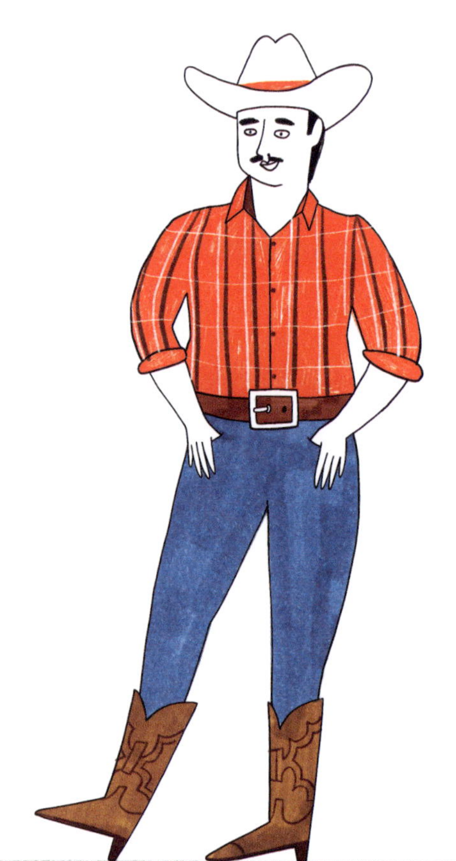

Fill this dance floor with rows of country line dancers. Who's in sync and who's ahead or behind the steps? Dress each character in a patterned plaid shirt, denim, hat, and boots! Yeehaw!

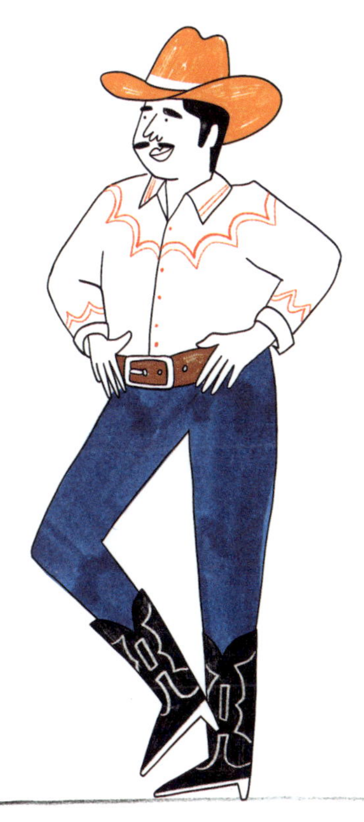

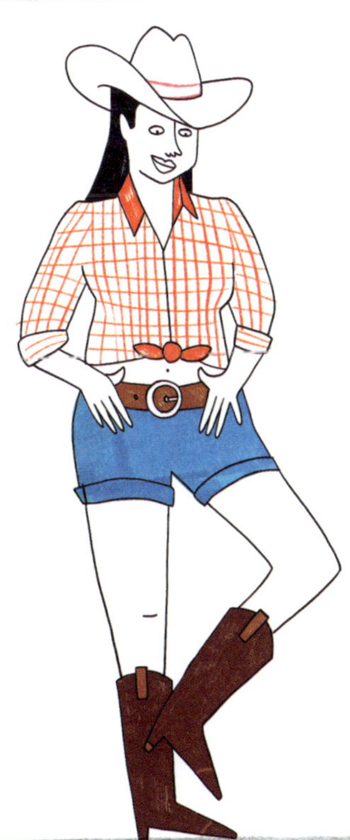

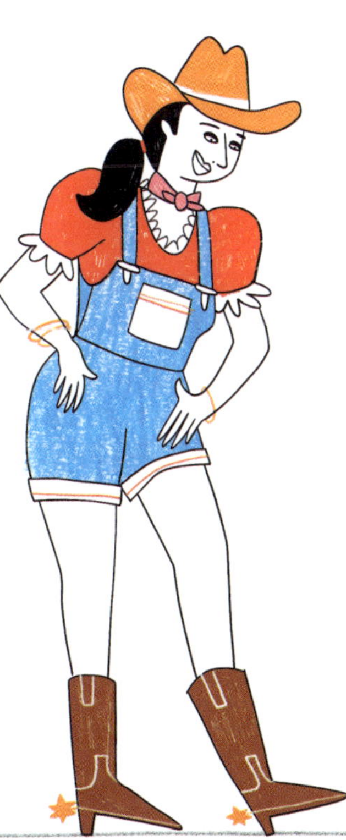

DRAW A PERSON IN PROFILE

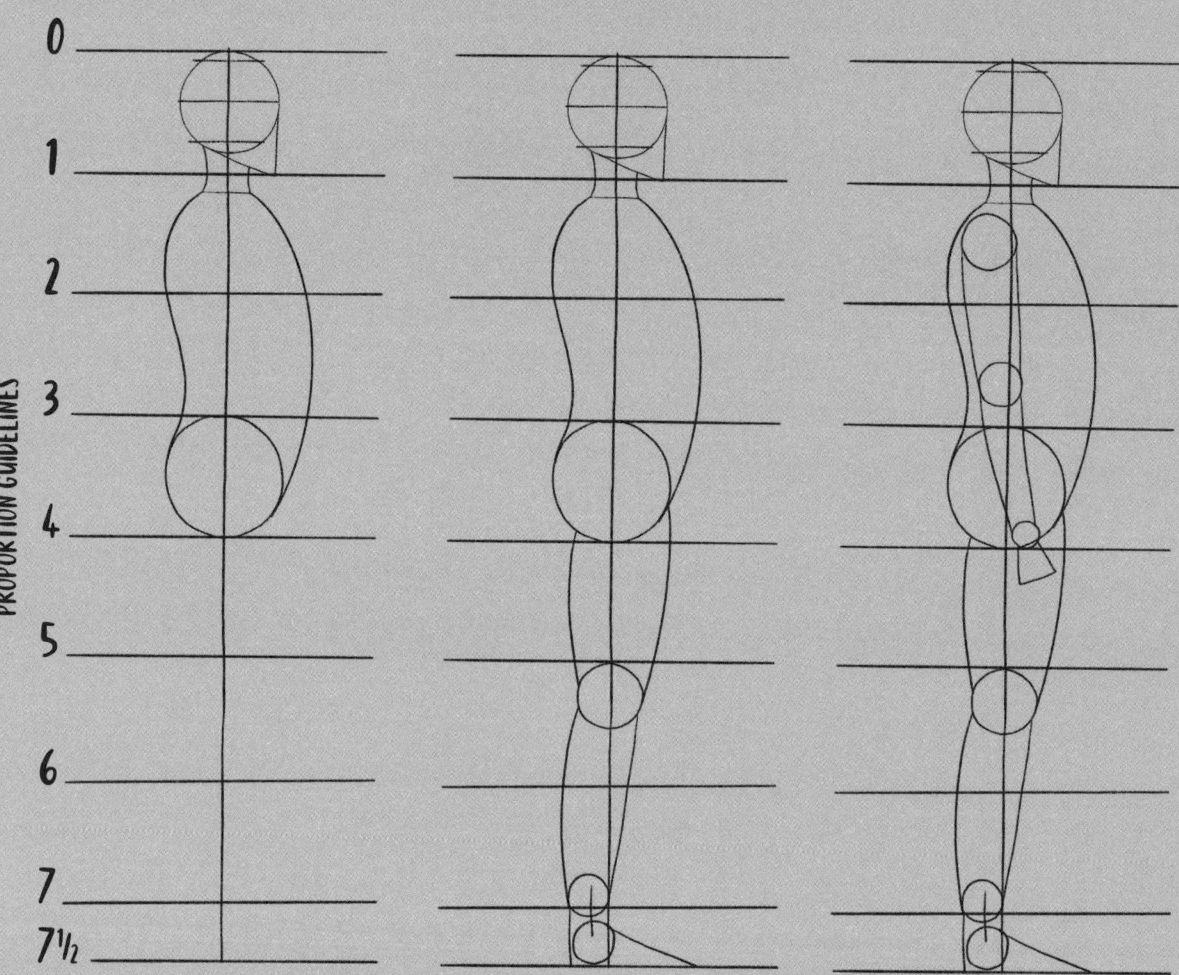

1 Sketch your character's head following the earlier tutorial. Continue the central line down to the bottom. Draw the neck one-third its length Add a circle for the pelvis and buttocks between the third and fourth line. Join with a kidney-like shape for the torso and chest.

2 Human legs aren't perfectly straight, they curve a little. Draw a circle for the knee on the center line. Add rectangles that curve slightly at the outer edges, as shown, with the calf leaning behind the center line. Then draw the feet, following the earlier tutorial, if needed.

3 The shoulder starts closer to the back of the body. Place the joint to the left of the center line, the elbow joint farther forward, and the wrist right of the center line. Add cylinders for the upper and forearms. Draw the hands and fingers, following the earlier tutorial.

This exercise will show you some of the basics of drawing a person in profile by breaking the task down into a few easy steps. Using reference material will make this exercise much easier.

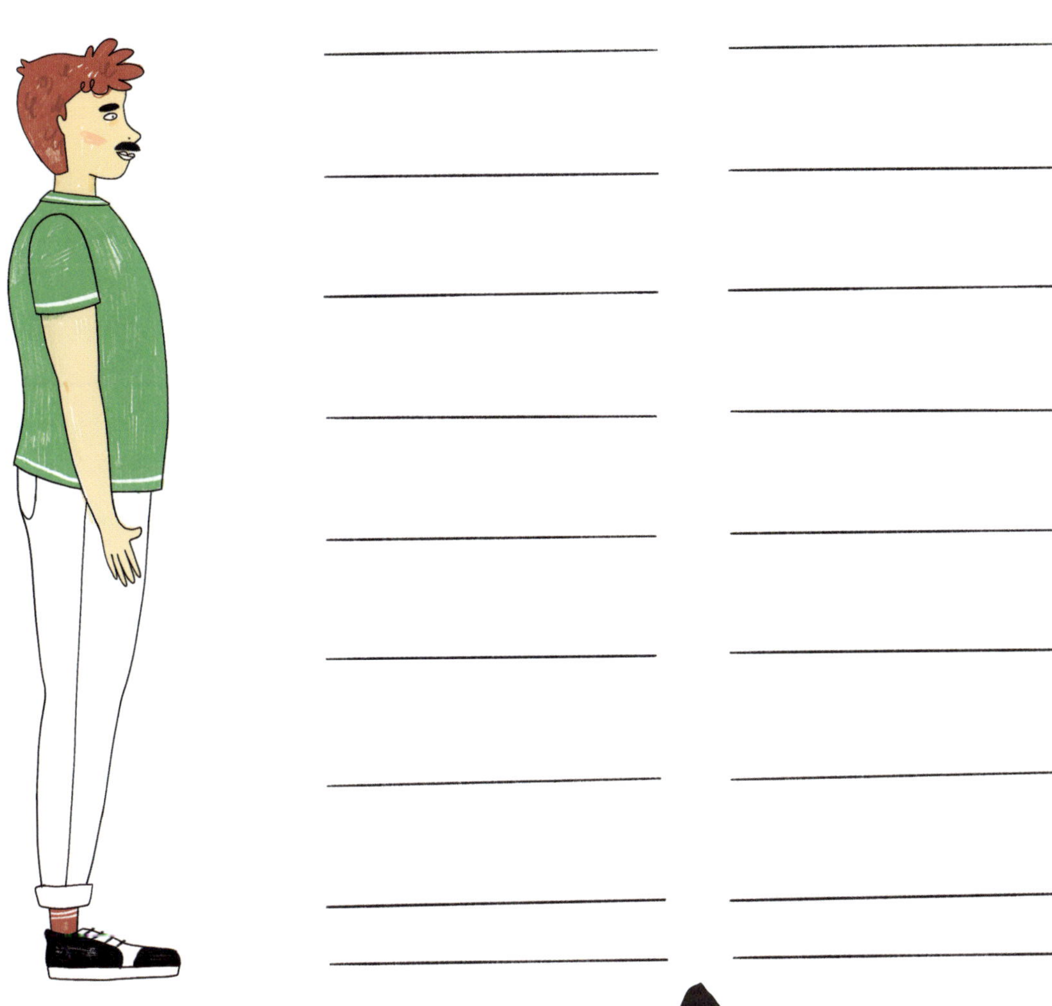

4 With a fineliner, draw over your pencil work, adding in the person's characteristics and style. When the pen has dried, finish by rubbing out your pencil lines.

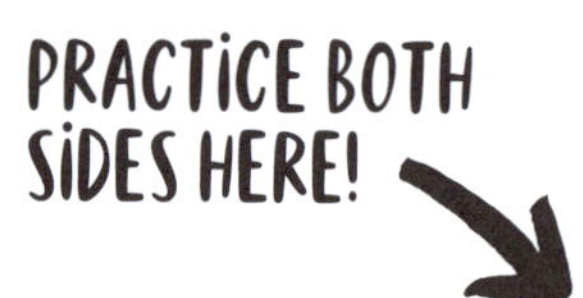
PRACTICE BOTH
SIDES HERE!

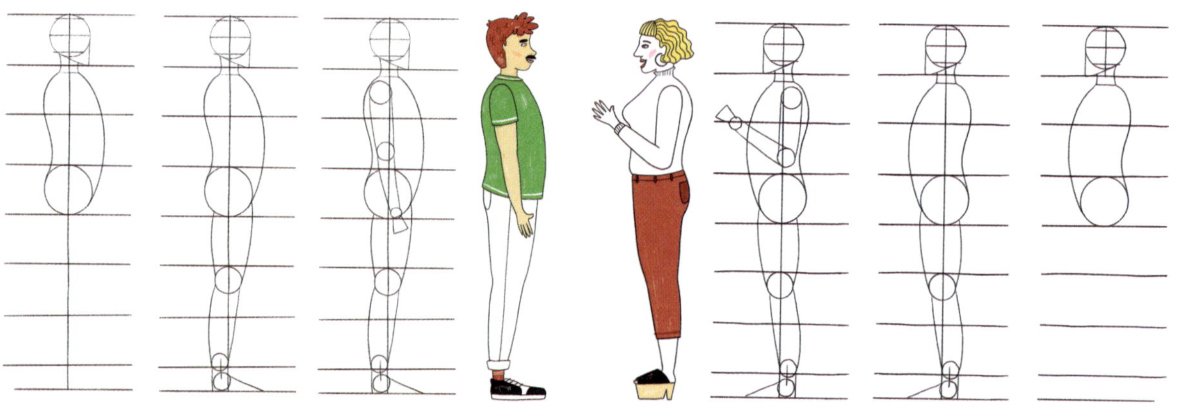

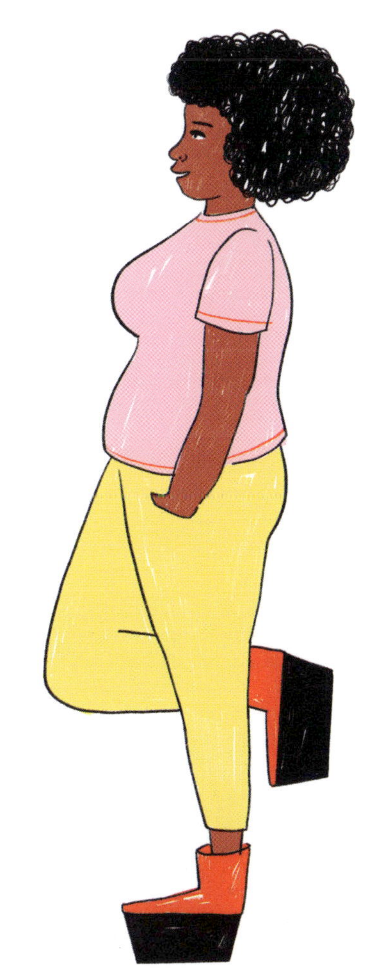

NOW, TRY DRAWING DIFFERENT POSITIONS!

WHAT'S ON THE MENU?

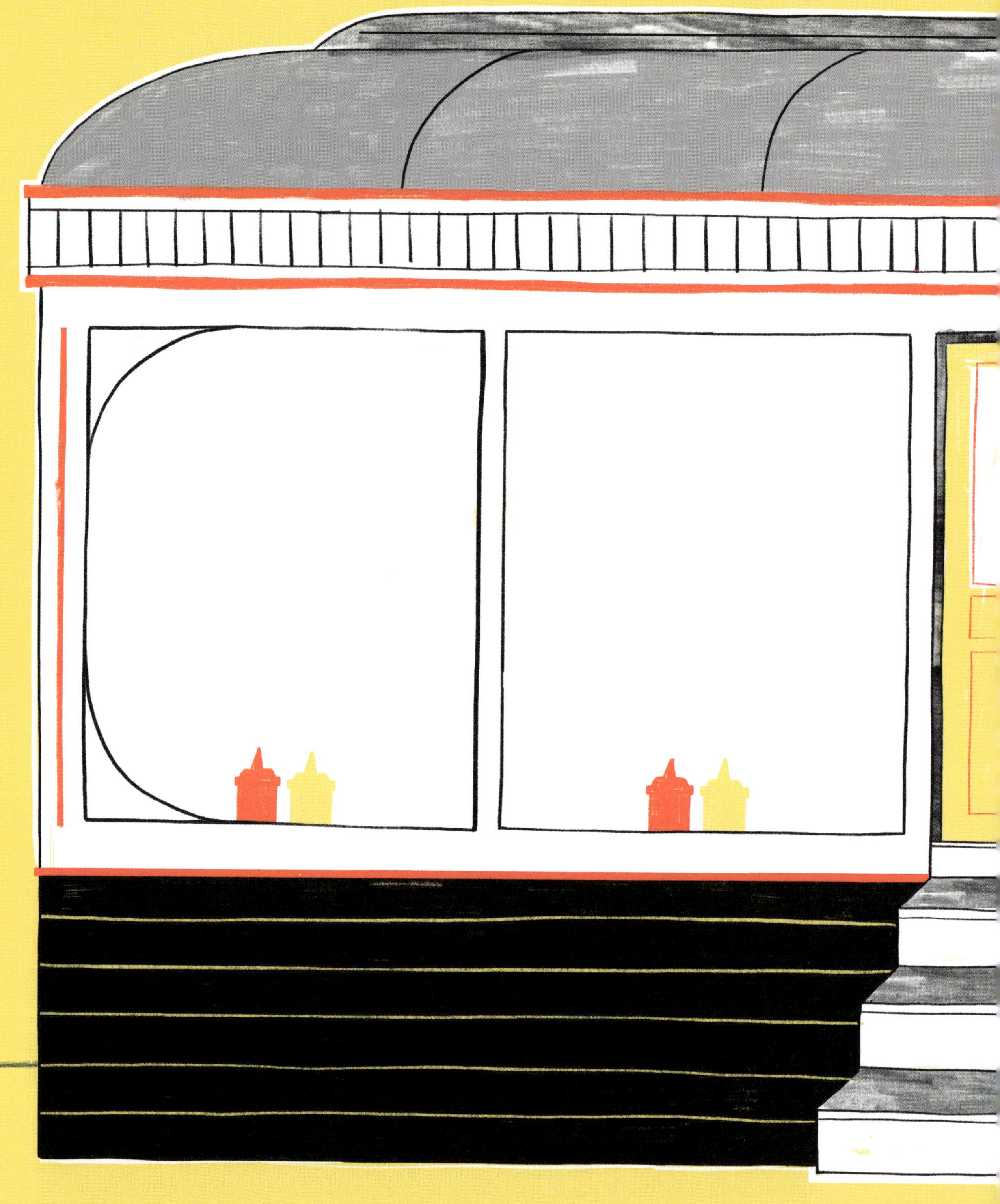

The diner is open and customers are sitting down in the booths ordering their lunch. Fill the windows with people enjoying their favorite food.

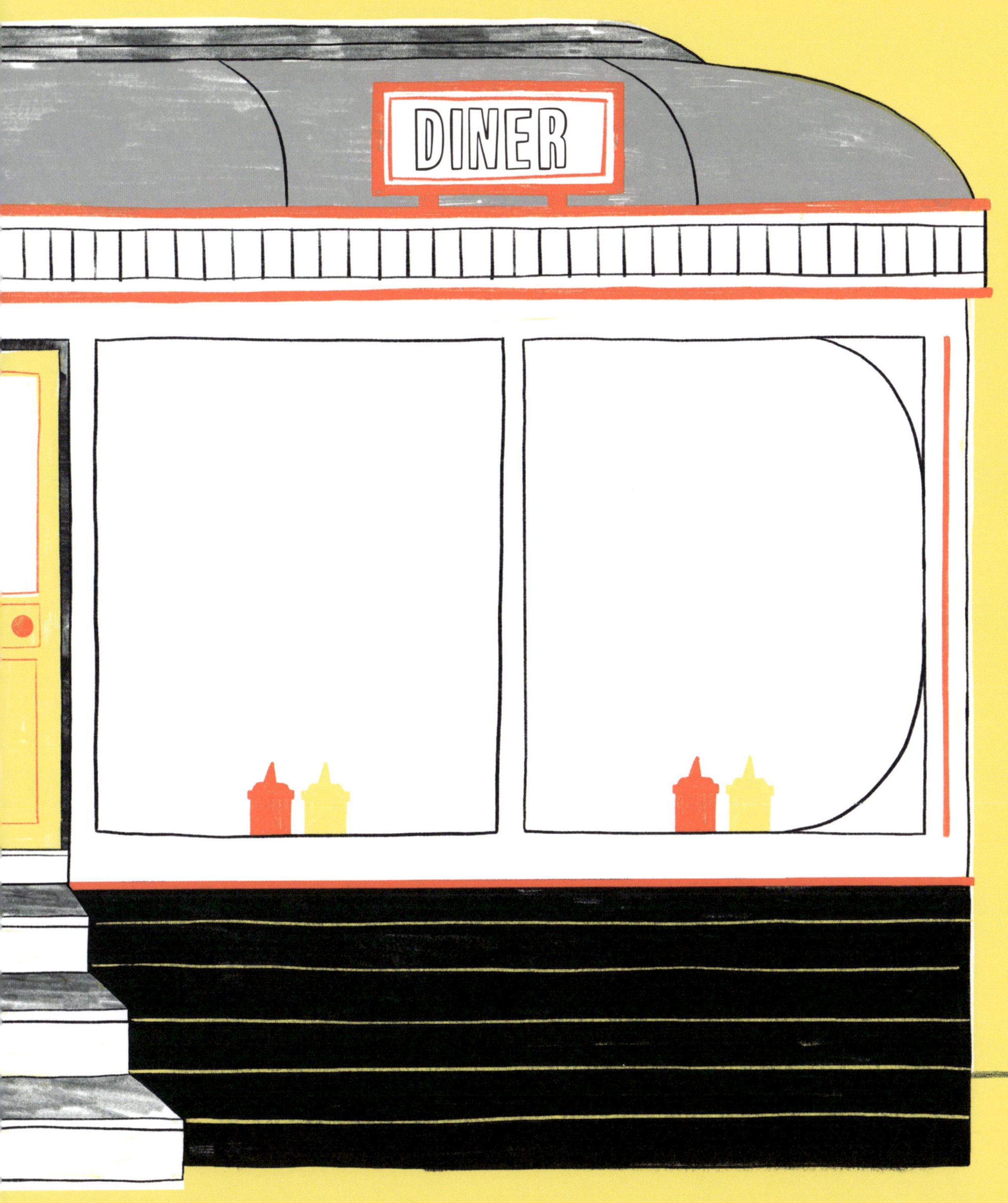

PIAZZA PERSPECTIVE

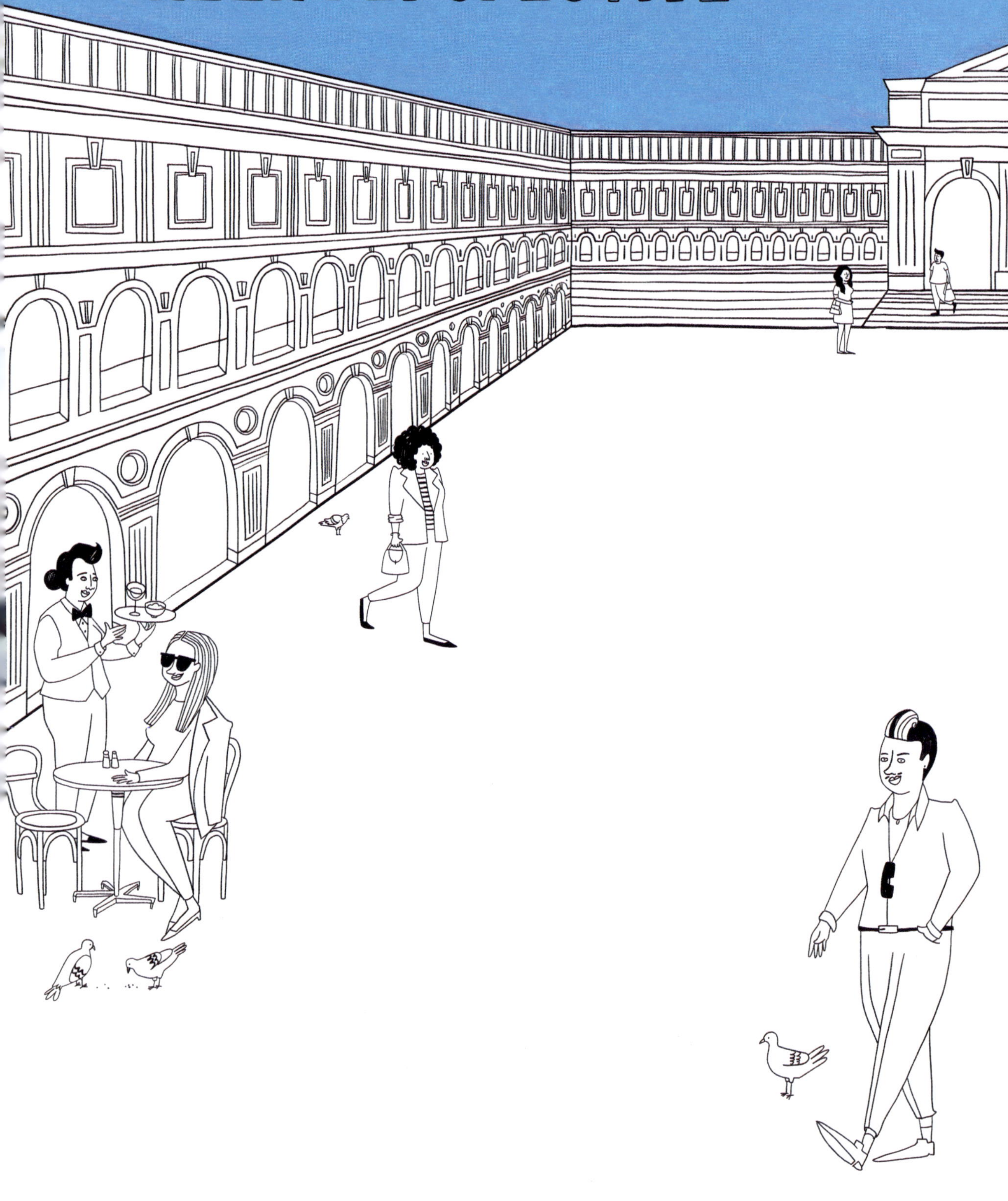

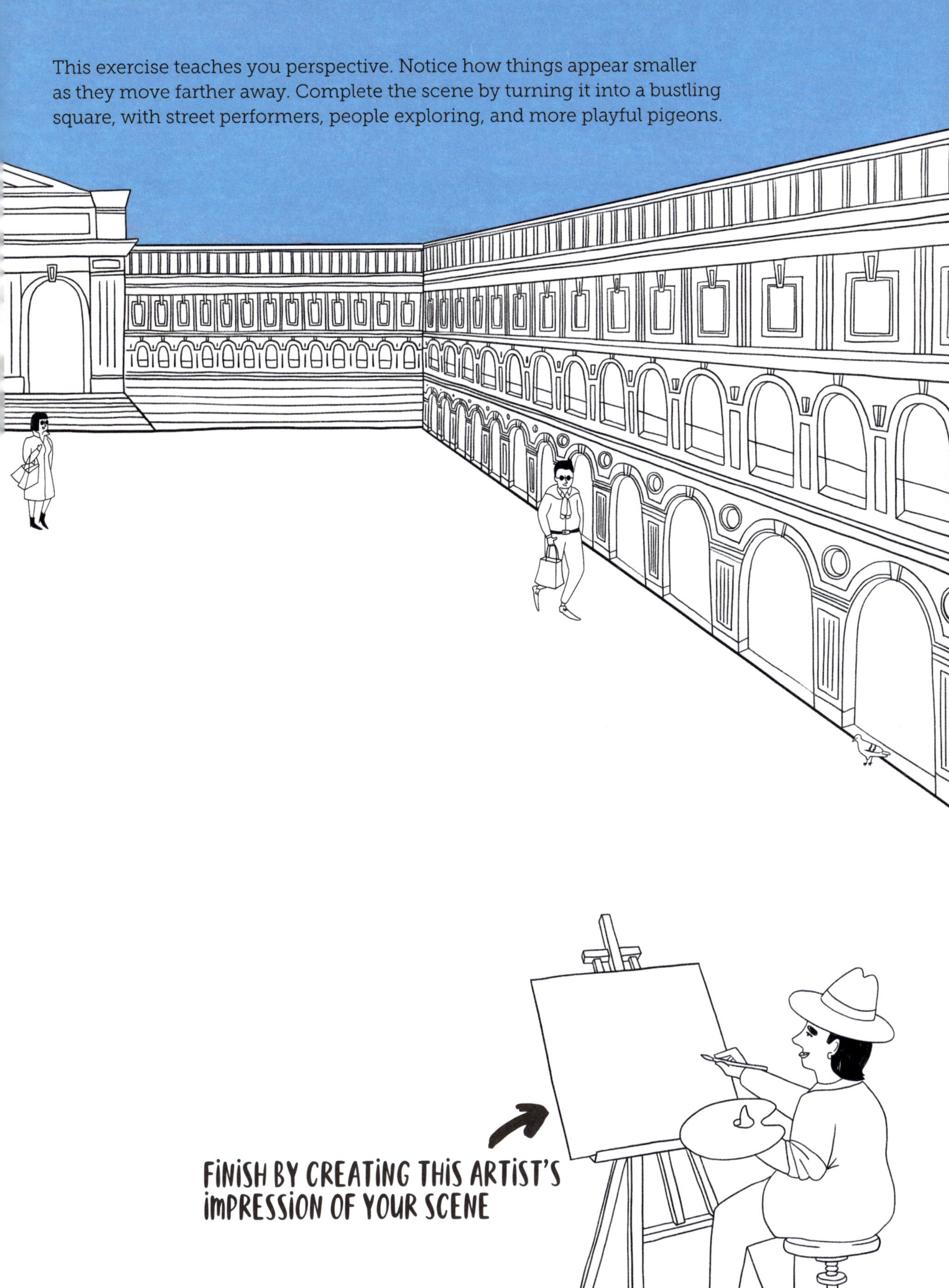

This exercise teaches you perspective. Notice how things appear smaller as they move farther away. Complete the scene by turning it into a bustling square, with street performers, people exploring, and more playful pigeons.

PAINTED FACES

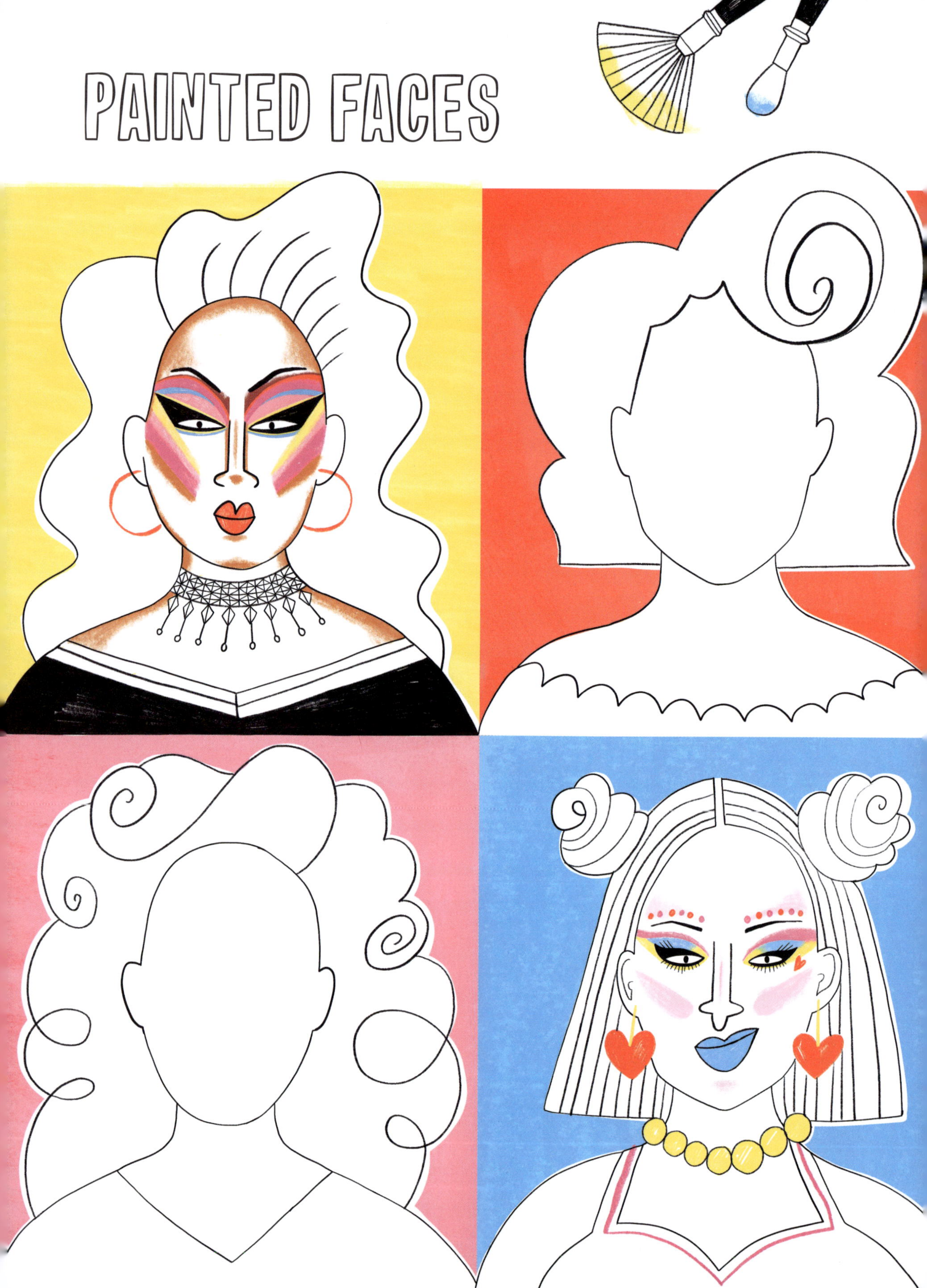

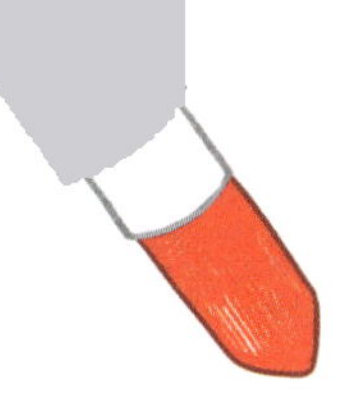

Explore using makeup as another form of painting by coloring in these characters. From drag queens to ravers, go all-out with bold colors and strong contouring. Discover how makeup can express a person's identity.

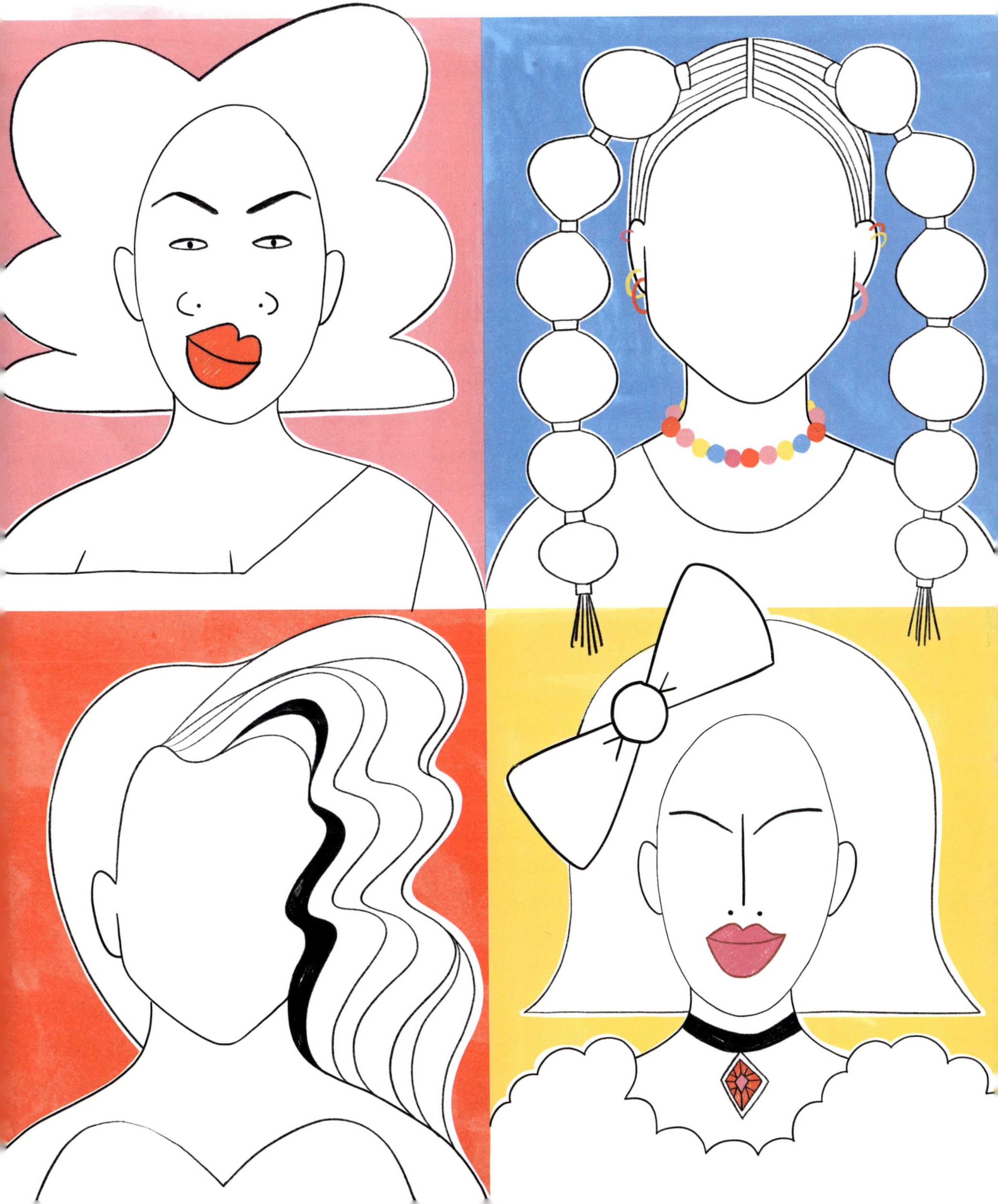

TINY CHALLENGES

Fill this grid with a series of tiny challenges, completing each one in under 15 minutes. Use them as quick warm-up exercises or miniature creative explorations, perfect for when you don't have much free time.

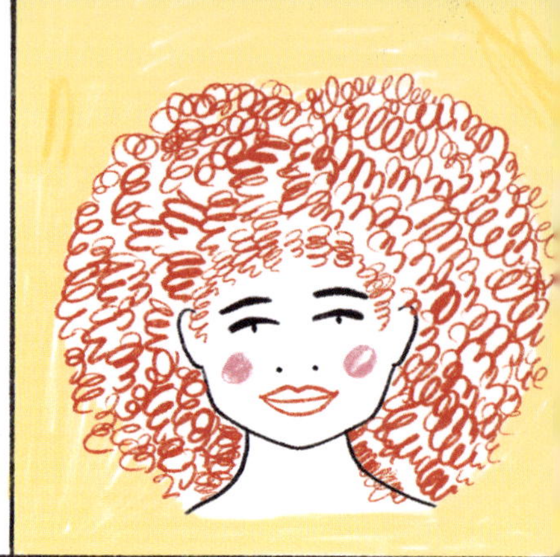

SKETCH SOMEONE WITH CURLY HAIR

DRAW A PROFILE USING NEGATIVE SPACE

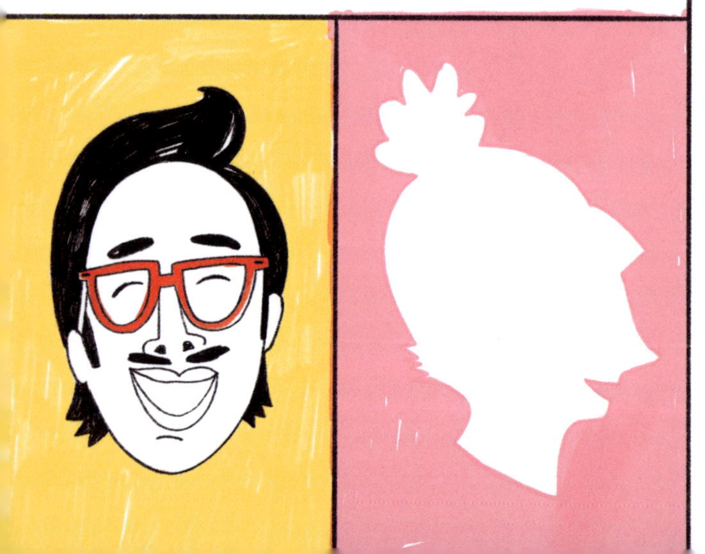

ILLUSTRATE SOMEONE LAUGHING

SKETCH A CHARACTER WEARING A HUGE HAT

DRAW A GROUP OF TINY PEOPLE CELEBRATING

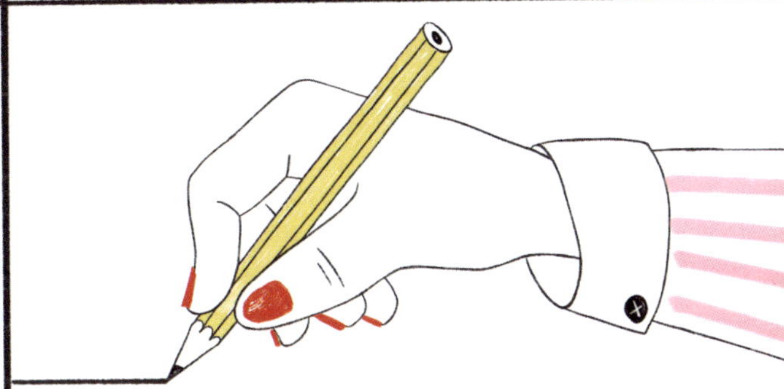

ILLUSTRATE SOMEONE JUMPING FOR JOY

DRAW A HAND HOLDING A PENCIL

OCCUPATIONS

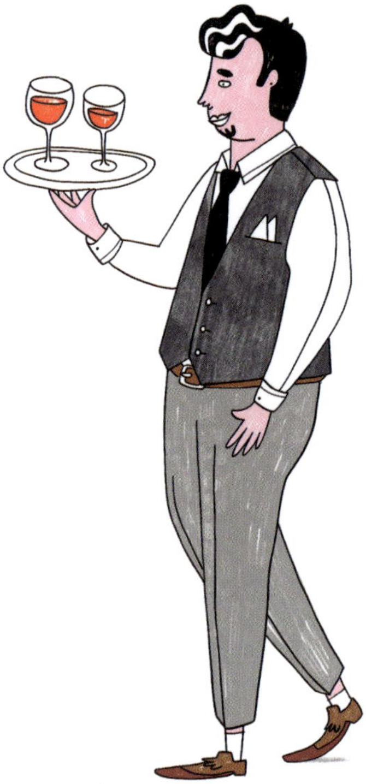

WAITER

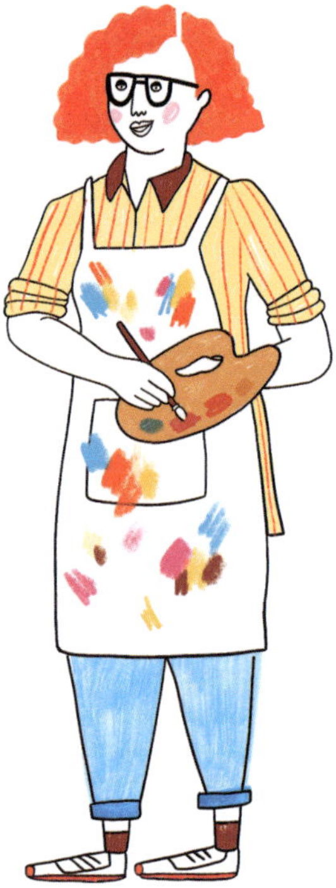

ARTIST

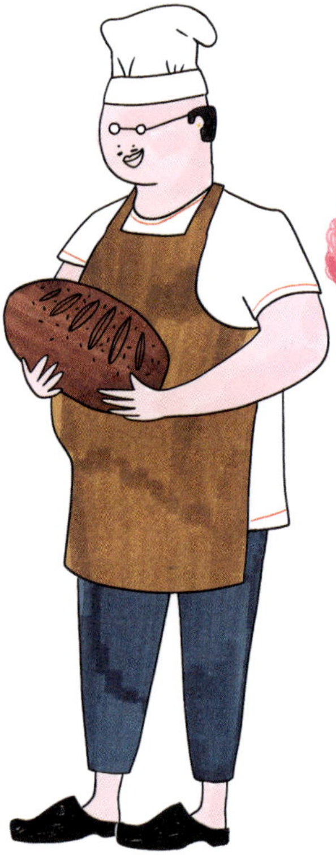

BAKER

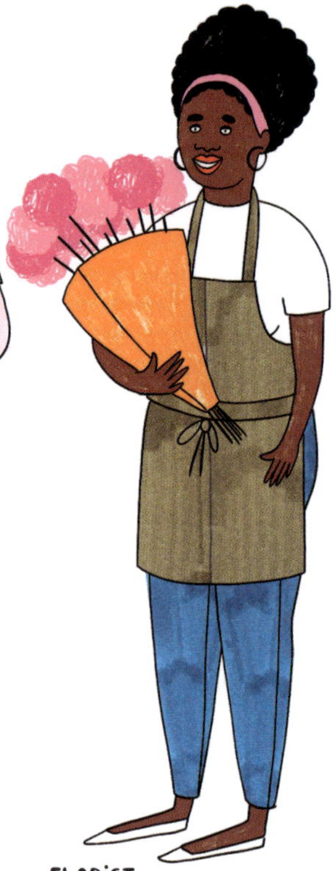

FLORIST

MUSICIAN

MECHANIC

FARMER

PHOTOGRAPHER

When drawing characters, you want the audience to be able to identify who they are through subtle cues, such as what they are holding or wearing, not just their facial expressions and gestures. Develop your own characters that would suit these jobs.

FLIGHT ATTENDANT

DOCTOR

BUILDER

DANCER

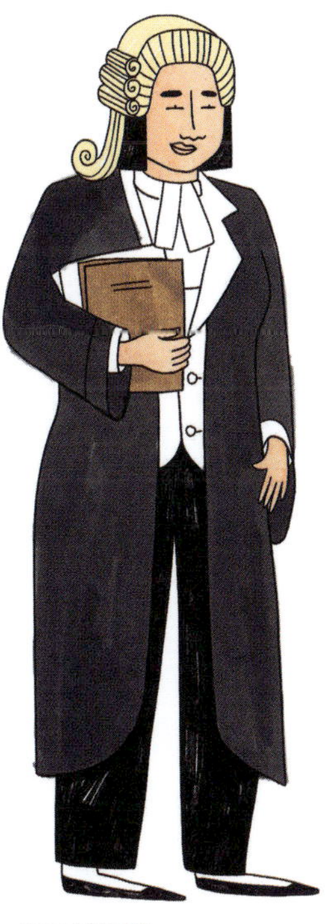

POLICEMAN

PILOT

BARRISTER

YOUR DREAM OCCUPATION!

TAKING A LINE FOR A WALK

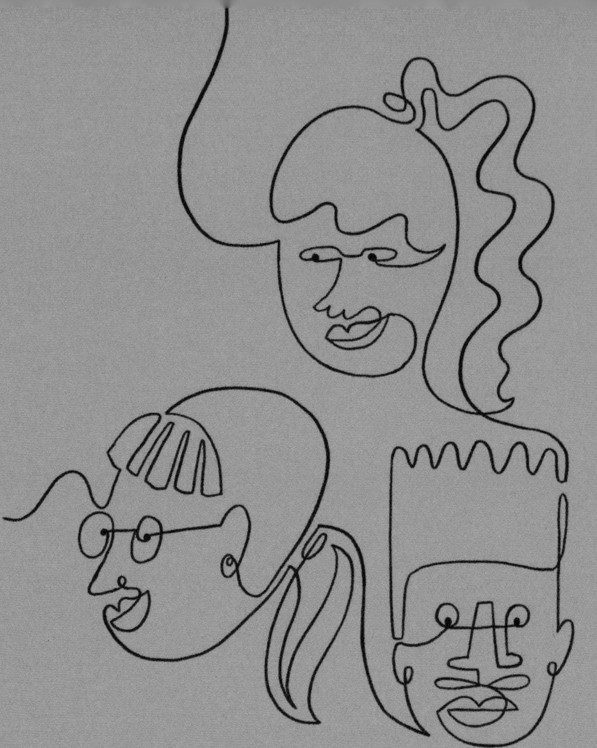

Known as continuous line drawing, the challenge is to keep your drawing
tool on the page the entire time, only lifting it up when you've finished.
Start on the left-hand page and, without lifing your pen, create your own
faces in a single line. Then, draw characters walking over this page.

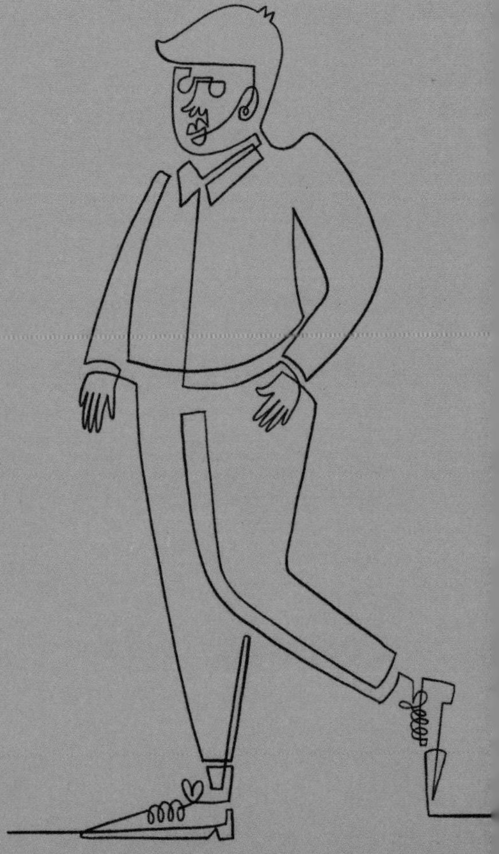

SUBCULTURES: GOTH

Add more characters to this page of goths, a style influenced by the Victorian and Edwardian eras, known for its black and dark colors, bold eyeliner, lace fabrics, and winklepicker shoes!

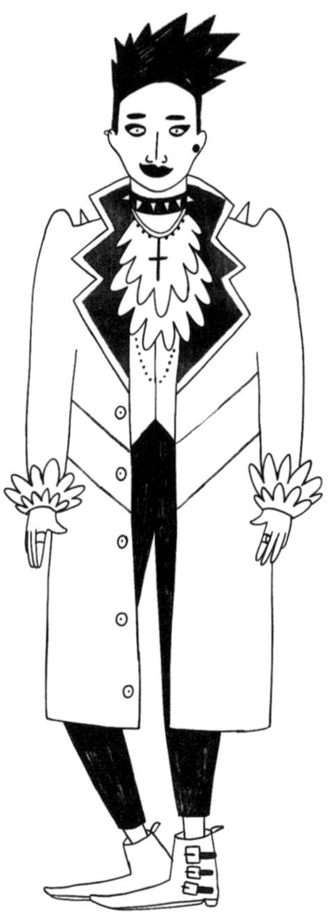

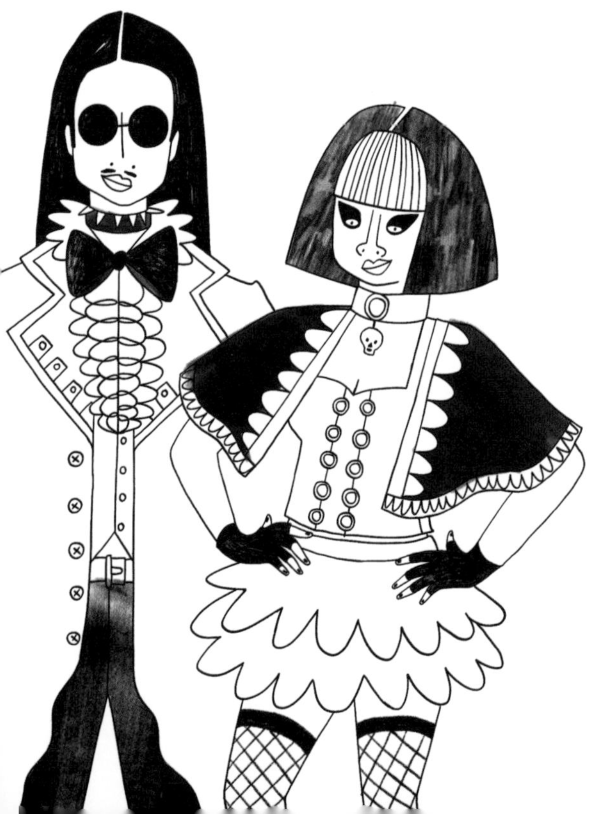

FINISH THE PORTRAIT

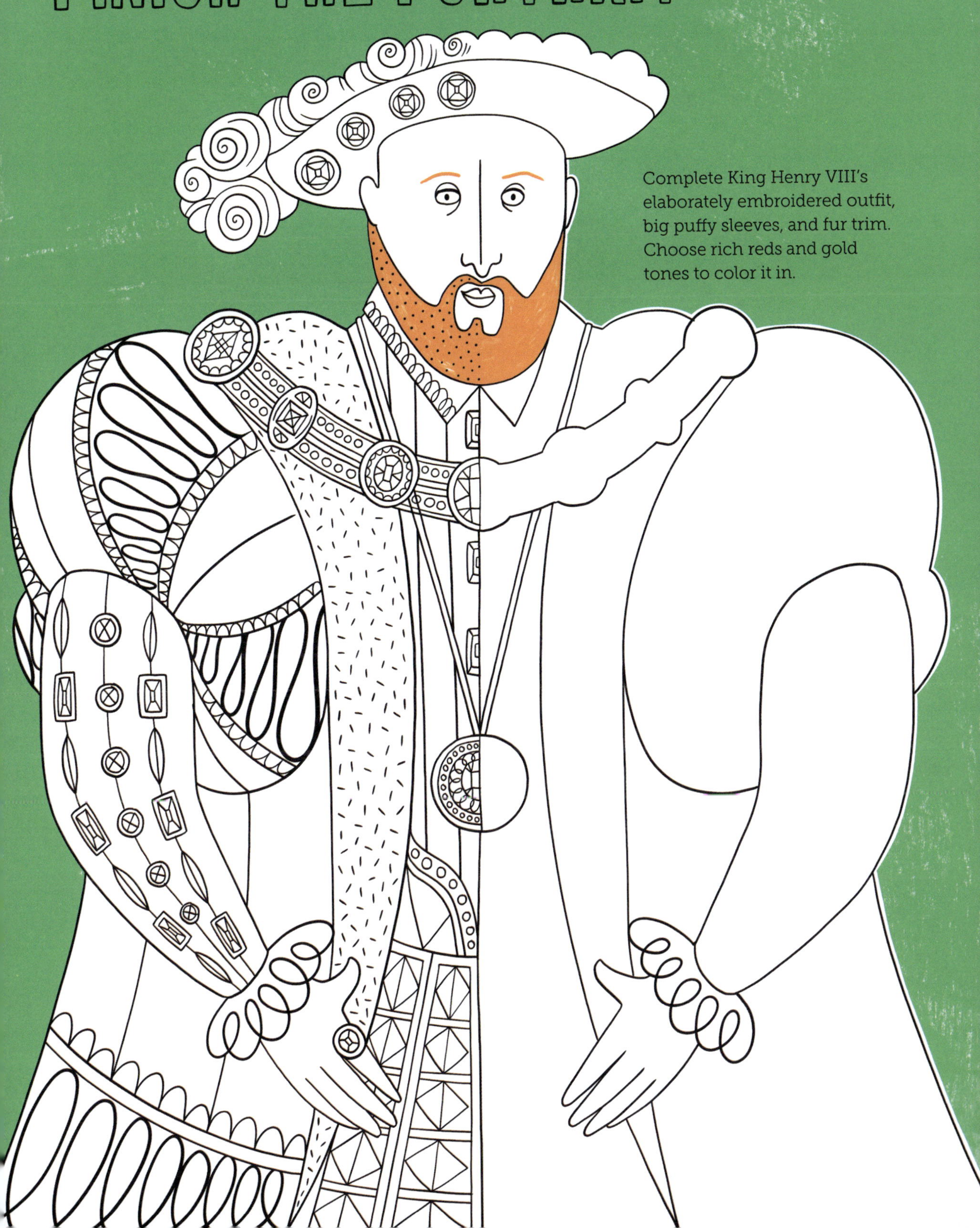

Complete King Henry VIII's elaborately embroidered outfit, big puffy sleeves, and fur trim. Choose rich reds and gold tones to color it in.

DAY OF THE DEAD

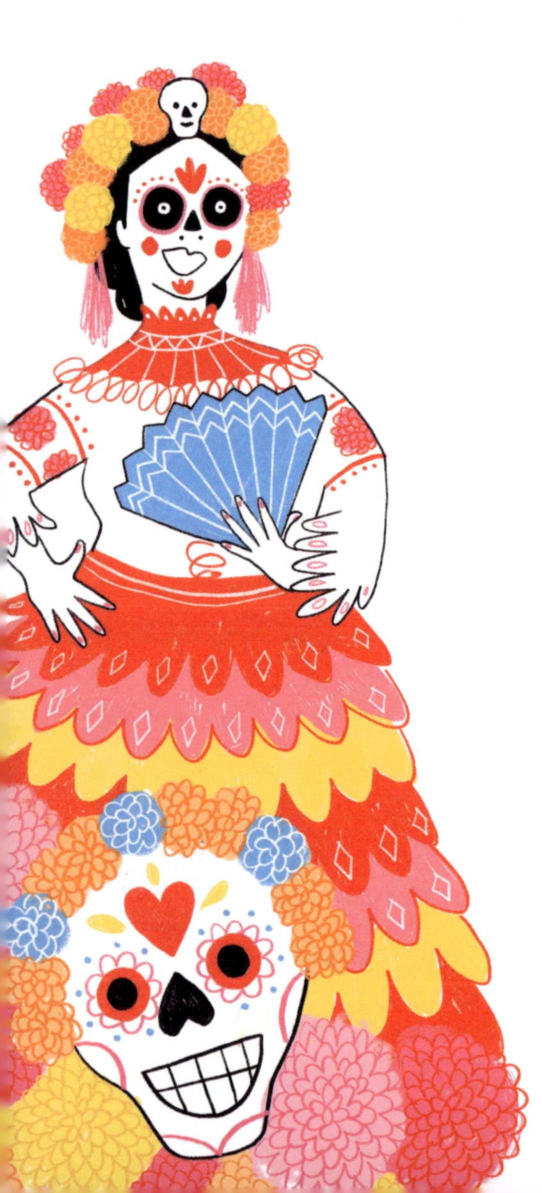

The Day of the Dead, also known as Día de Muertos, is a national holiday in Mexico. It's a joyful festival, full of vibrant colors, face painting, and costumes to celebrate deceased loved ones. Add more people and color to this page as they celebrate the people they love.

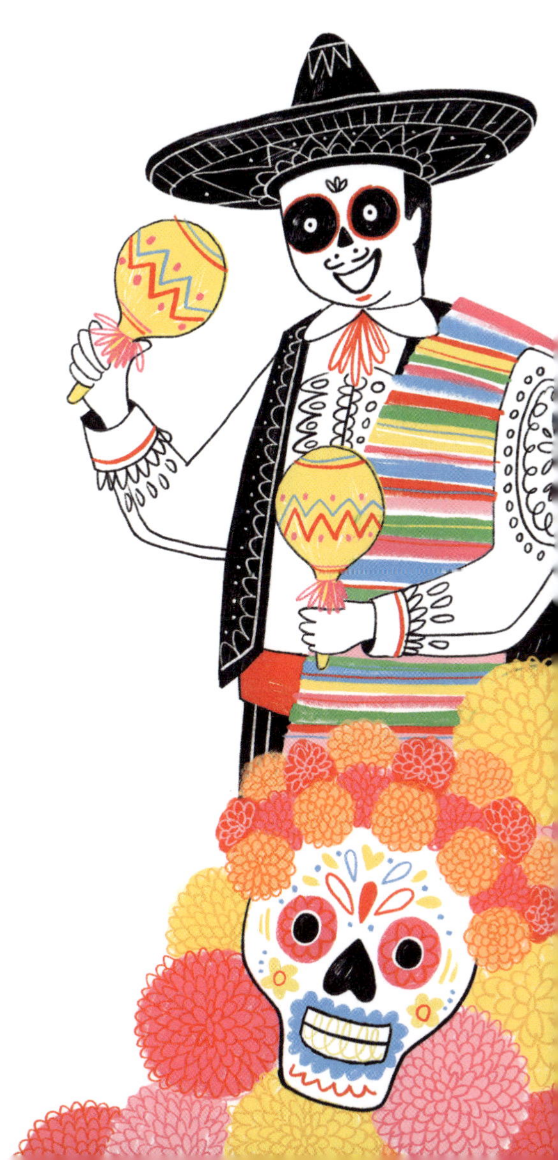

HAIR TYPES

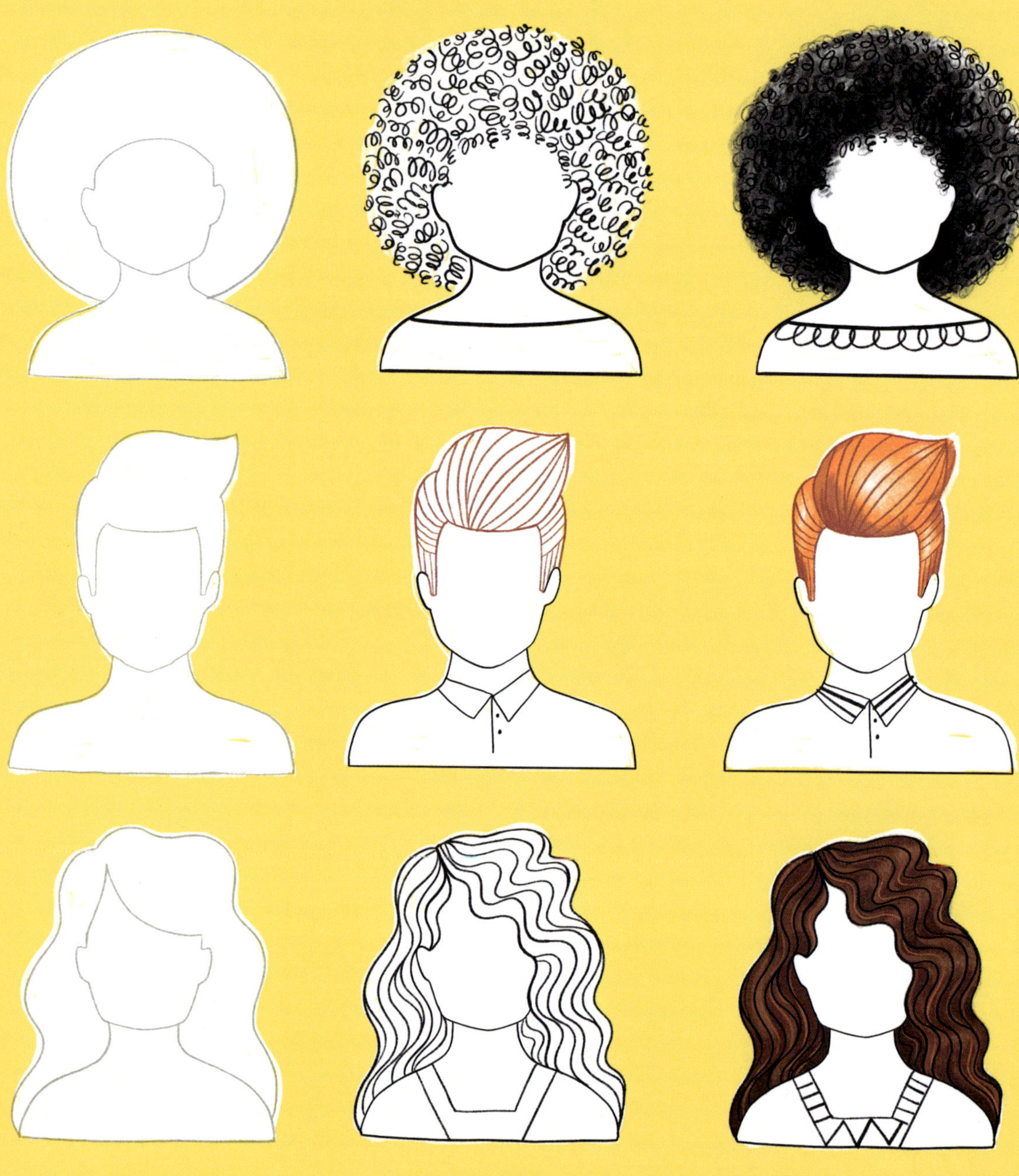

1 In pencil, sketch your character's face shape, then decide on what hairline and style of haircut suits that shape.

2 Hair doesn't tend to just fall straight down, it can go in every direction depending on the hair type. Use the direction of your lines to suggest movement and volume.

3 Next, pick a material that will compliment the natural texture of the hair you want to draw. Use tone to show the different shades of color.

Hair comes in many types, from straight strands to loose waves, and from soft bouncy curls to tight coils. This exercise focuses on a wide range of texture and shape. Practice these hair types below. If you want to include curly hair, follow the same process as coily hair, just loosening the curl.

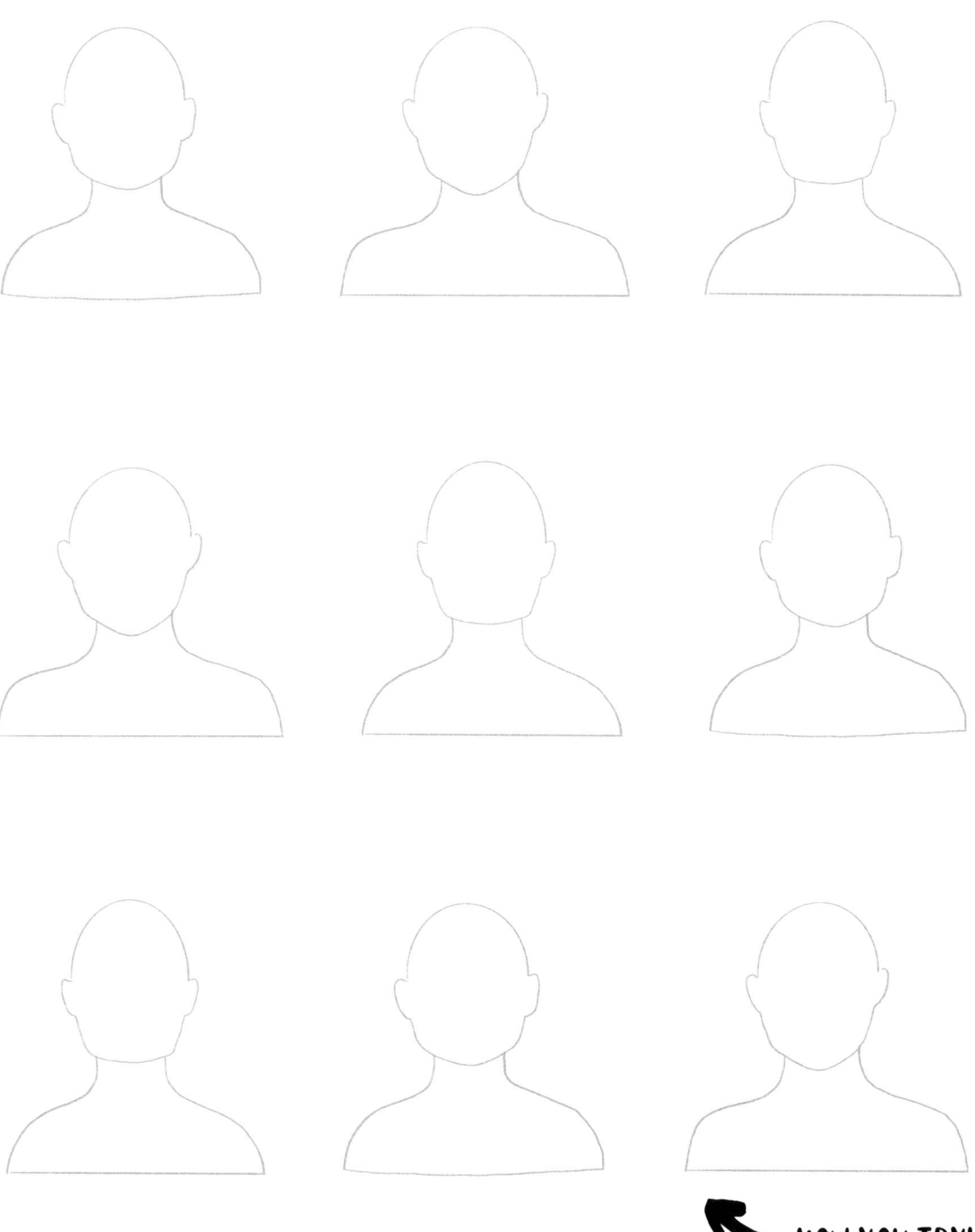

HAIRSTYLES

Now you have learned the different types and textures of hair, put those lessons into practice and create a range of hairstyles. Draw a character in each corresponding box. Who would choose which style?

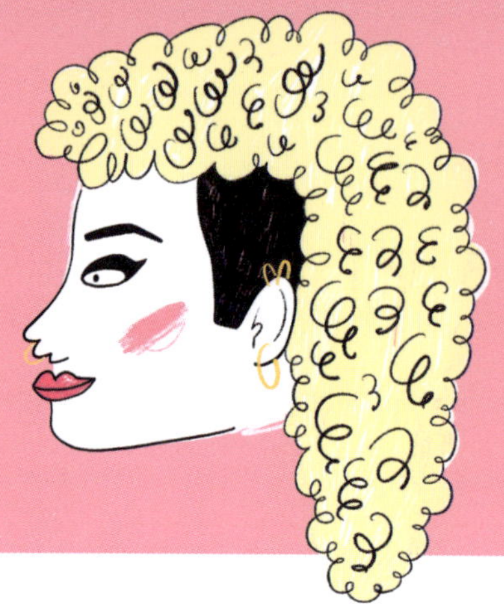

MULLET

BEEHIVE

BOB

AFRO

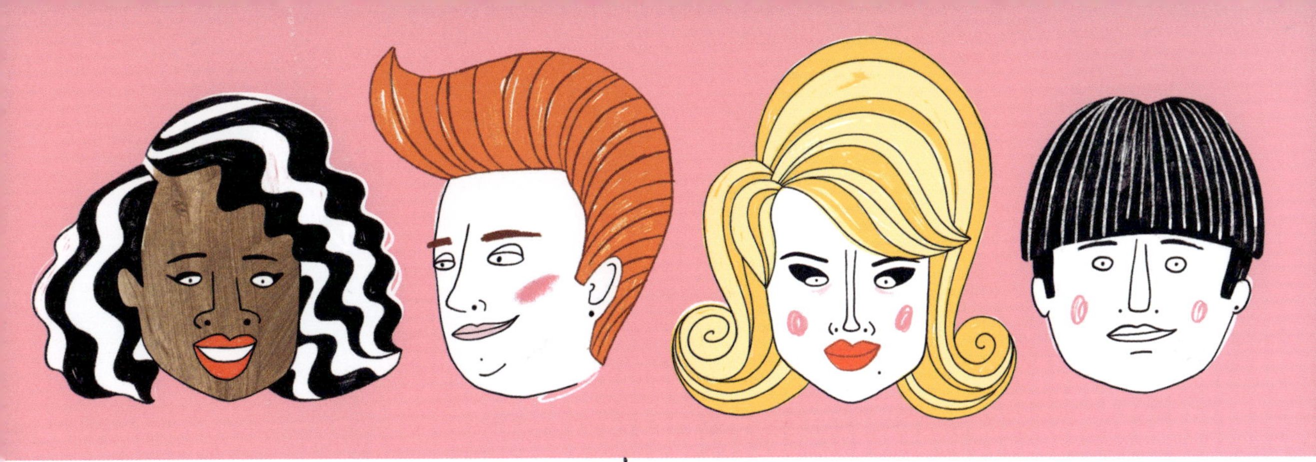

BOWL CUT

QUIFF

CURTAINS

BOUFFANT

CATCH OF THE DAY

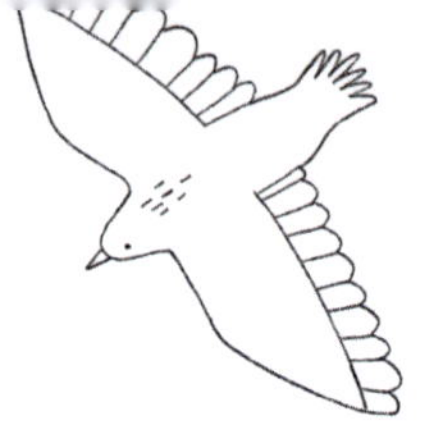

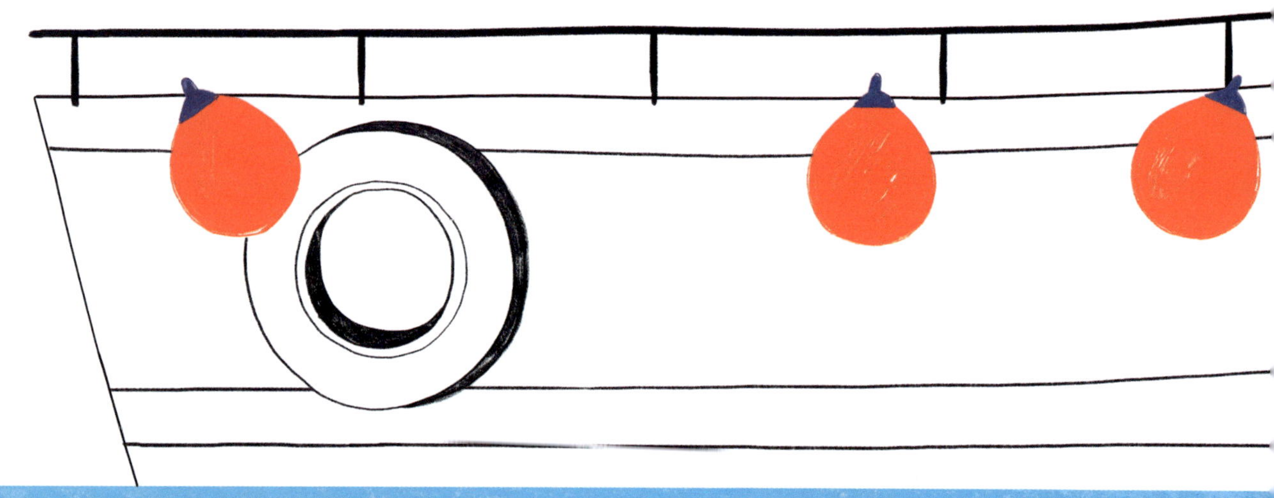

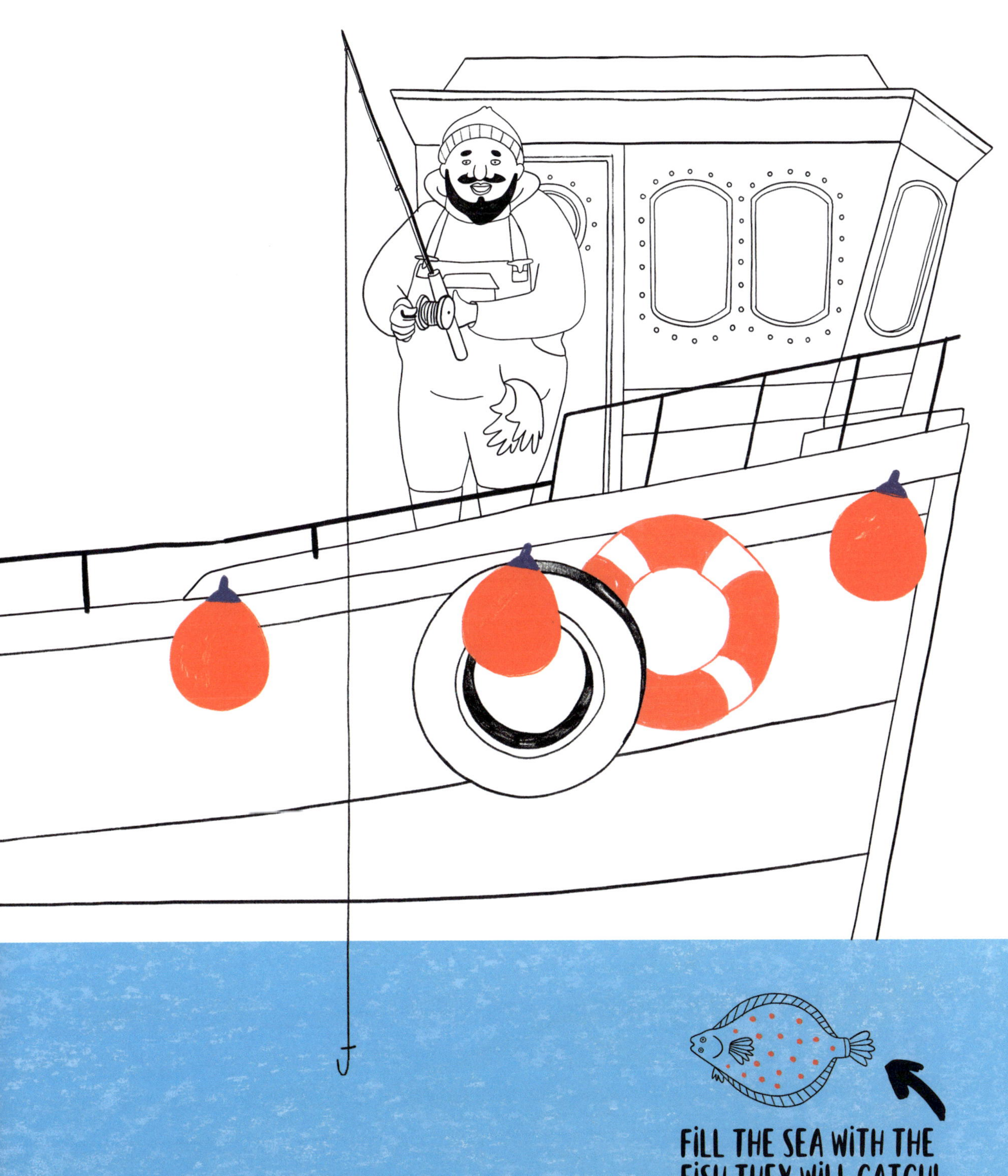

Draw people on this boat, alongside the skipper already on board, out for a fun day of fishing. Get them sea-ready in waterproof bibs, braces, and boots. Are there any more seabirds in the sky ready to dive down for their lunch?

CHAMPIONSHIP BEARDS

Celebrate flamboyant and fabulous facial hair by filling the page with the best beards and moustaches you can imagine! Whether it's a goatee, mutton chop, or a moustache like Dalí, let your imagination run wild. Start by giving these beards faces and coloring in the chaps on the page.

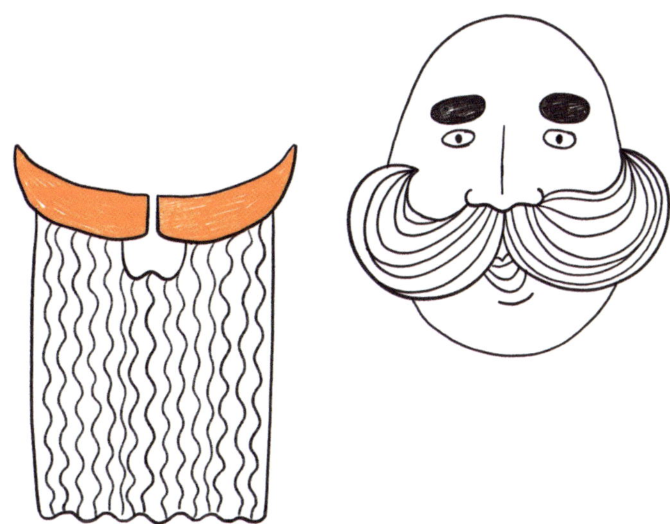

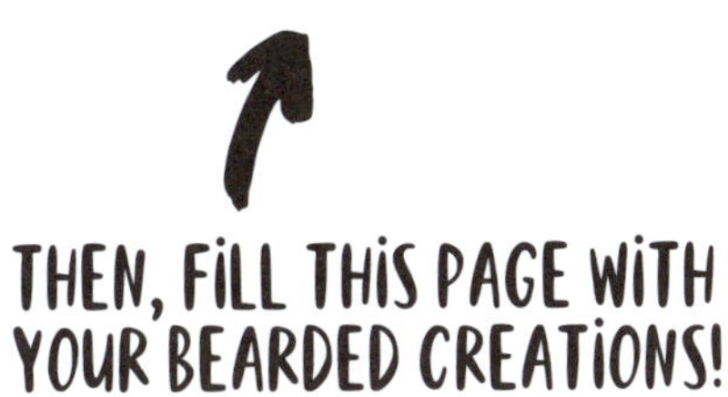
THEN, FILL THIS PAGE WITH YOUR BEARDED CREATIONS!

USING BODY LANGUAGE

JOY

CONFIDENCE

AMUSEMENT

SERENITY

CURIOSITY

Practice drawing people using their body language to express their emotions shown through facial expressions, gestures, and eye contact.

RELIEF

SURPRISE!

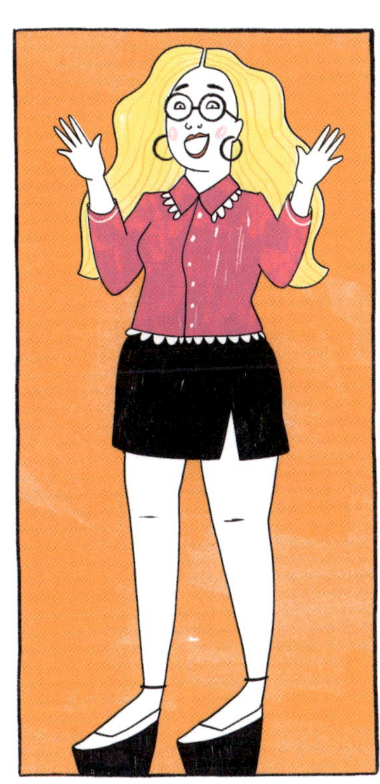

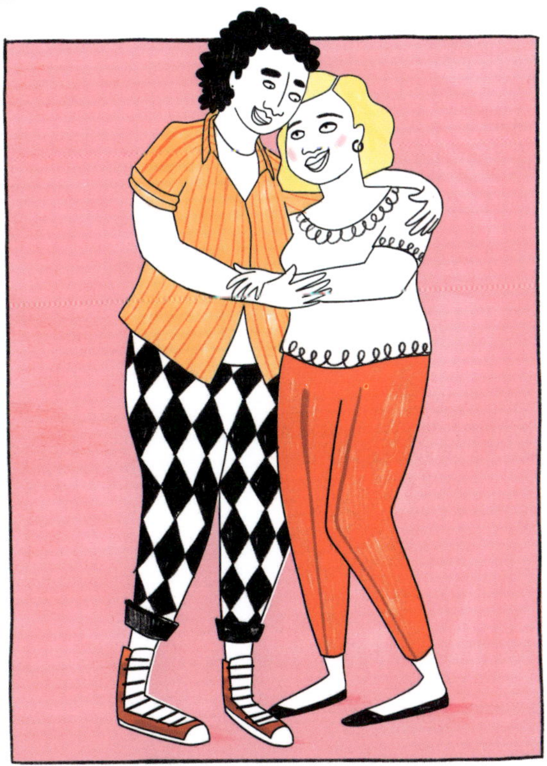

TWO PEOPLE IN LOVE

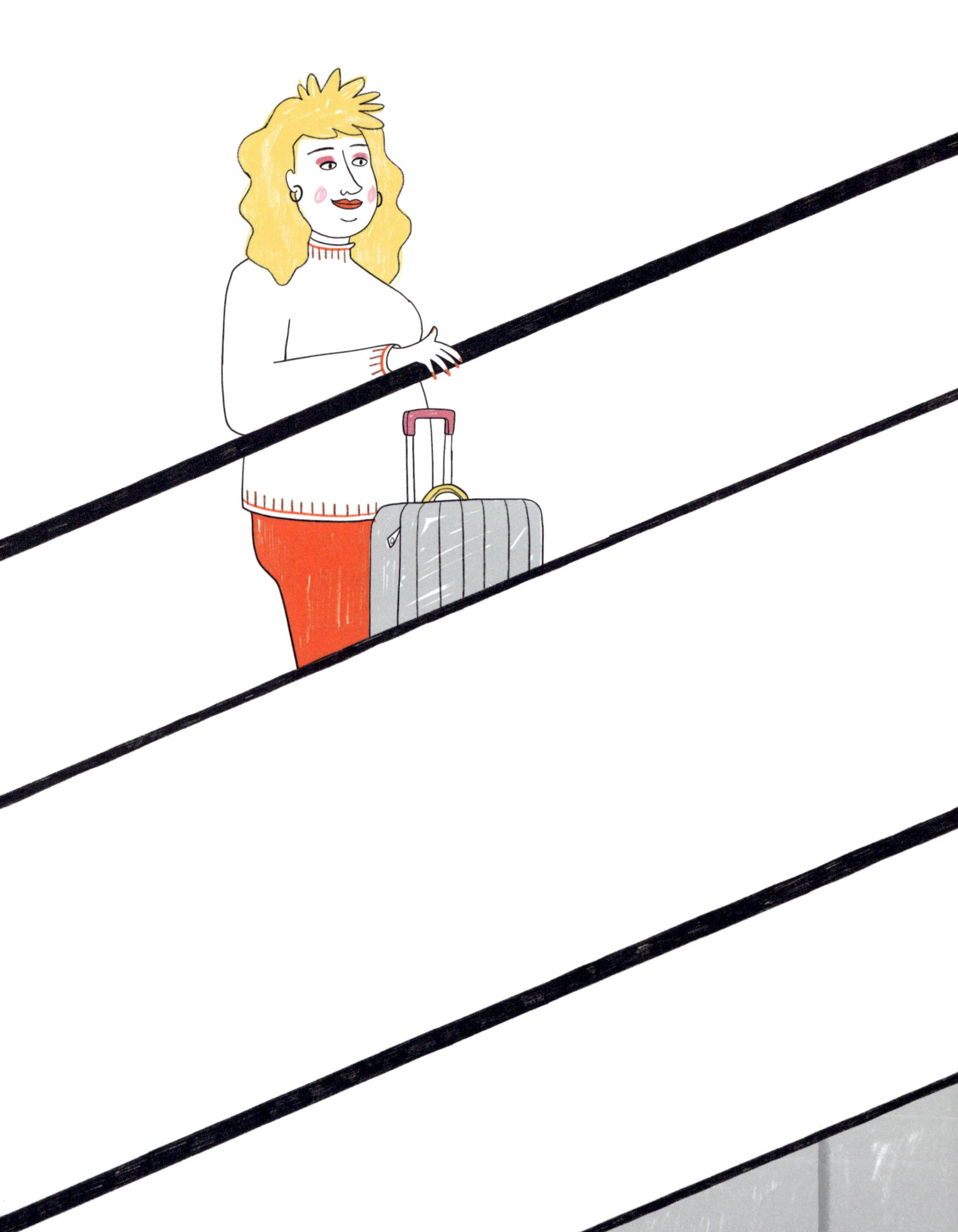

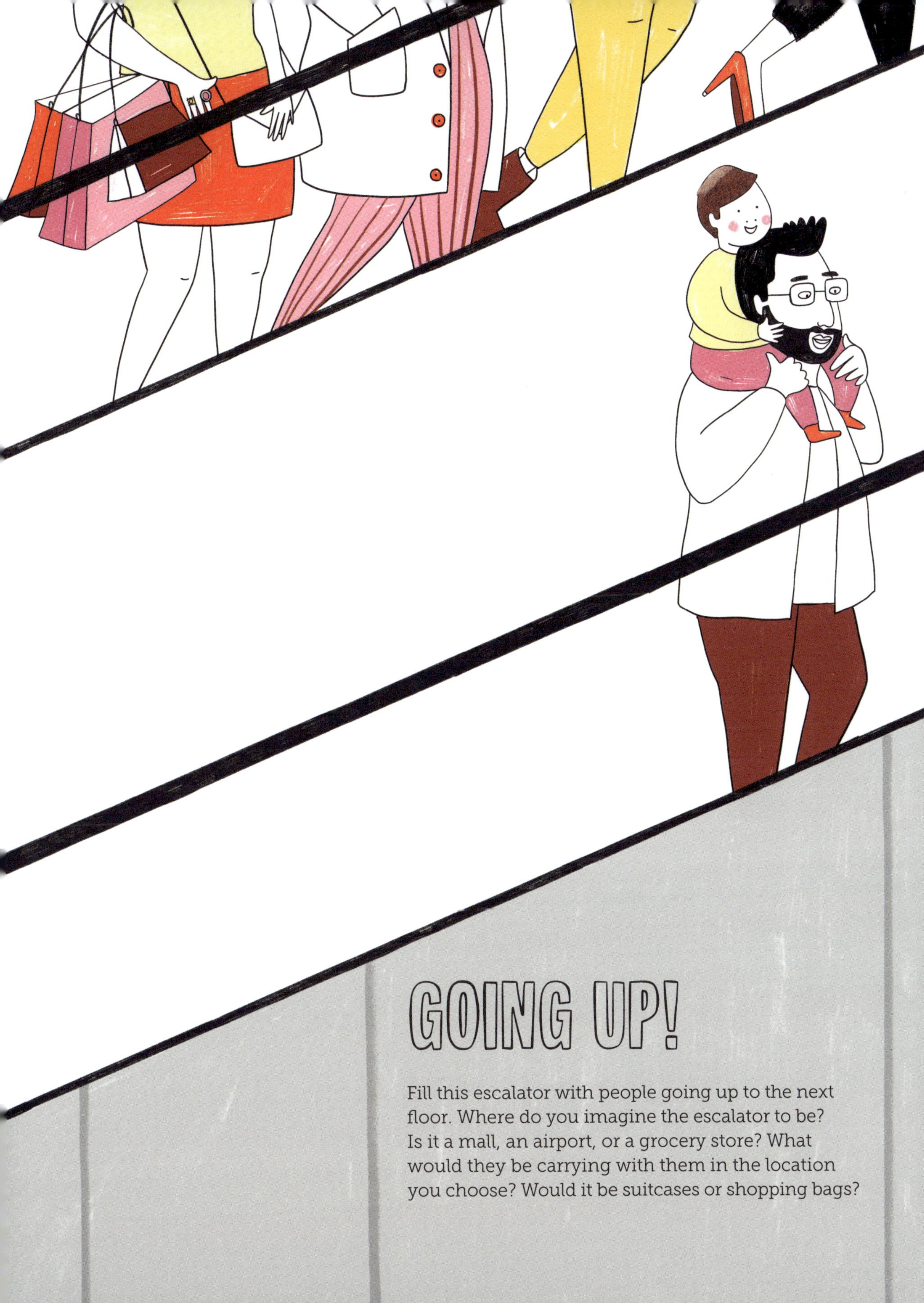

GOING UP!

Fill this escalator with people going up to the next floor. Where do you imagine the escalator to be? Is it a mall, an airport, or a grocery store? What would they be carrying with them in the location you choose? Would it be suitcases or shopping bags?

SEASONS: SUMMER

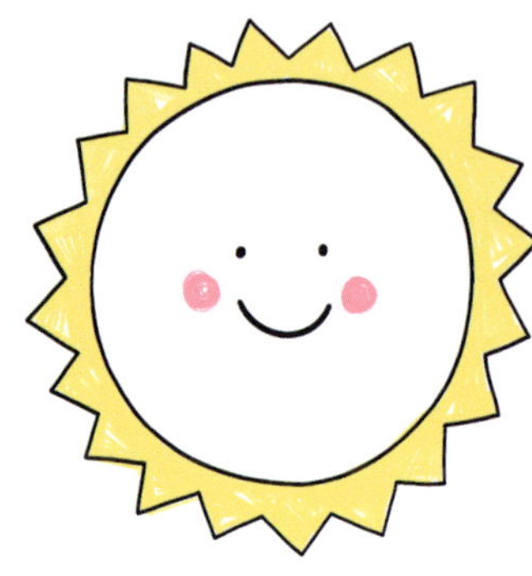

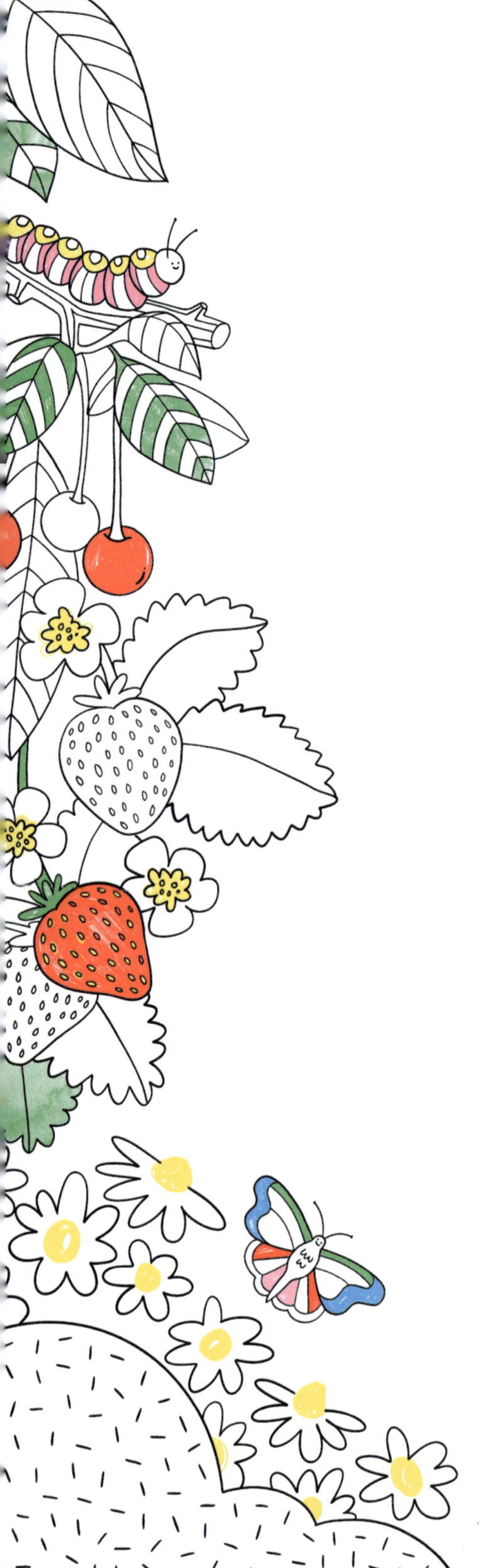

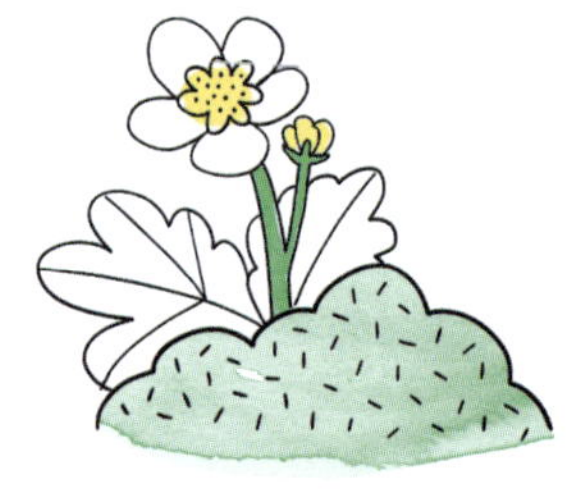

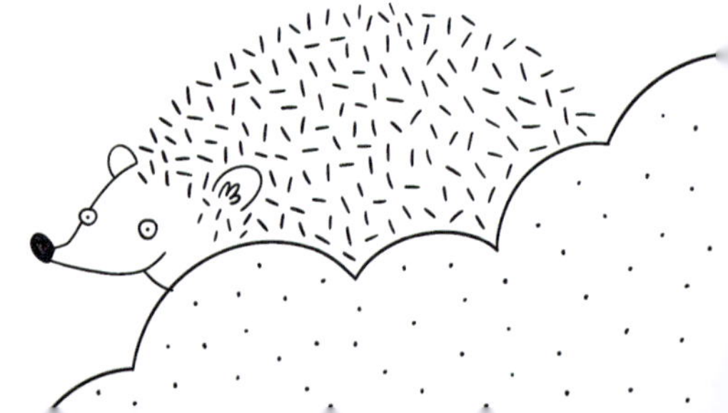

It's hot and sunny during the summer and many people go on vacation.
Using a bright, bold color palette, draw people out and about, dressing
them in clothes to keep them cool, and giving them hats and sunglasses.

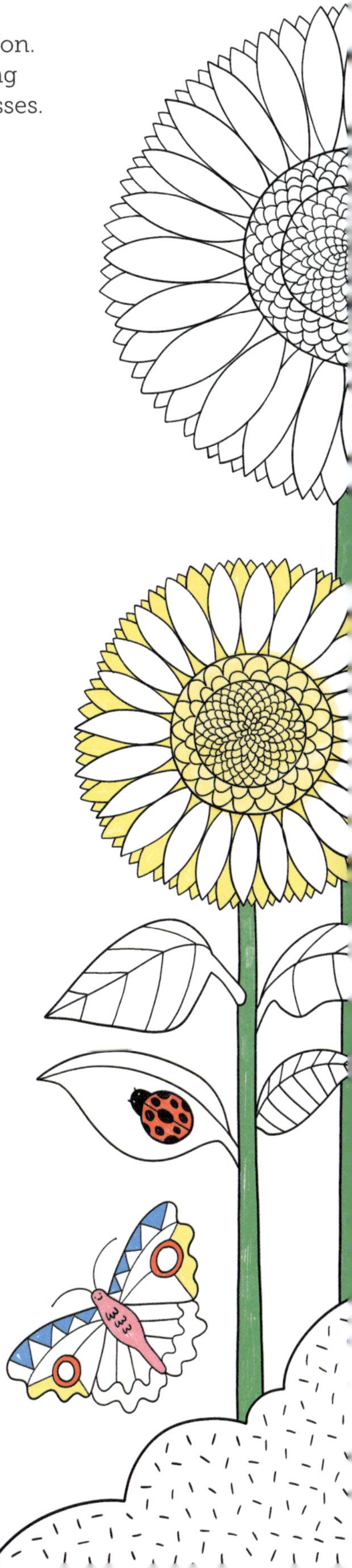

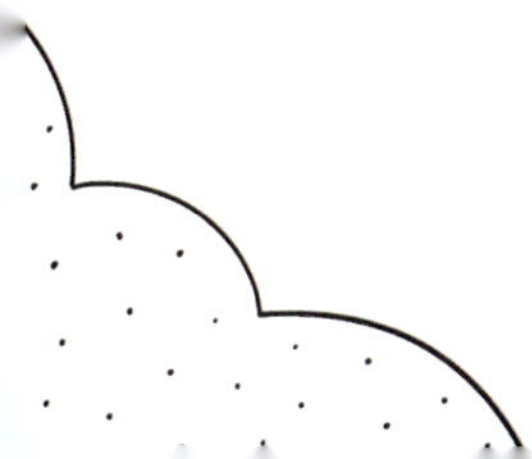

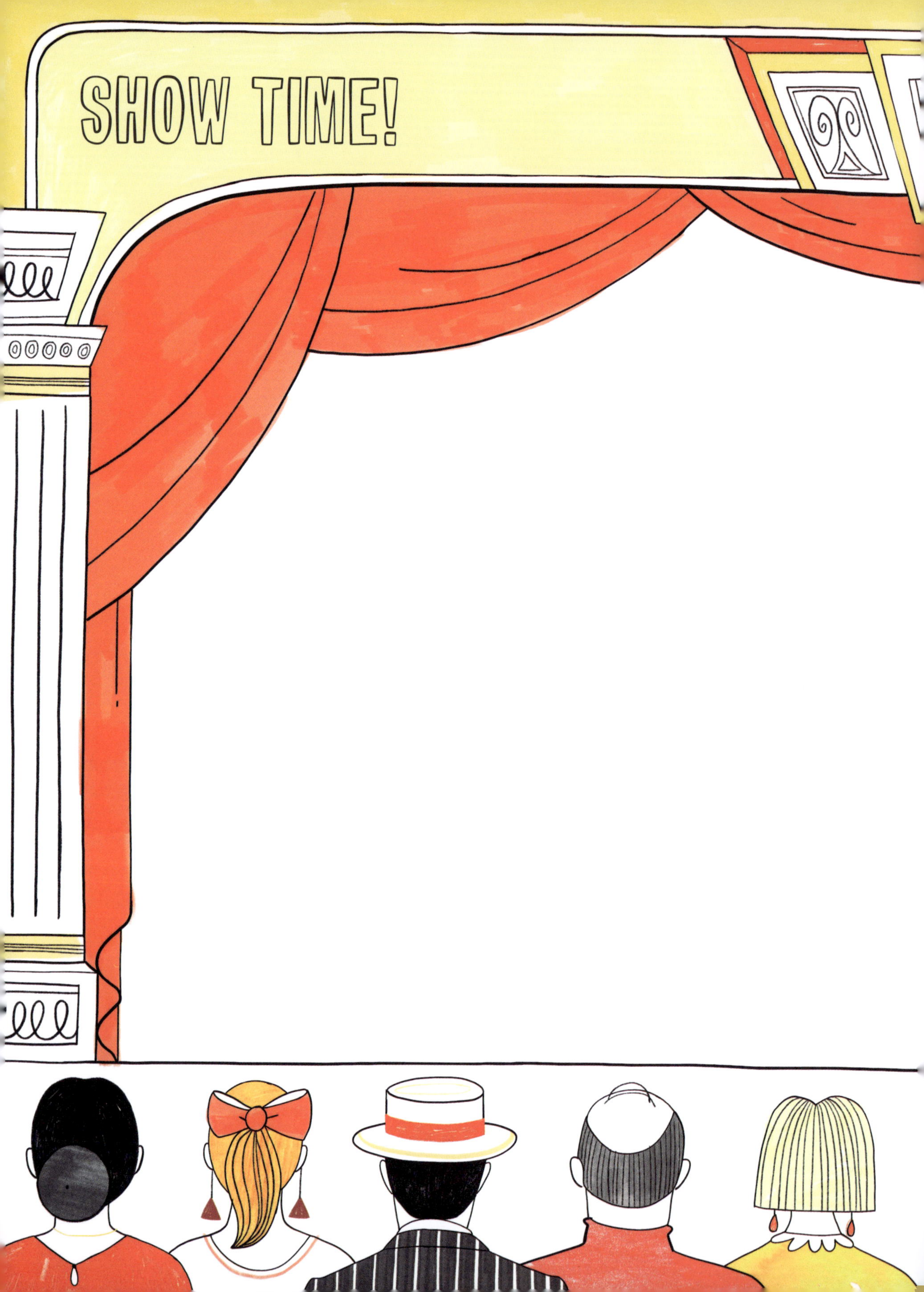
SHOW TIME!

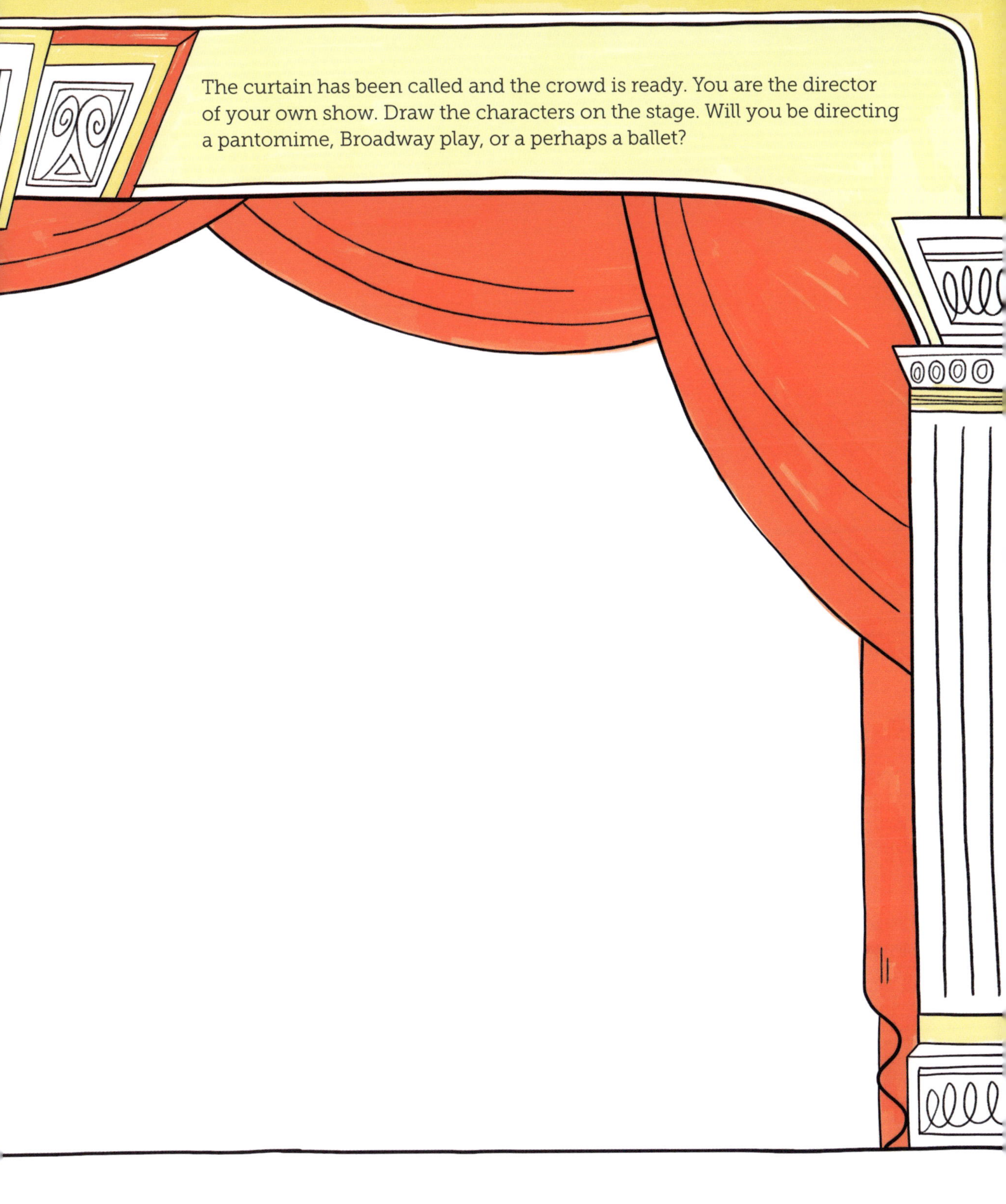

The curtain has been called and the crowd is ready. You are the director of your own show. Draw the characters on the stage. Will you be directing a pantomime, Broadway play, or a perhaps a ballet?

DRAW THE REST OF THE AUDIENCE!

DARE TO BE DIFFERENT!

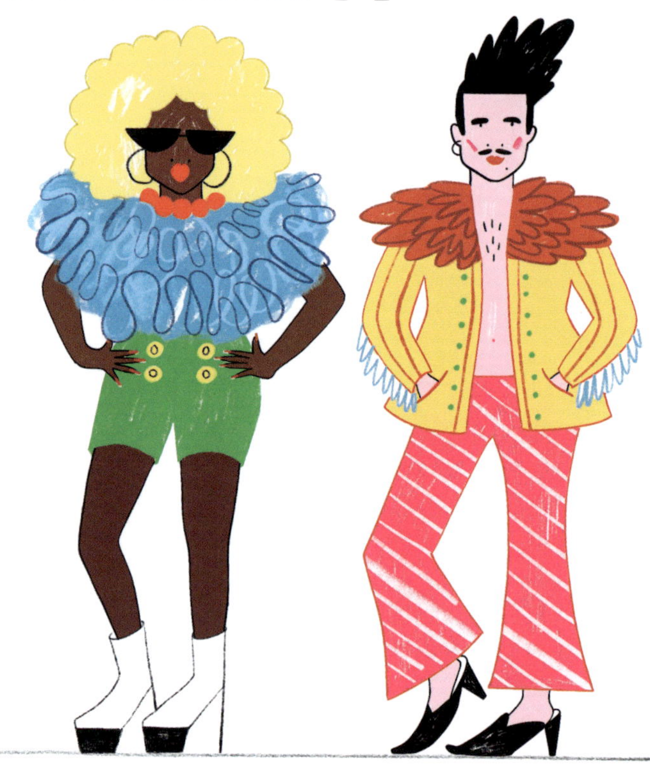

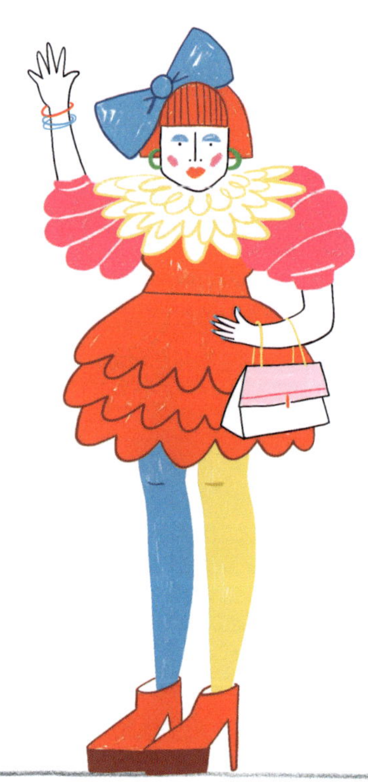

Let's celebrate being different. The world is a more interesting and kinder
place when we embrace everyone's unique qualities. Create characters that
use their clothes as a flamboyant, colorful canvas to express themselves.

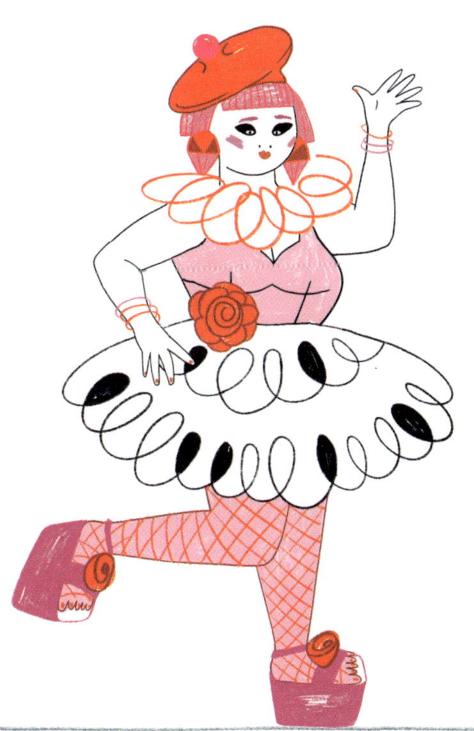

DRAW A PERSON SITTING

These steps will teach you the basics of how to draw a person sitting down. Observe where each limb is positioned and how it connects to the others. Then, place the limbs at different angles to change the character's position.

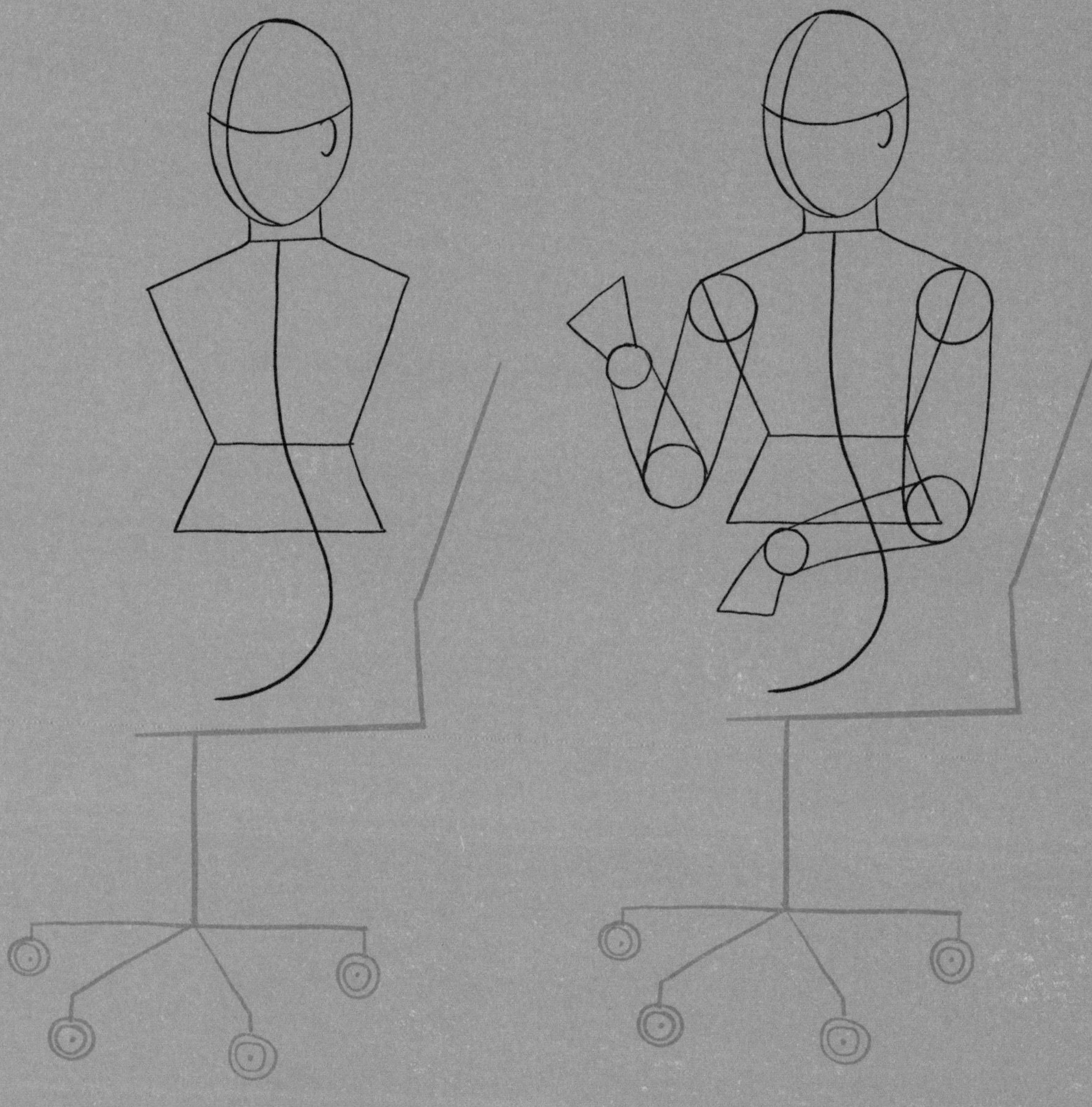

1 Sketch the head at a slight angle; add the neck. For the chest, make a shape similar to a trapezium with the top points pointing upward for the shoulders. Add a smaller trapezium for the torso. Create a curve for the spine.

2 Add two circles for the shoulders as shown. Draw rectangles for the upper arms, add one forearm pointing upward and one tilting slightly downward. Add circles for the wrists and a rough shape outline for the hands.

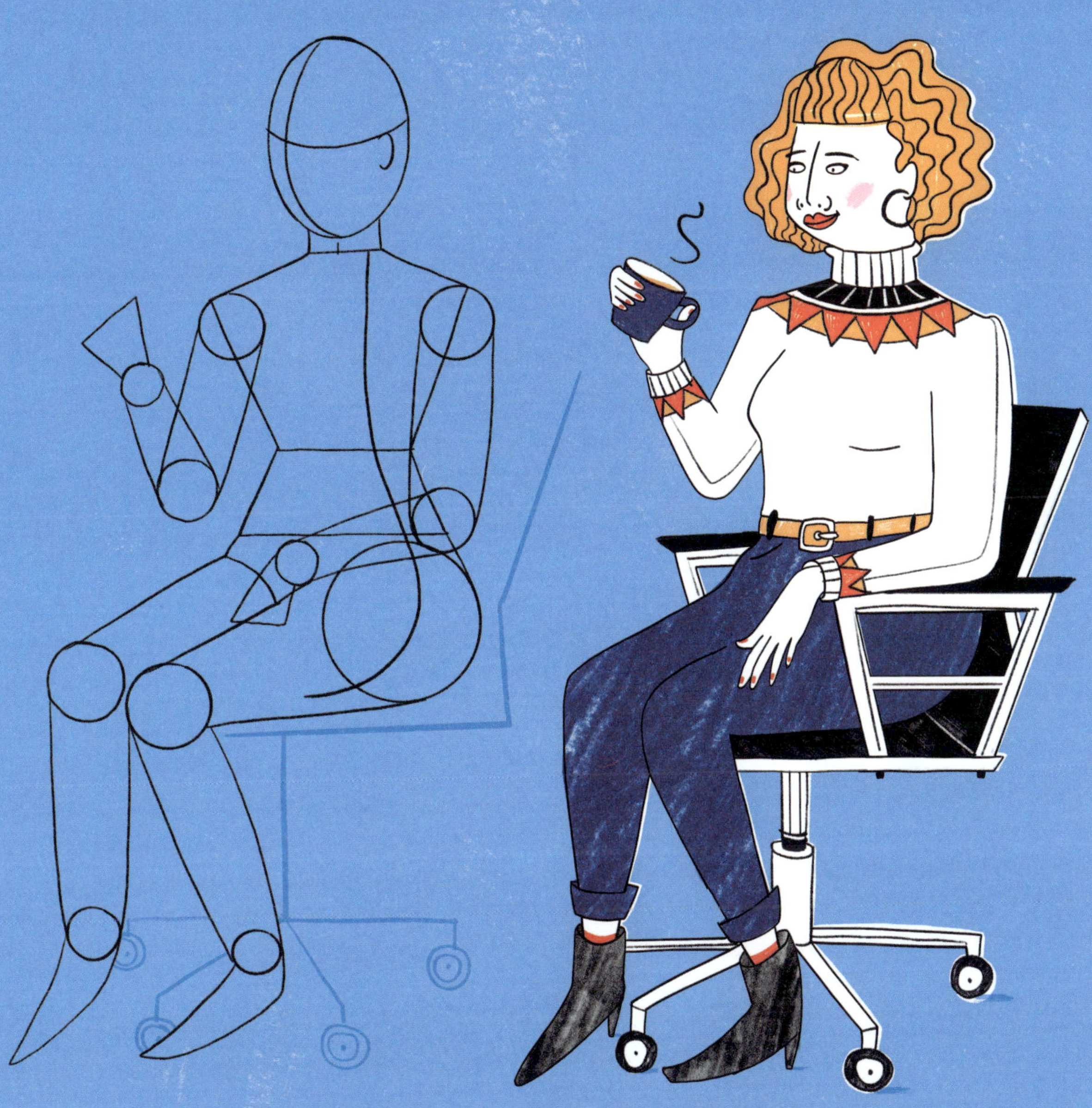

3 Draw a large circle for the buttocks, adding a shape similar to underwear for hips. Sketch two rectangles for the upper legs tapering toward the knees with circles for the knees. Add two rectangles tapering toward the ankles and two circles for the ankles. Draw the feet outline.

4 Now, add the fun details! Using a fineliner, draw over your sketch adding in the character's details and style. Finish by rubbing out your pencil marks.

TURN OVER TO PRACTICE ➡

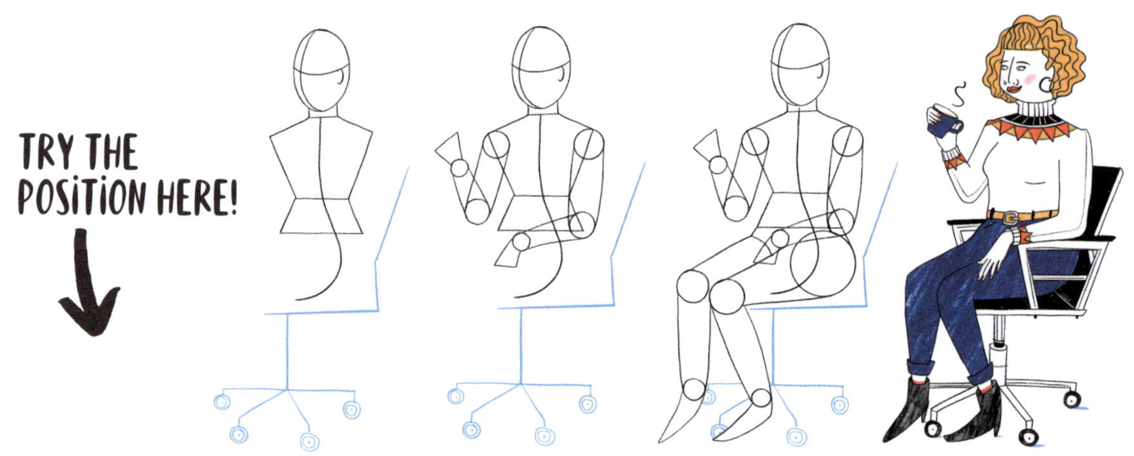

TRY THE
POSITION HERE!

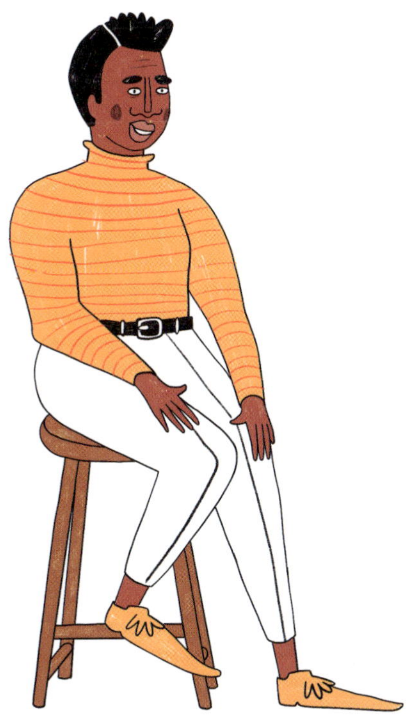

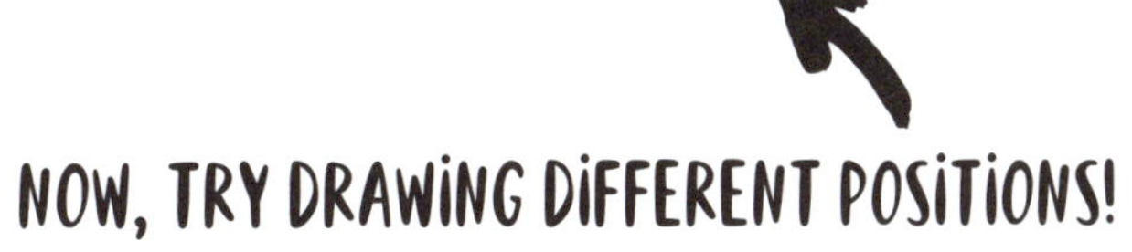
NOW, TRY DRAWING DIFFERENT POSITIONS!

SERVICE PLEASE!

This head chef needs her team of sous-chefs to join her in the kitchen. Draw them in and choose what they will be serving on today's menu!

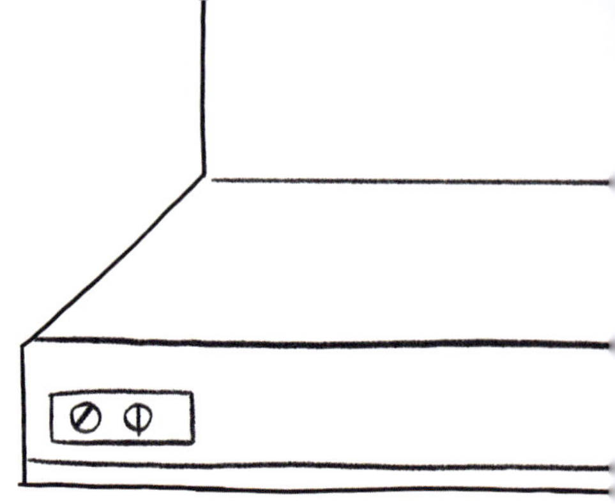

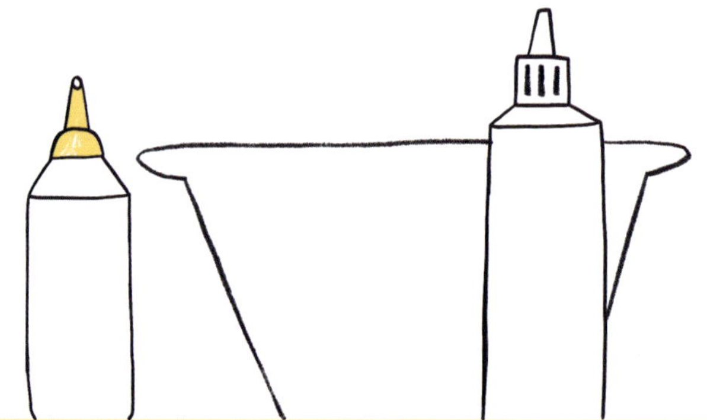

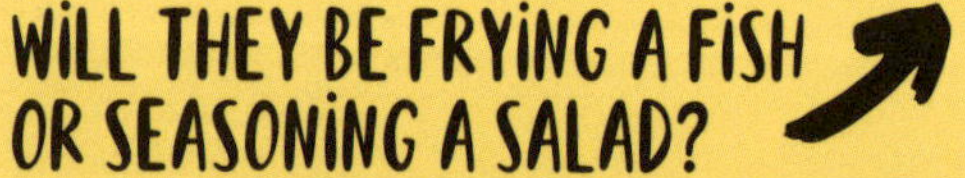

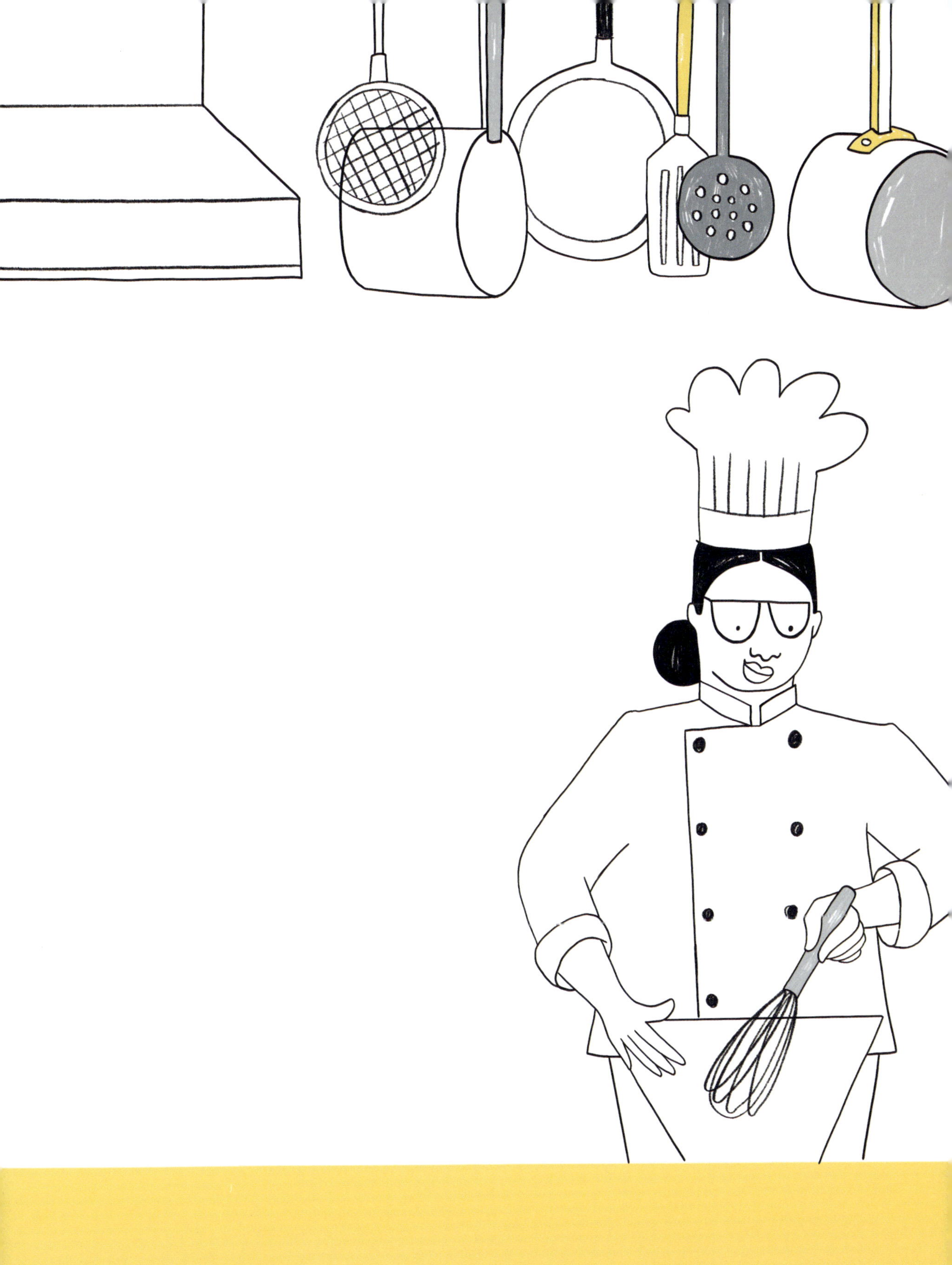

SUBCULTURES: ROCKABILLY

Add your own characters to this trio of rockabillys in their trademark leather jackets, quiffed hair, and polka dot or striped accessories. Keep to their iconic black, white, red, and blue colors.

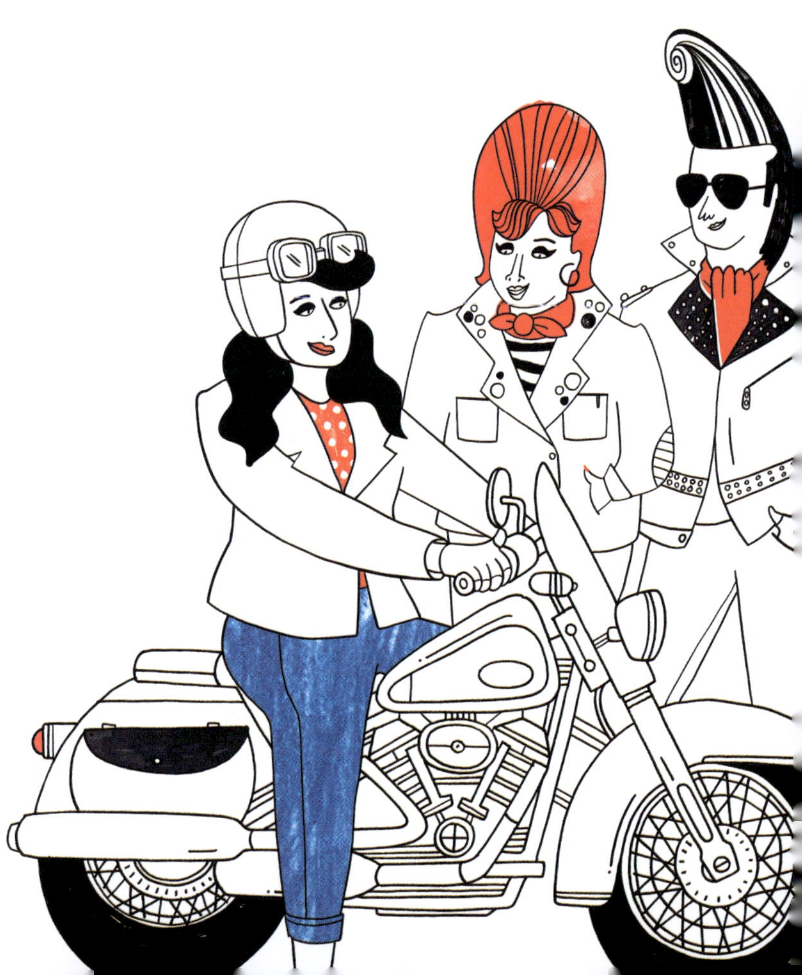

FINISH THE PORTRAIT

Complete Genghis Khan's traditional Mongolian clothing. Add in the details of his long embroidered robe, known as a deel, and finish his beard and hat. Then color in the portrait in warm, rich colors.

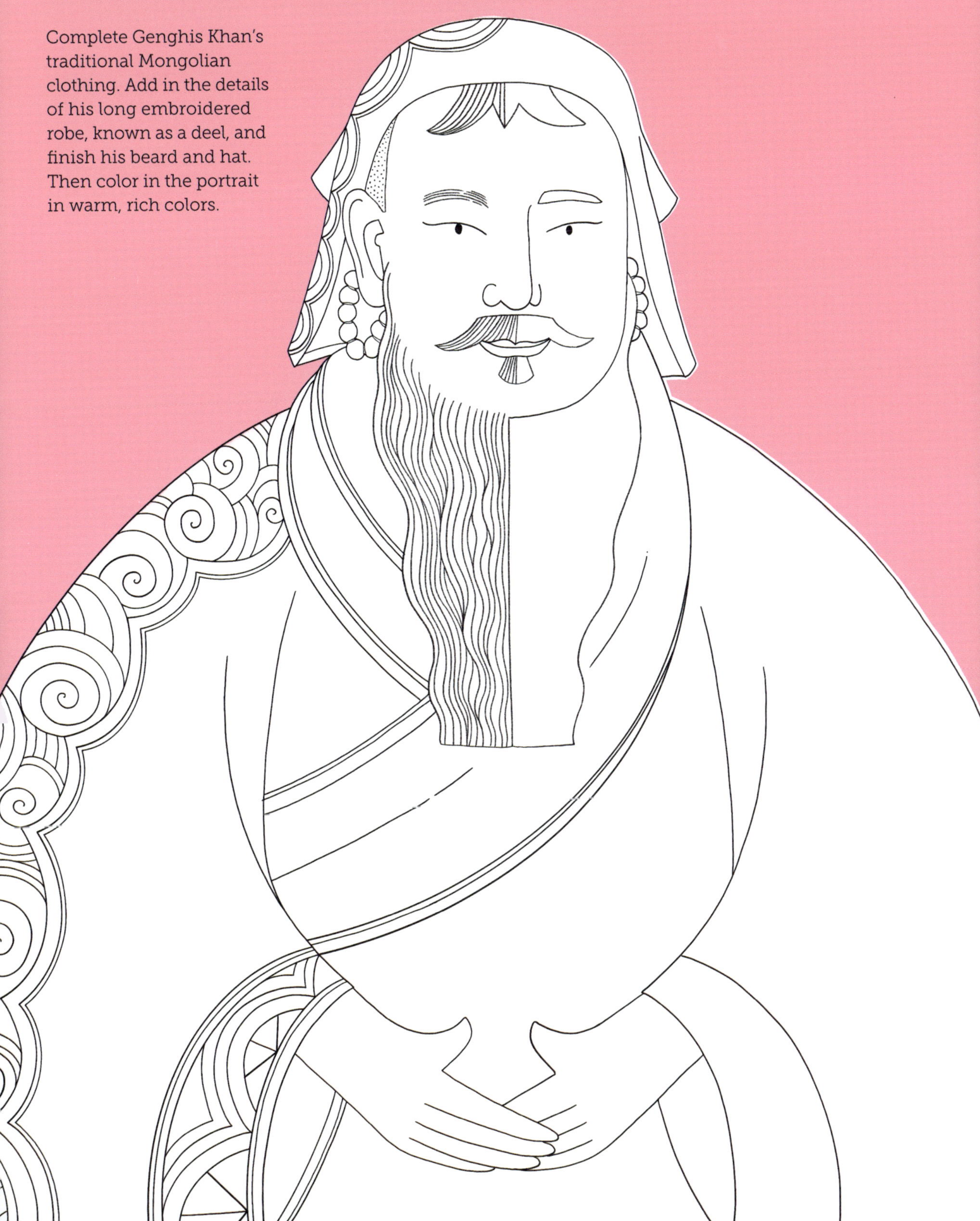

ERAS: 1920S

Fill this page with fashion from the roaring Twenties. From the famous flapper dresses, bobs, pearls, and cloche hats to men's Fedora or flat cap hats and tailored suits, design a set of outfits and characters to suit that era.

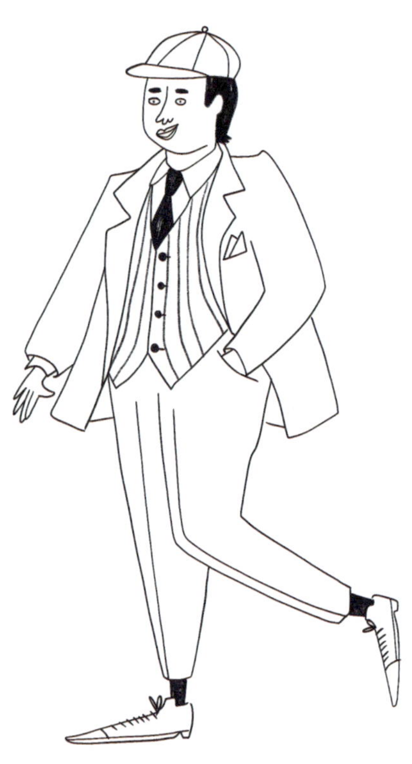

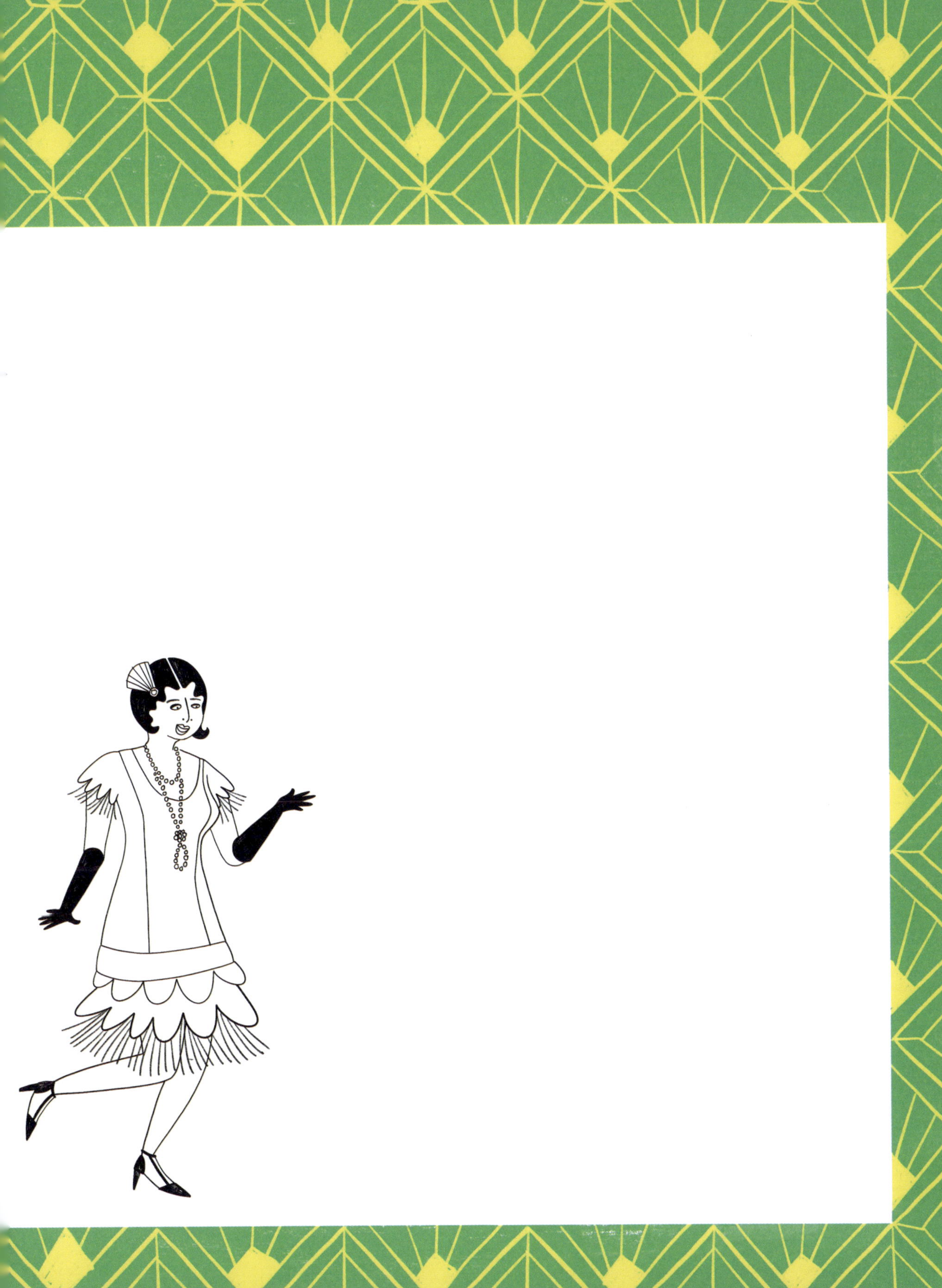

PRECIOUS METALS

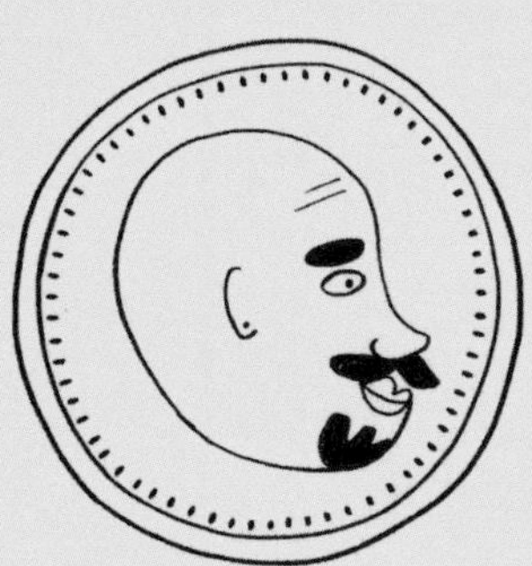

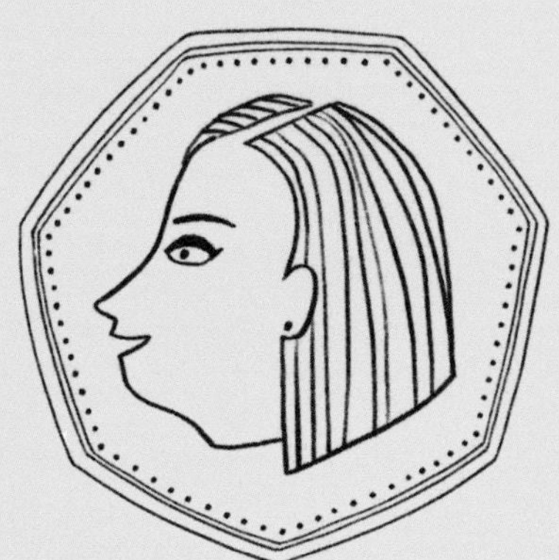

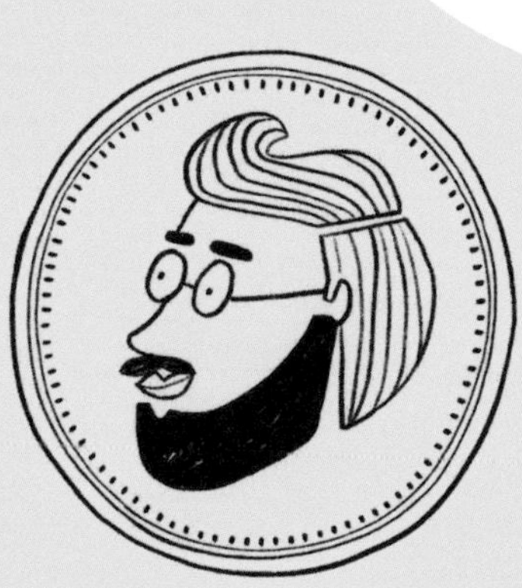

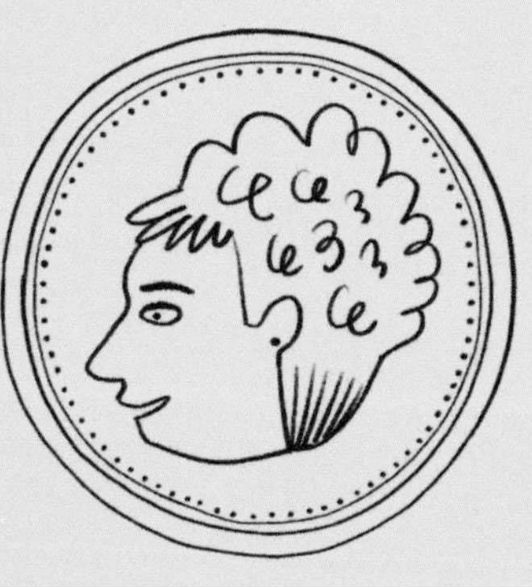

Turn your most precious people into gold, making your own unique set of commemorative coins. Draw each character in a side profile, then color them in either gold, silver, or copper tones.

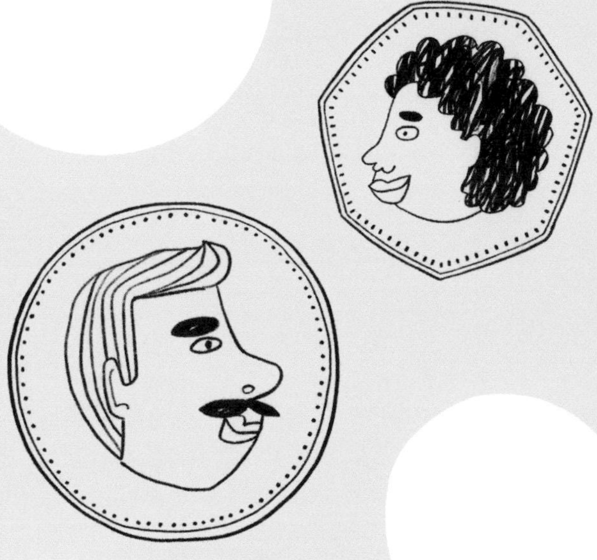

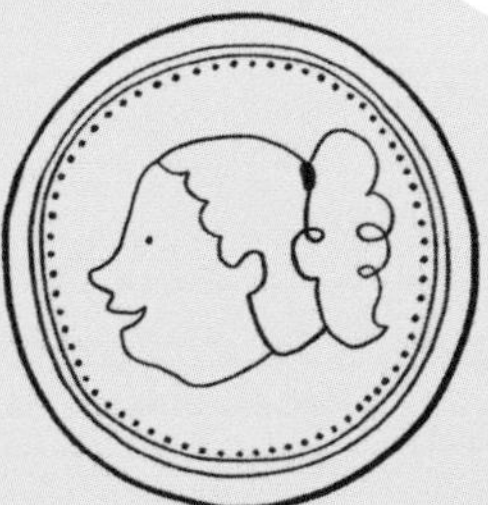

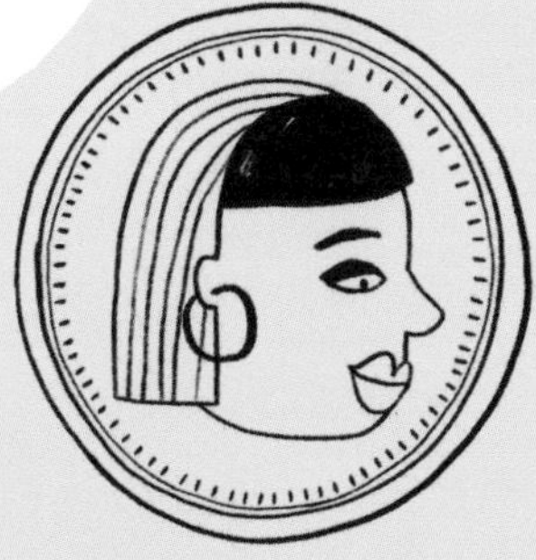

HAPPY HALLOWEEN

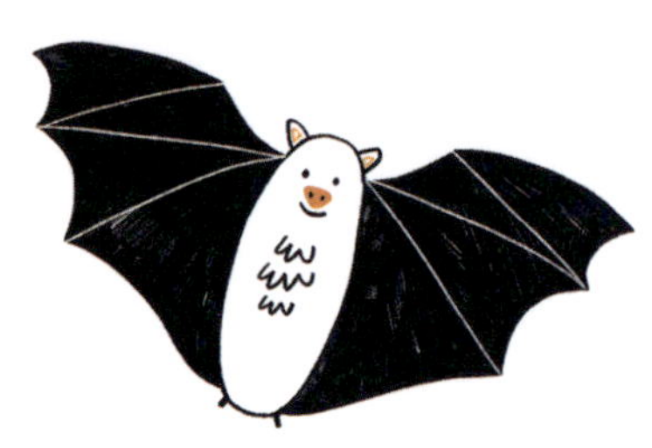

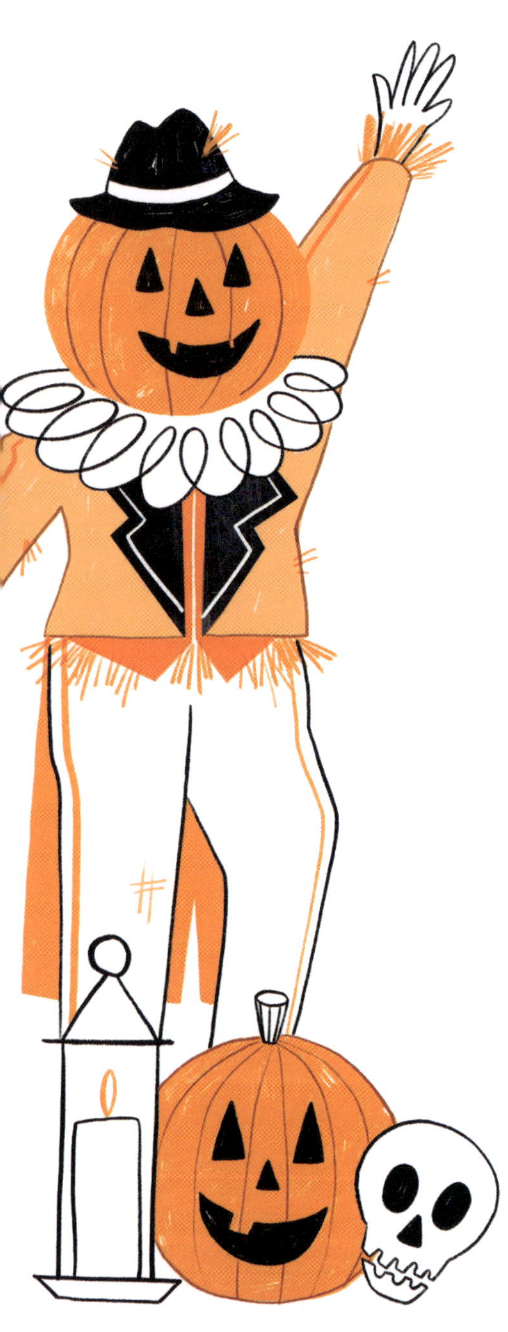

Decorate this page with spooky people celebrating Halloween in all their wonderful costumes, turning it into a busy parade. From mummies to monsters and witches, give each character a costume! Challenge yourself to use a color palette of just orange and black.

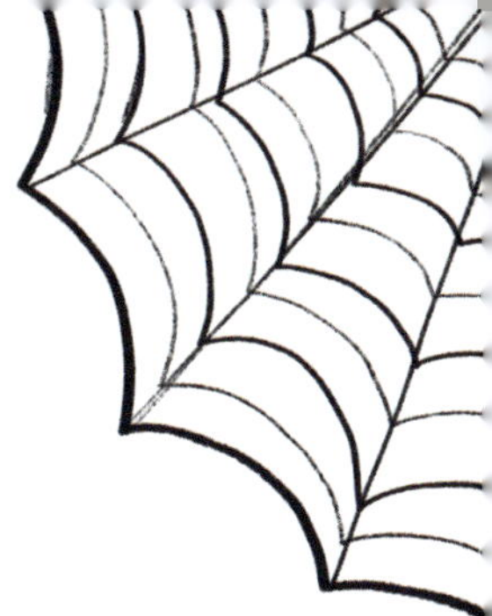

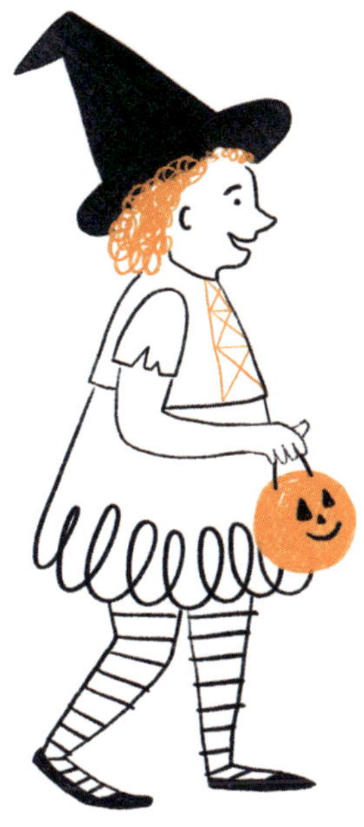

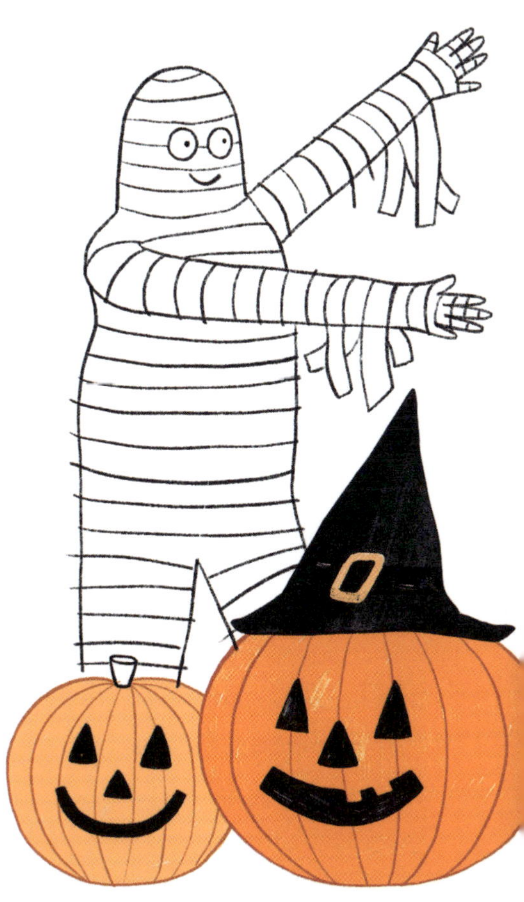

SEVEN-DAY CHALLENGE

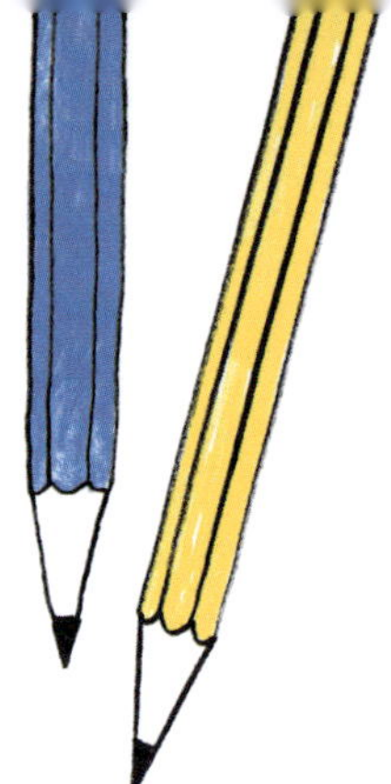

Choose this page when you have time to commit to this small but mighty activity. Spending a short amount of time, such as 20 minutes, on a daily basis will have a big impact on your development over time. Trust the process, but don't be too hard on yourself if you miss a session—just pick up your pencil the next day and carry on.

DRAW YOURSELF SMILING

SKETCH YOUR NONDOMINANT HAND

SKETCH A TONAL PORTRAIT

DRAW A SIDE PROFILE PORTRAIT

DRAW A PERSON CARRYING SOMETHING

SKETCH SOMEONE WITH AFRO HAIR

YOU CHOOSE!

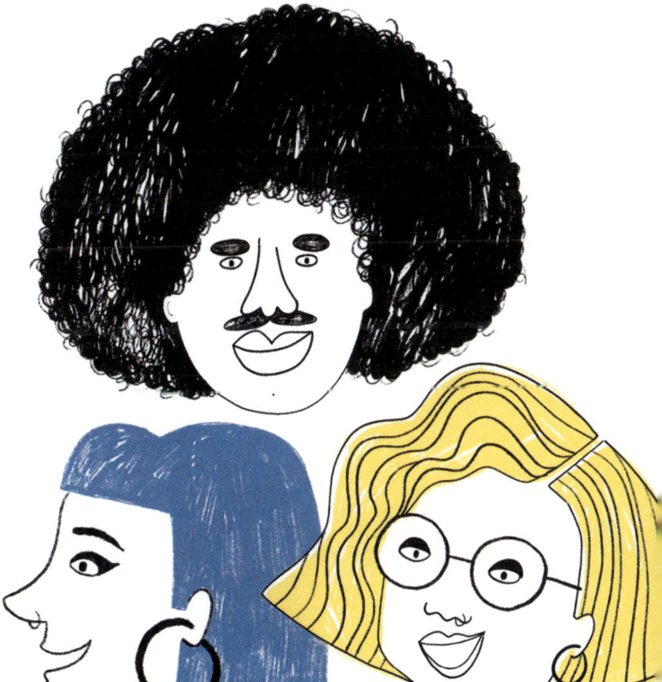

COMMIT TO A DAILY PRACTICE
AND YOU WILL SOON SEE RESULTS!

CULTURAL CLOTHING

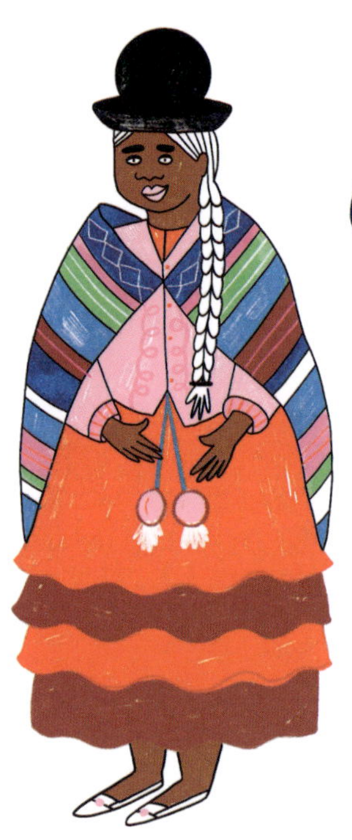

BOWLER HAT (BOLIVIA)

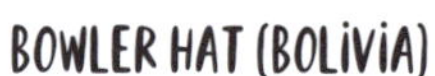

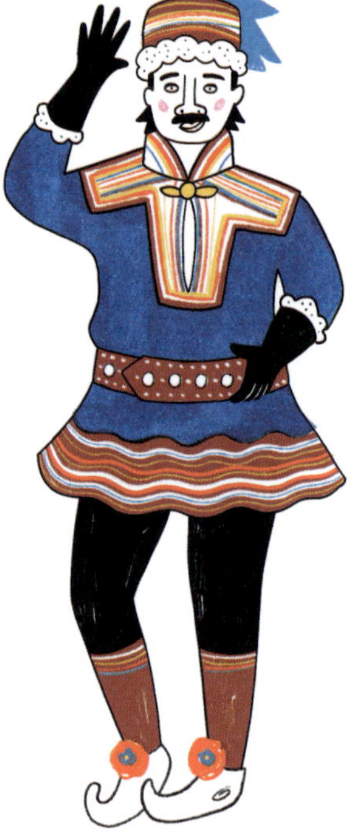

SÁMI GÁKTI (LAPLAND)

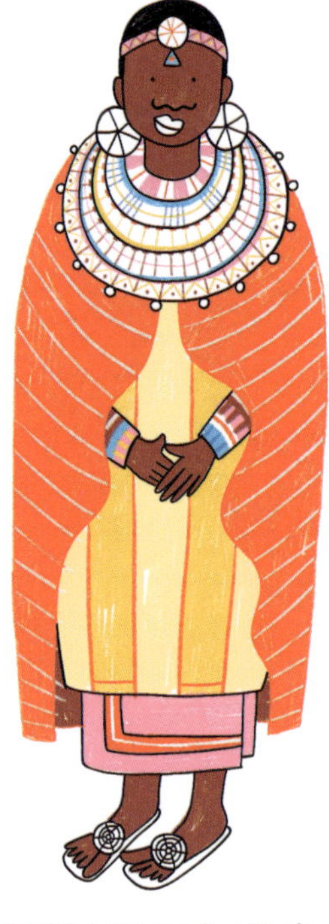

BEADS & SHUKA (MAASAI)

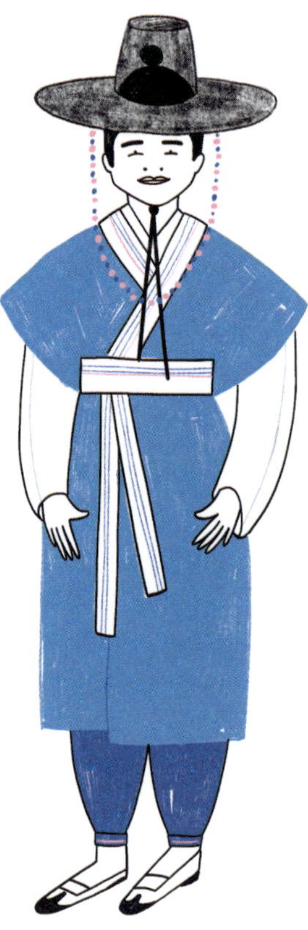

HANBOK (SOUTH KOREA)

PONCHO (PERU)

BUNAD (NORWAY)

FLAMENCO DRESS (SPAIN)

LEDERHOSEN (BAVARIA)

Explore the traditional everyday wear and celebratory dress found throughout the world. From the bowler hat in Bolivia to the Stetson, an iconic symbol of the American West. Fill this page with people showcasing the way they dress to express their culture.

KIMONO (JAPAN)

ÁO DÀI (VIETNAM)

STETSON (TEXAS)

SARI (INDIA)

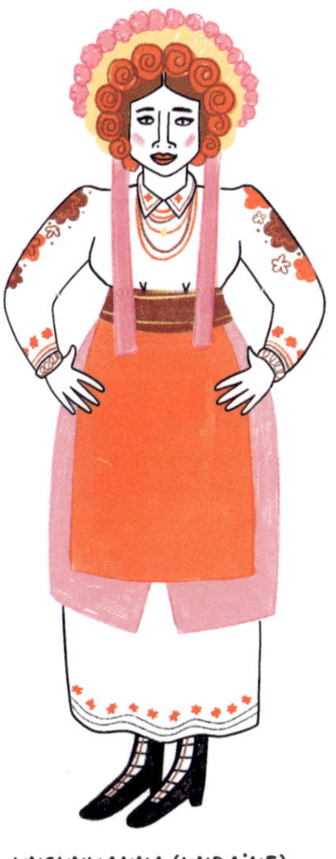

DASHIKI (WEST AFRICA)

KILT (SCOTLAND)

HERERO (NAMBIA)

VYSHYVANKA (UKRAINE)

ART ON THE WALLS

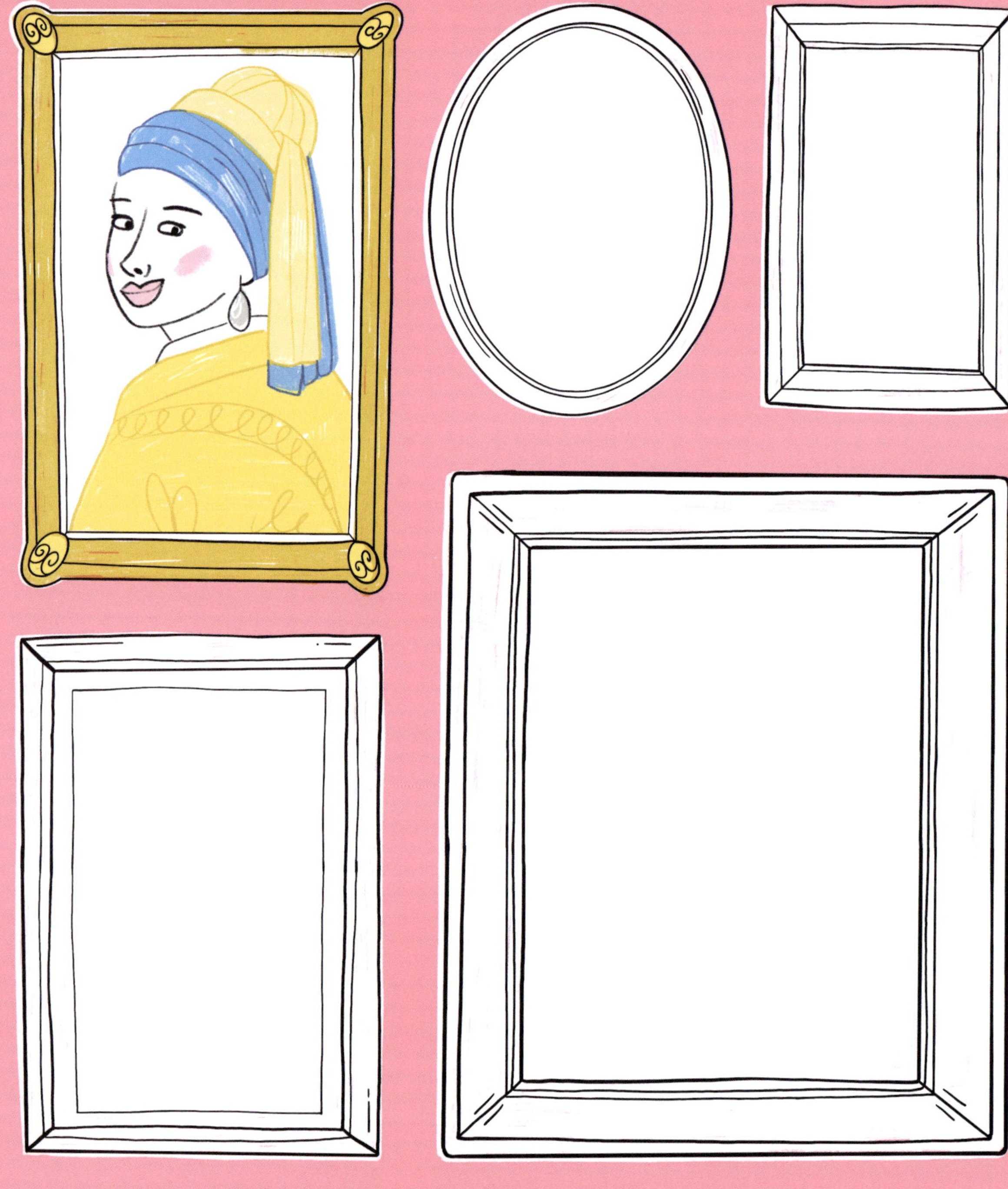

Today, you are the curator of your own portrait exhibition. Will you choose to celebrate the classics, showcasing iconic paintings, or fill the walls with your own masterpieces?

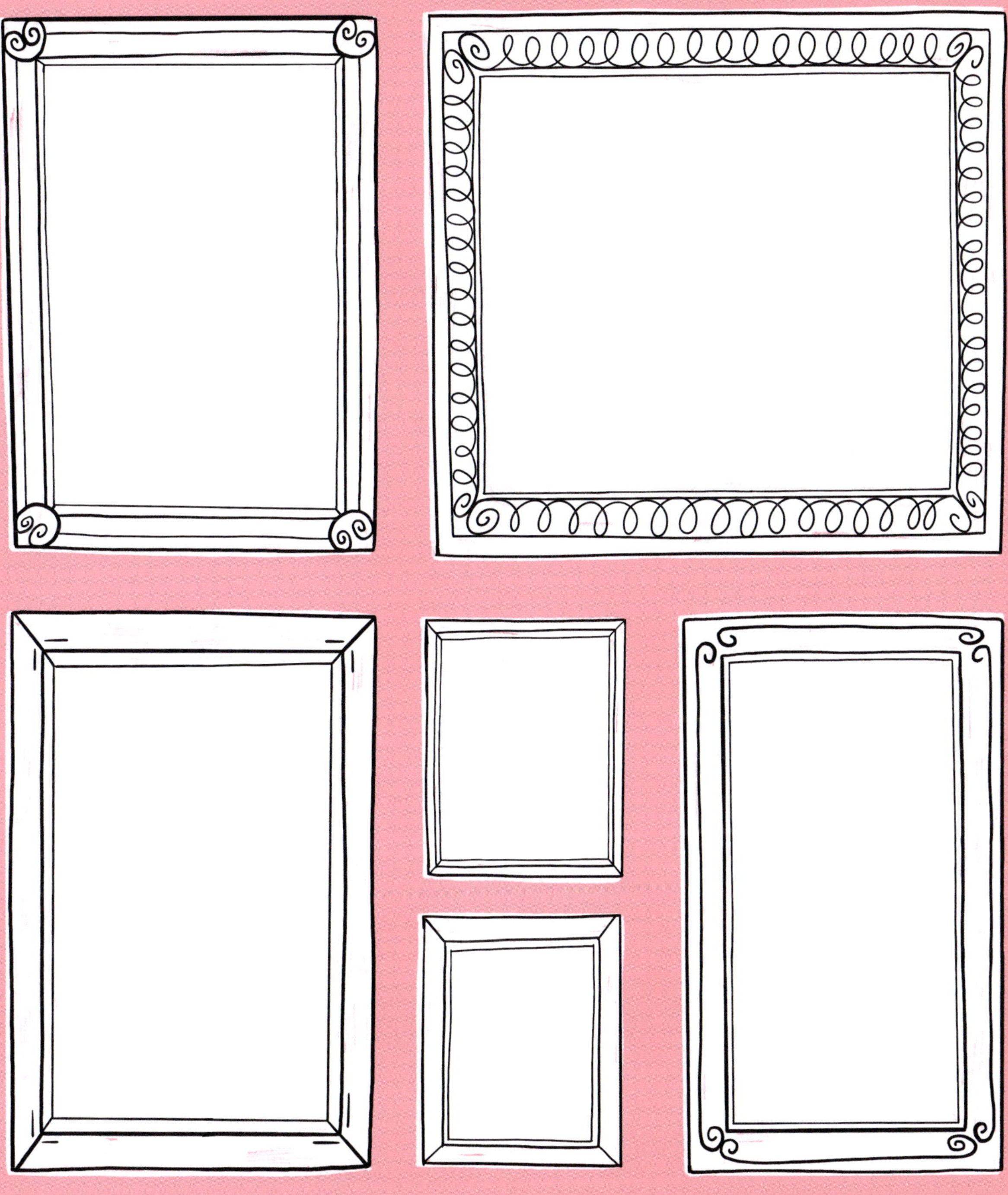

WALKING SEQUENCE

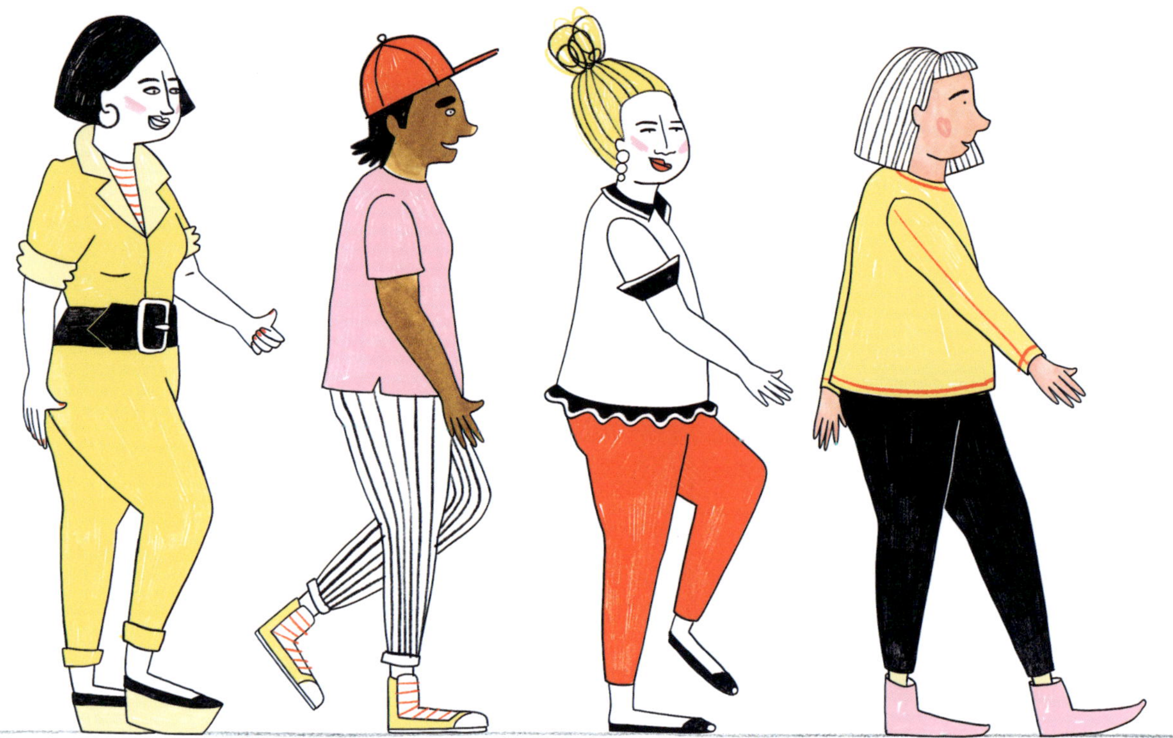

Here you will learn to illustrate a walking sequence, broken into eight steps. Observe the movements of the people walking on the top line, then create your own characters wandering across the page on the line below.

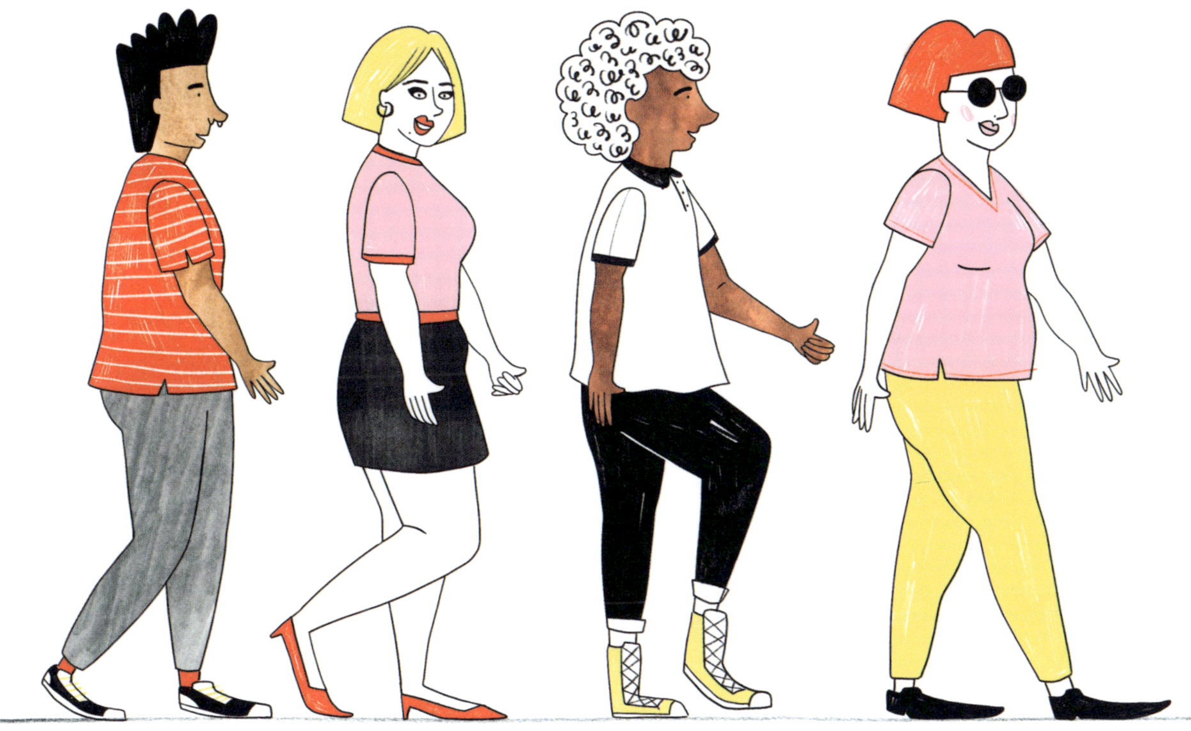

ROLLER DISCO

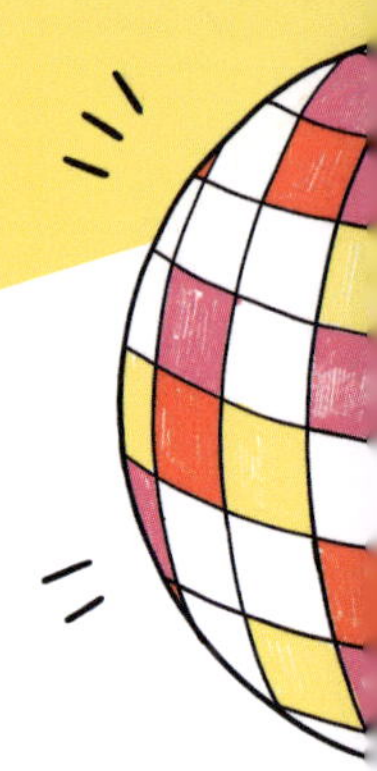

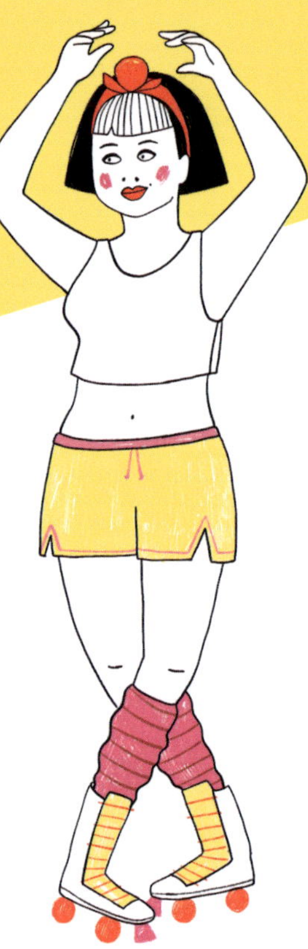

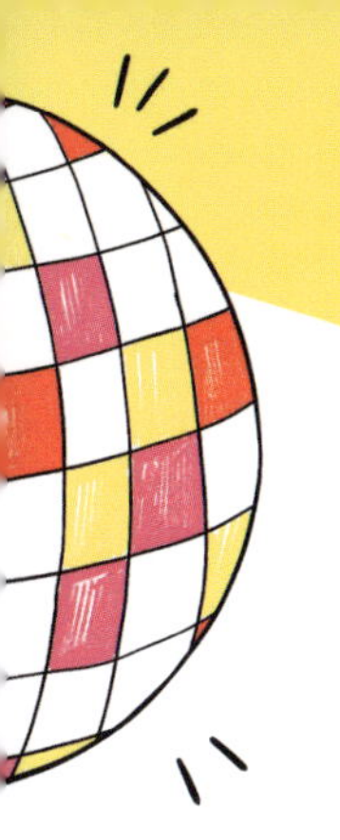

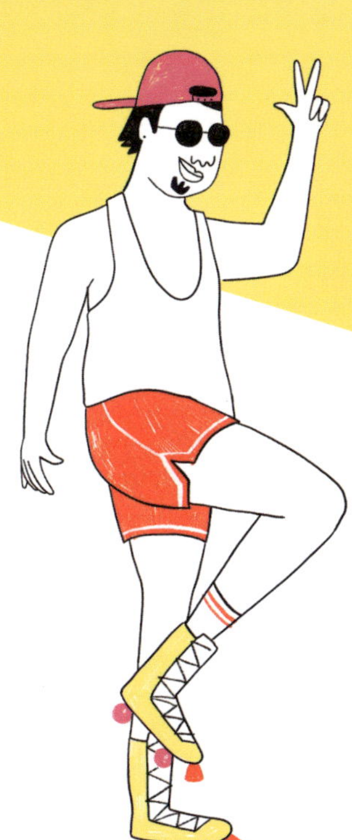

Join in the fun at the roller disco. Finish the scene by coloring in these characters and adding more of your own. Experiment with shape and movement as your characters practice different tricks and dance moves.

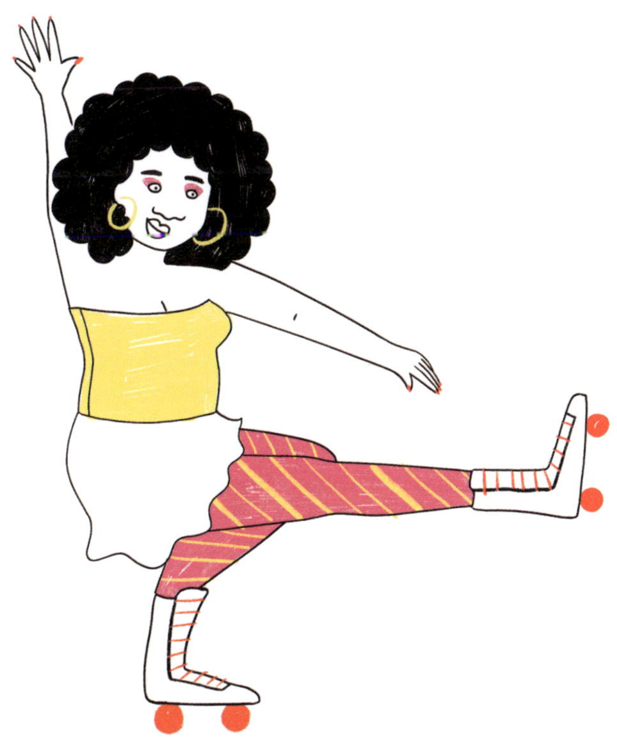

TINY ICONS

Create a set of stamps featuring icons throughout time. You could choose your favorite artists, authors, sports personalities, or scientists. Pick people and genres that you find inspiring.

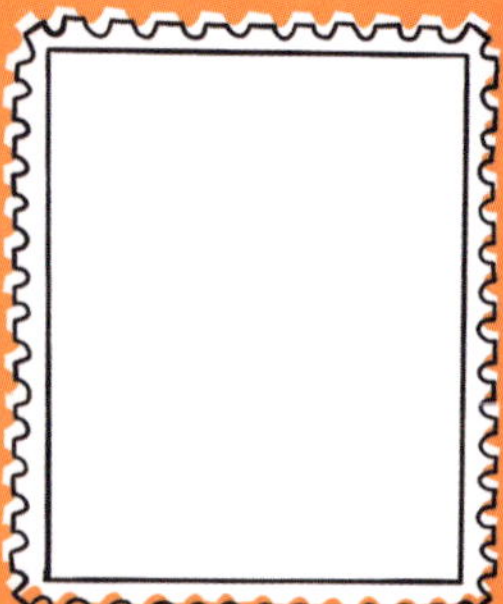

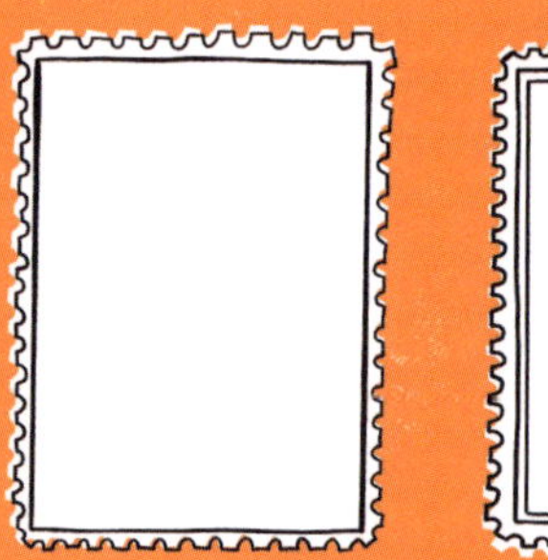

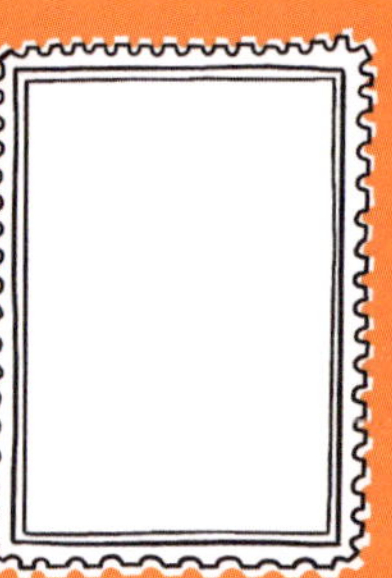

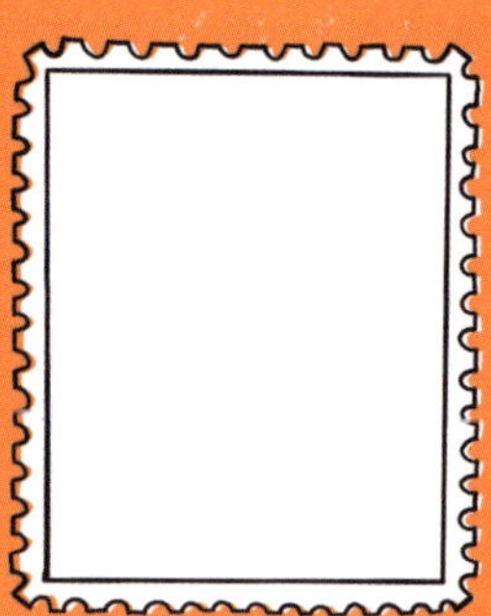

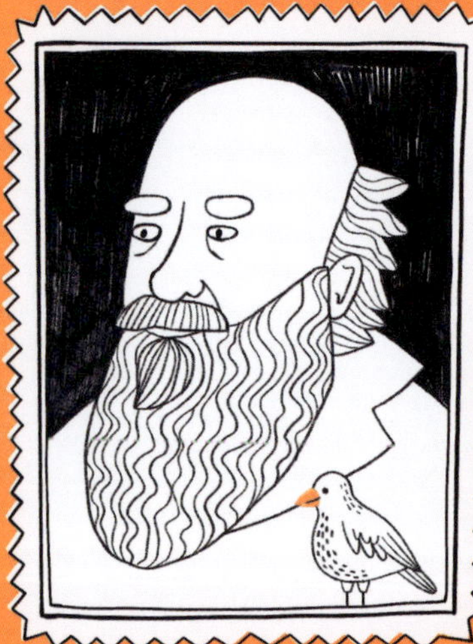

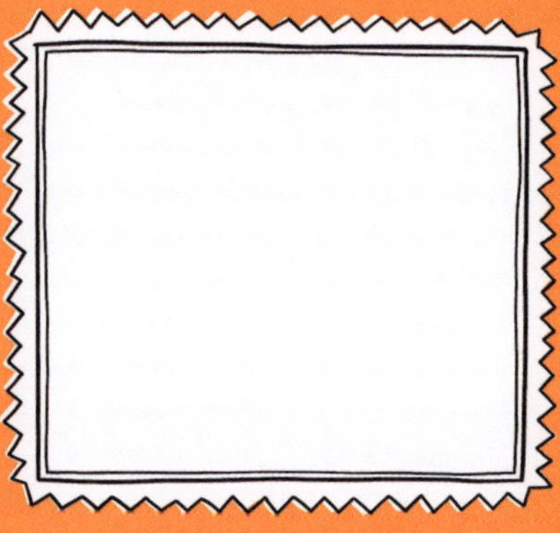

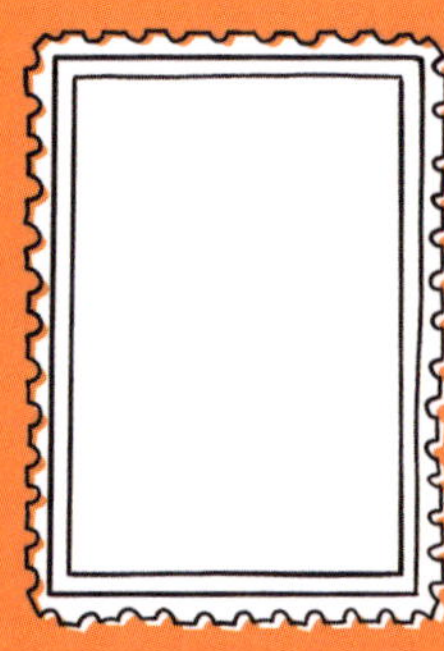

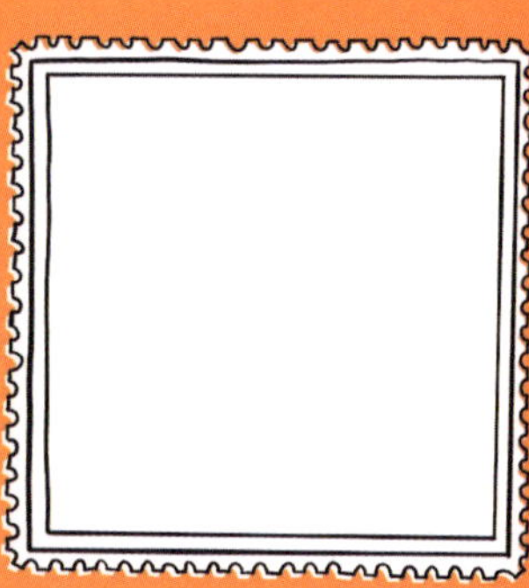

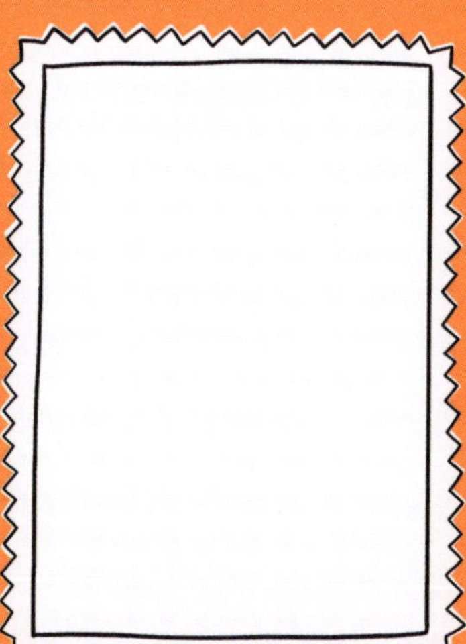

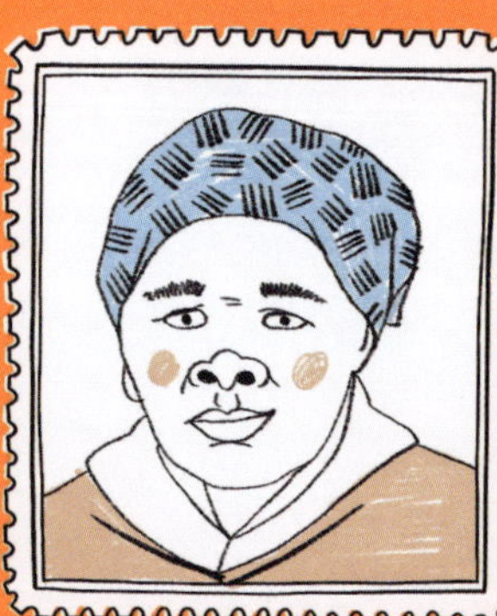

PRIDE CELEBRATIONS

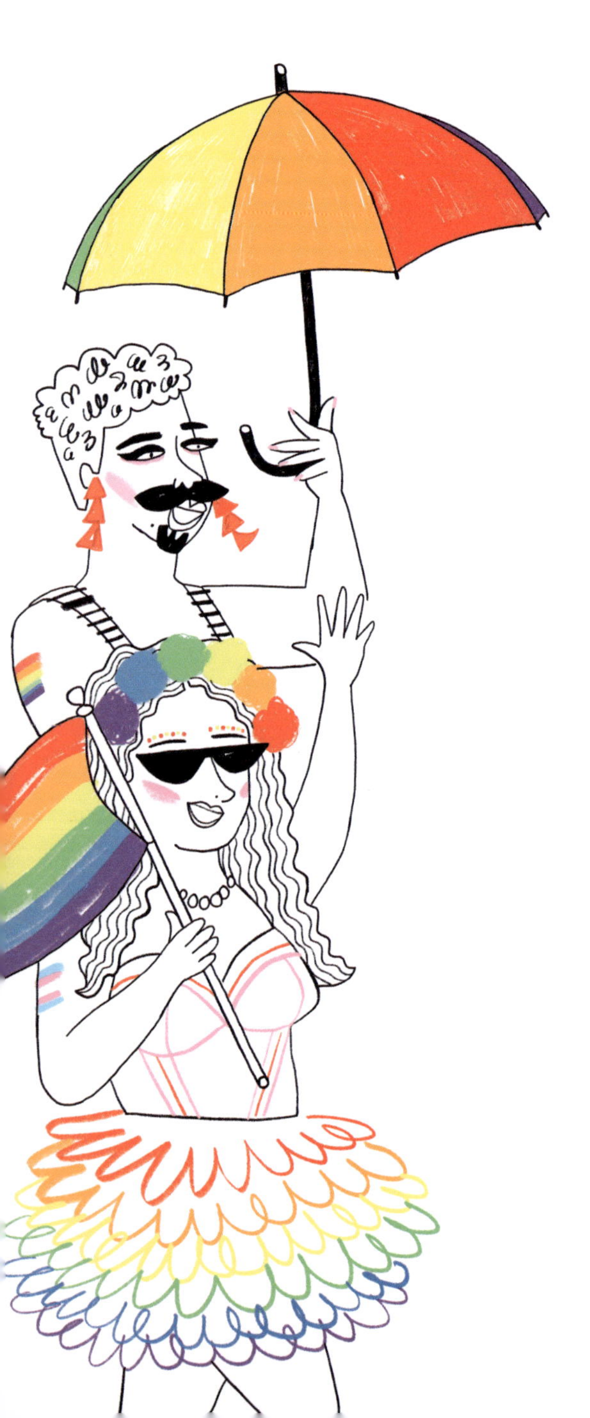

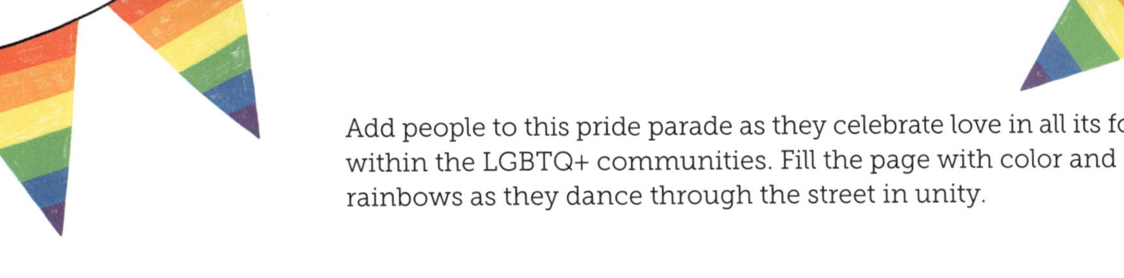

Add people to this pride parade as they celebrate love in all its forms within the LGBTQ+ communities. Fill the page with color and rainbows as they dance through the street in unity.

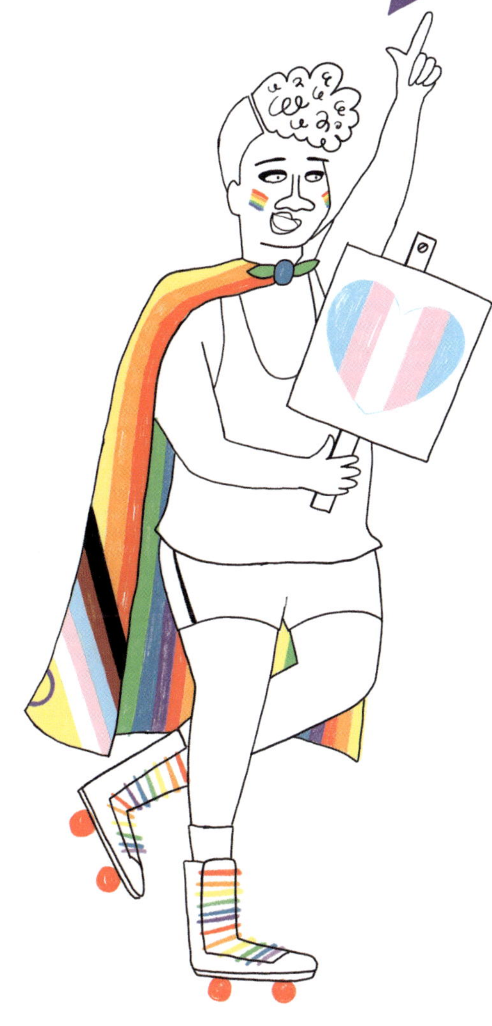

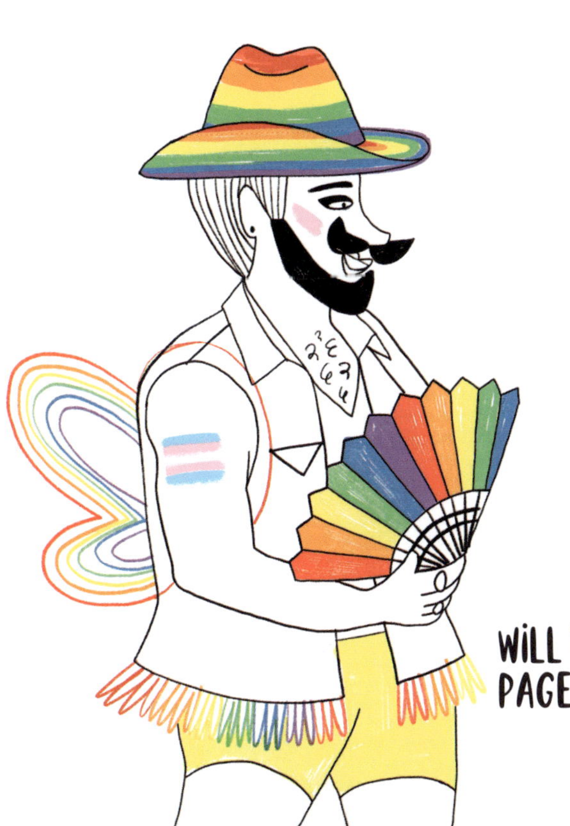

WILL YOU DESIGN A FLOAT MOVING ACROSS THE PAGE OR IS THE STREET BURSTING WITH PEOPLE?

PETS AND THEIR OWNERS

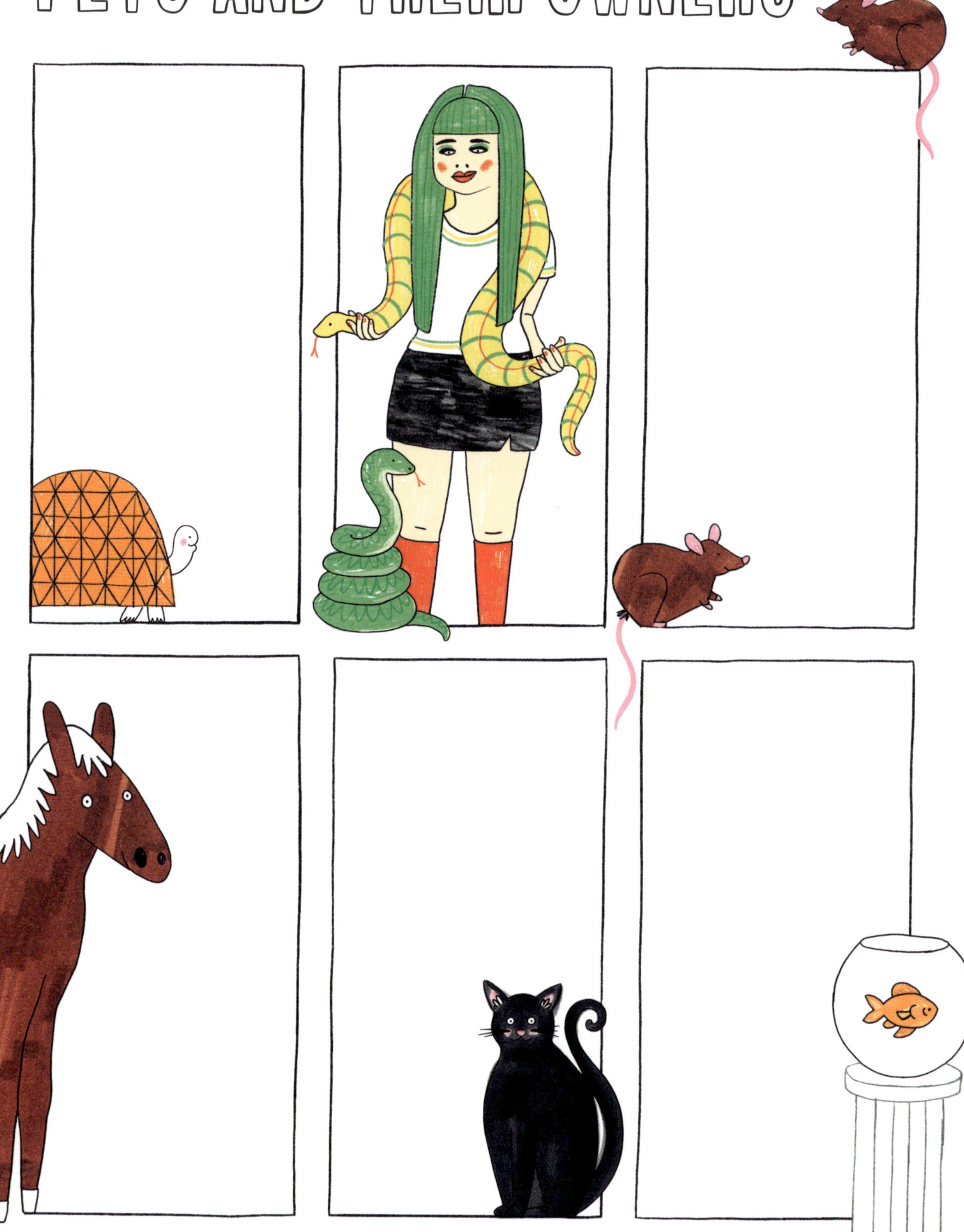

They say people can look like their pets and share some personality traits. Draw the owners to these fine pooches, feline friends, reptiles, and rodents.

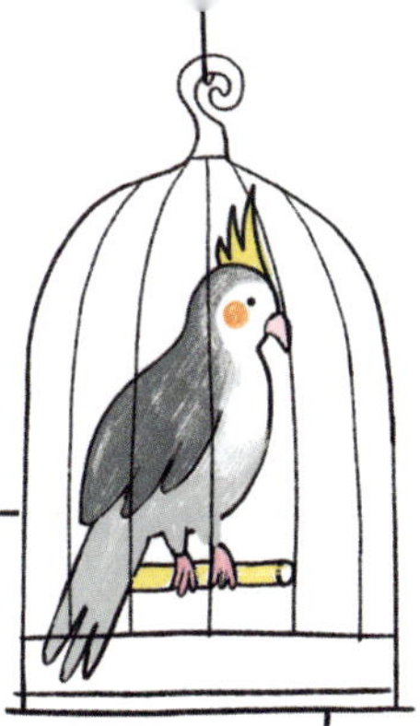

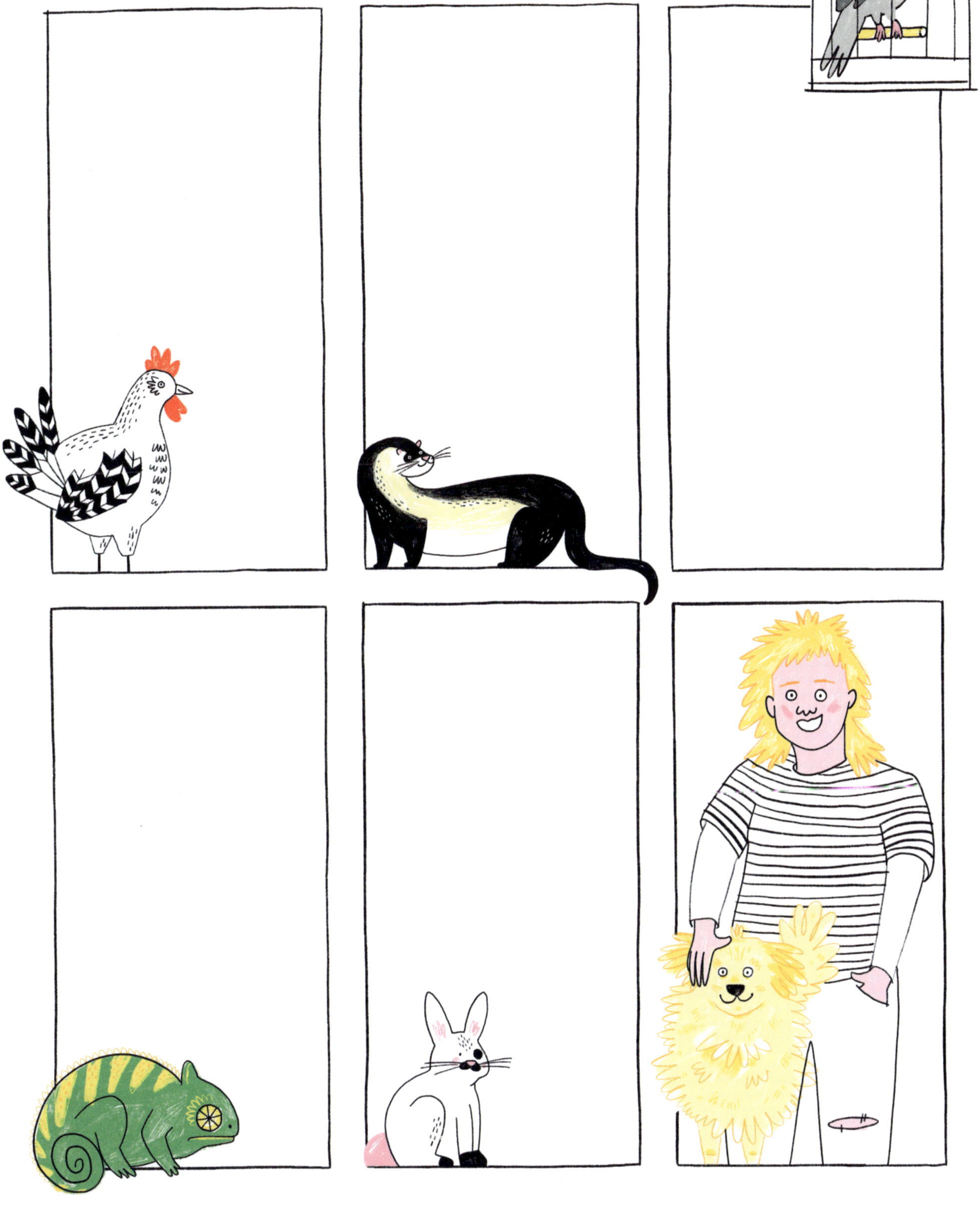

SUBCULTURES: GLAM ROCK

Add more characters to this gathering of glam rockers. Popular in the 1970s and known for their platform boots, sequinned flares, spandex jumpsuits, and bold, expressive makeup.

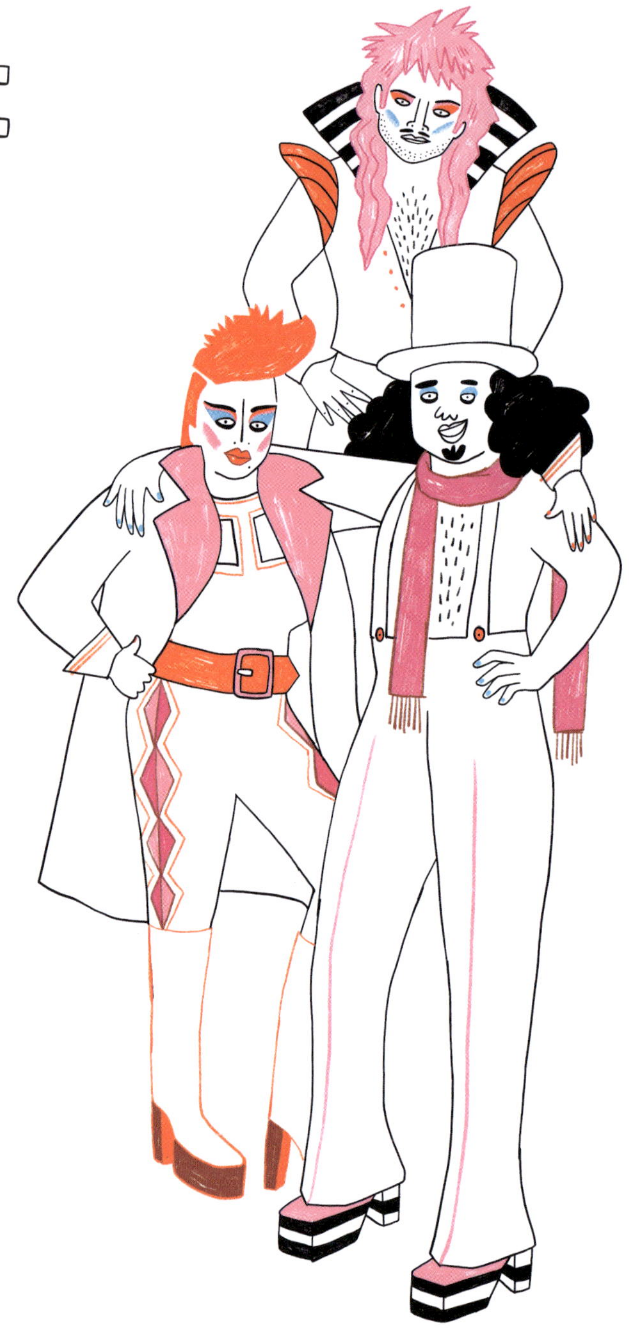

FINISH THE COSTUME

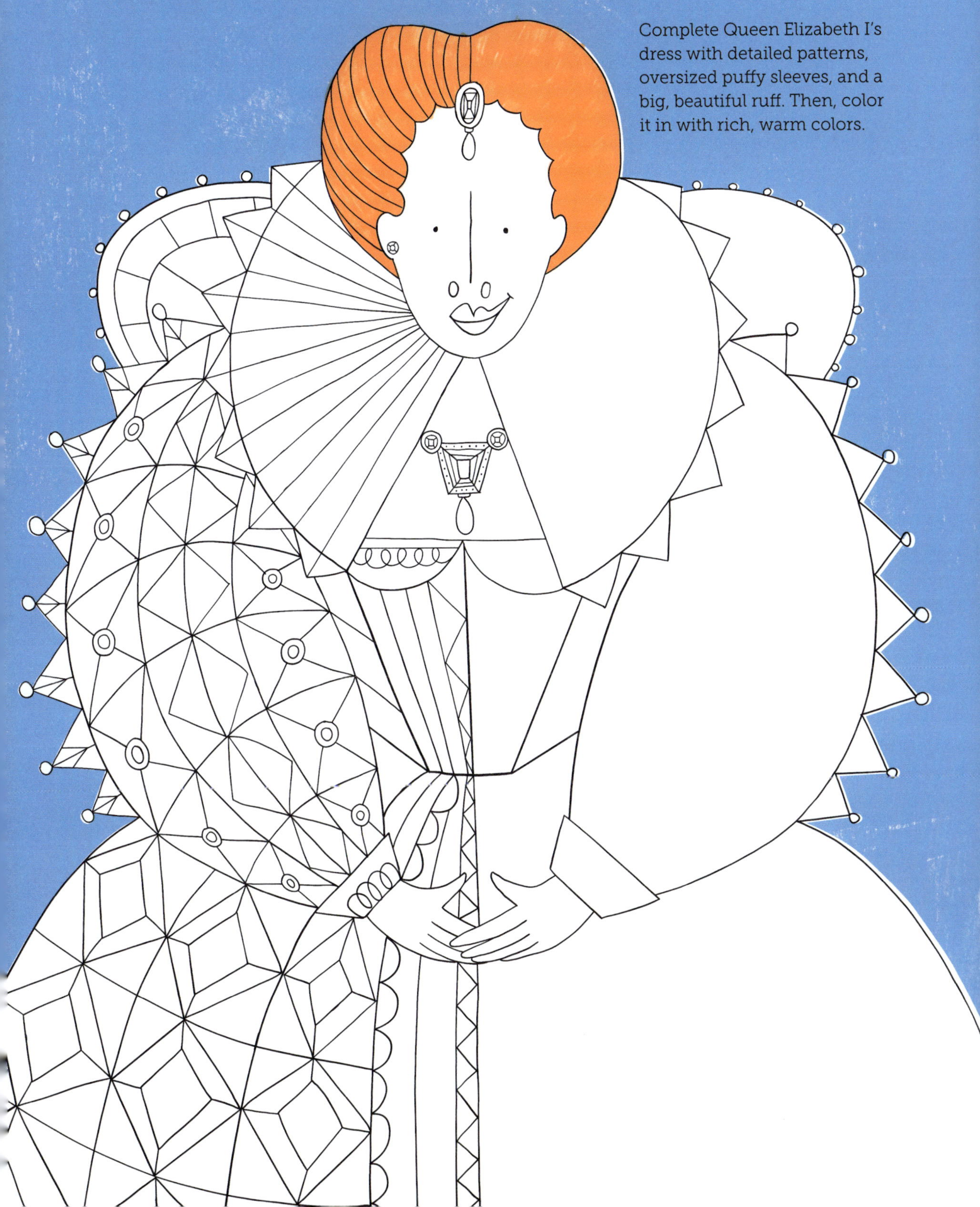

Complete Queen Elizabeth I's dress with detailed patterns, oversized puffy sleeves, and a big, beautiful ruff. Then, color it in with rich, warm colors.

HAPPY HOLI

Holi is a festival in India that celebrates love and the end of winter. It is also known as the festival of color, as people joyfully throw colored powder over each other! Draw people in black fineliner dancing over the top of this page covered in chalk pastels.

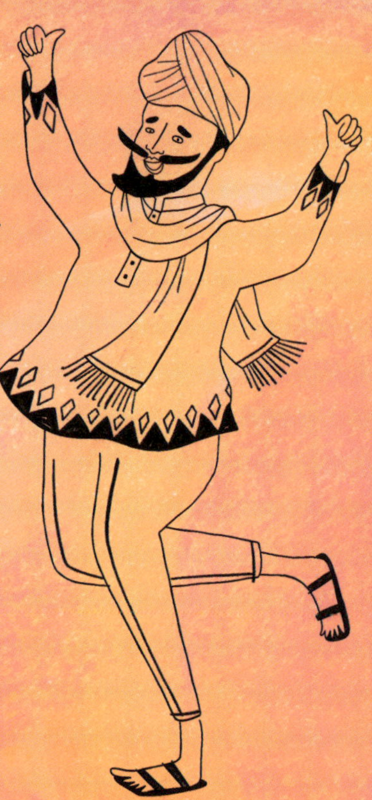

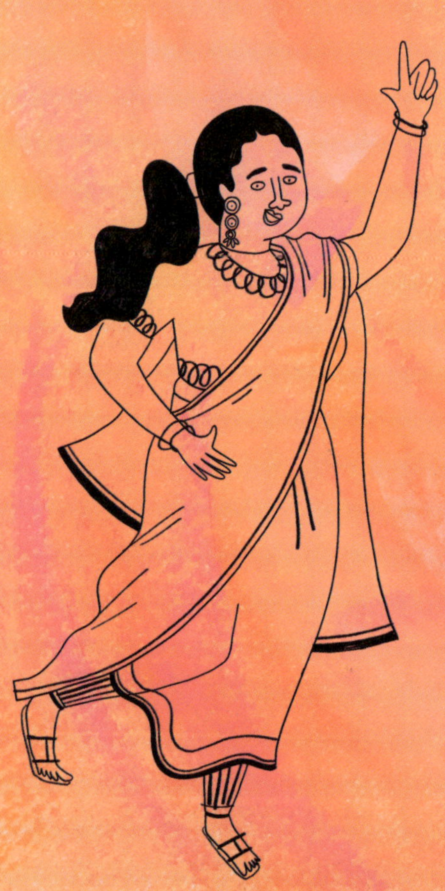

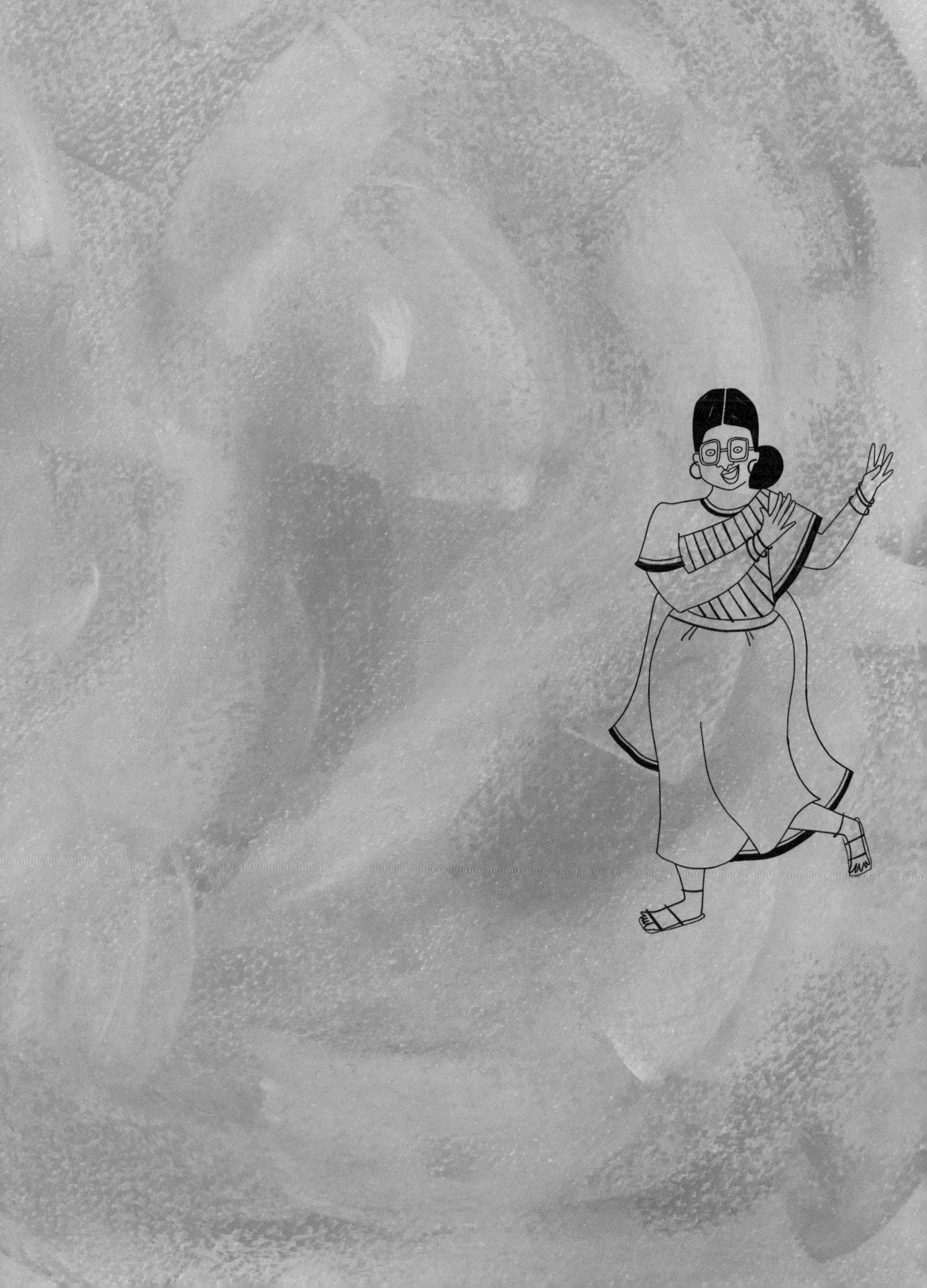

TIMED POSES: FACES

Ask your friends and family to pose for you, then draw them in the boxes below in the time allocated in each box. The quick poses are a great way to loosen up, while the longer pose is a good opportunity to explore tone (the range of light and shadow), by using shading to define their form.

3 MINUTES

5 MINUTES

10 MINUTES

20 MINUTES

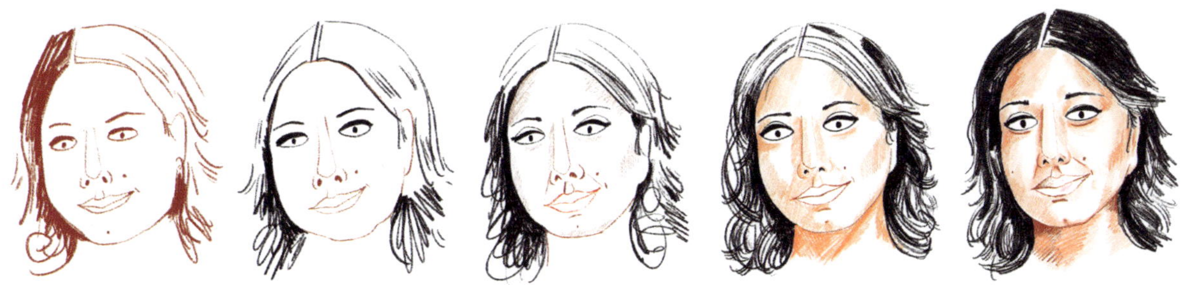

30 MINUTES

EVERYDAY STYLE

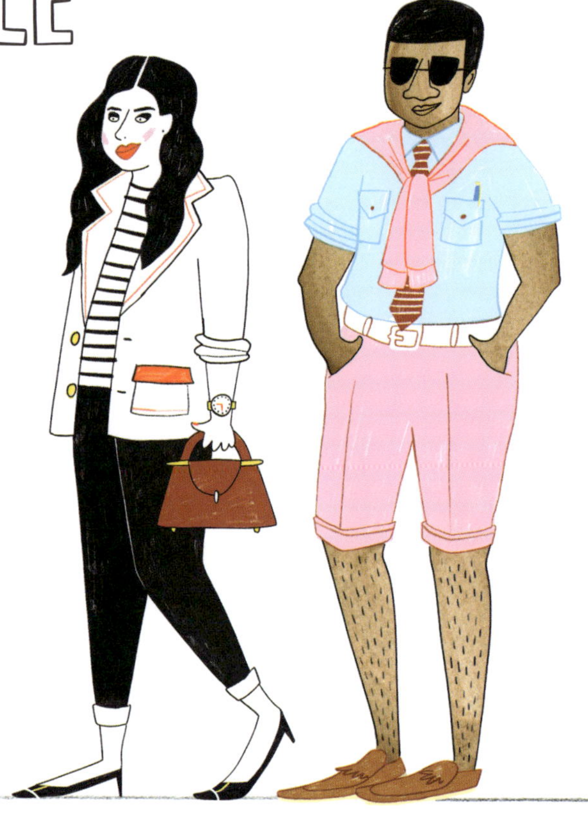

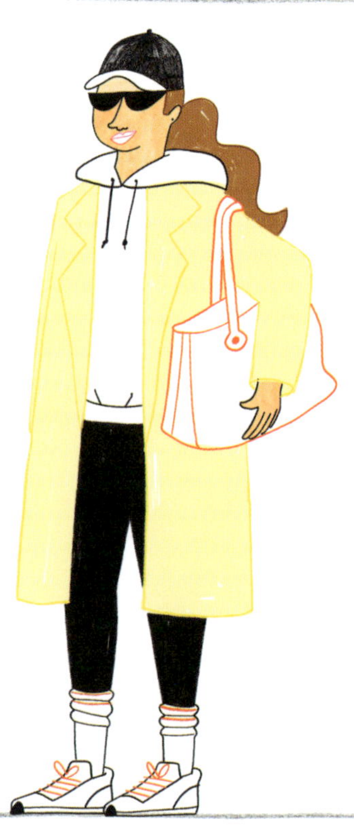

Design the outfits you see out and about every day, from the casual androgynous jeans and T-shirt, preppy chinos, and sweaters to the athleisure chic of sneakers and sportwear.

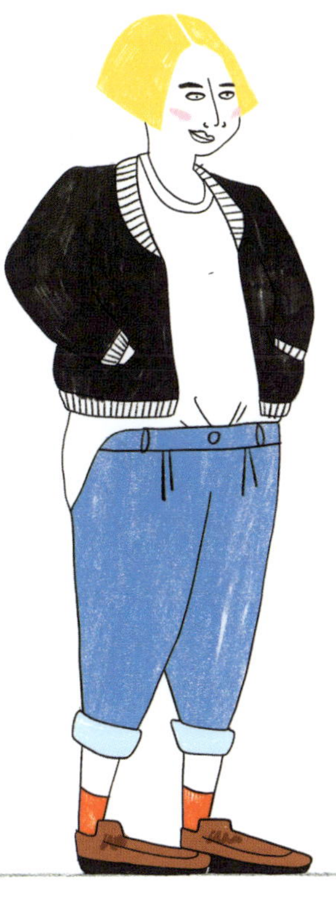

SEASONS: FALL

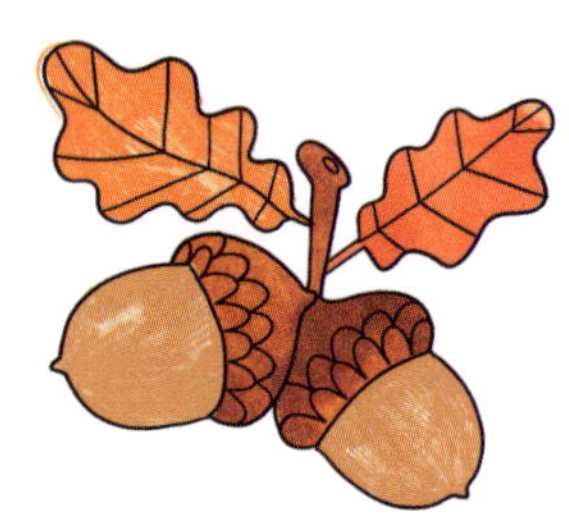

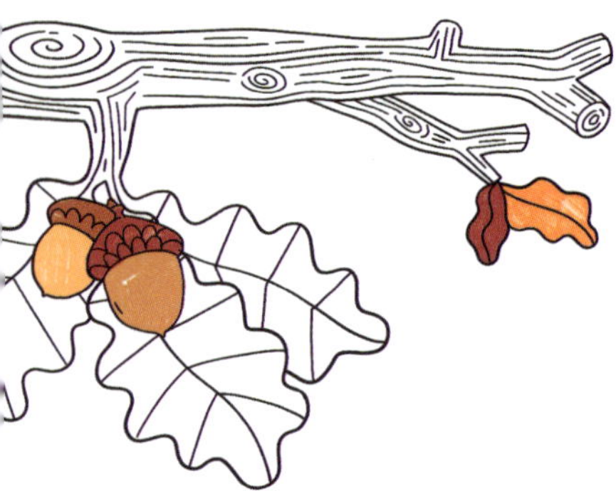

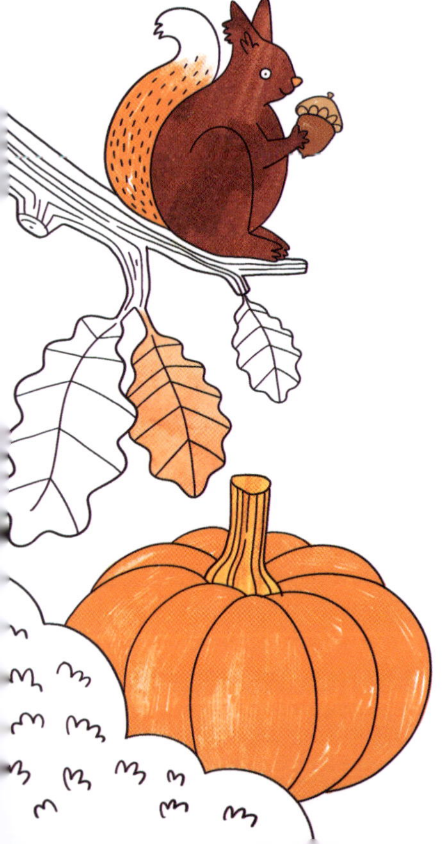

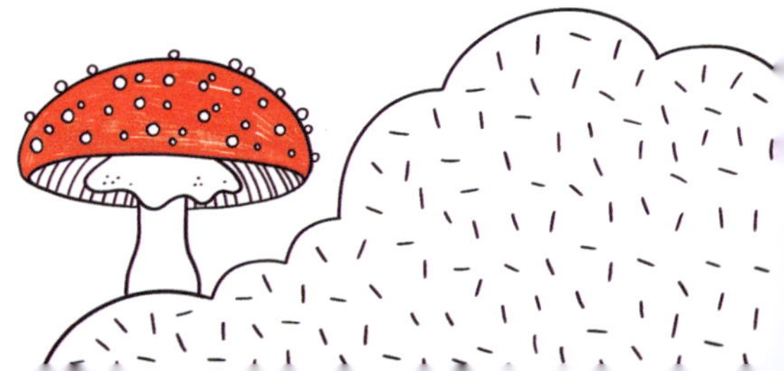

By the time fall comes, it's starting to become cooler and rain clouds begin to roll in. Using a warm color palette, draw people dressed appropriately for fall. It's time to get those chunky knits and coats out!

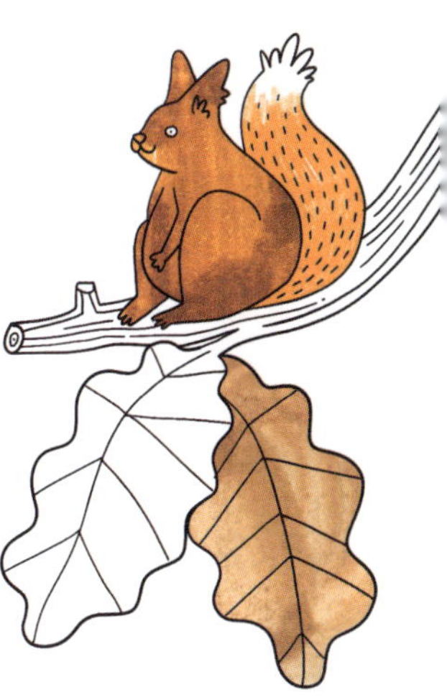

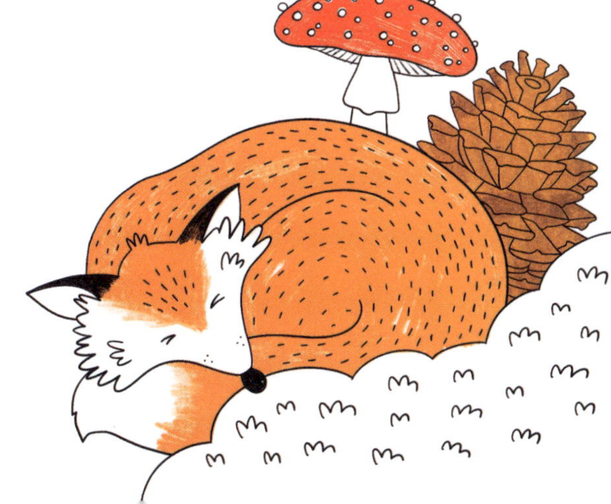

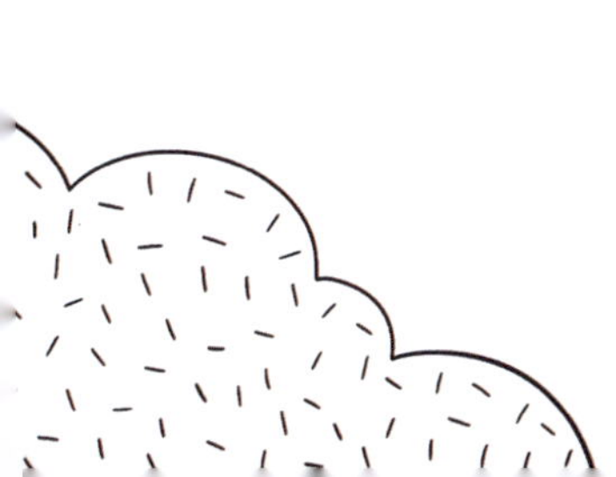

A DAY AT THE BEACH

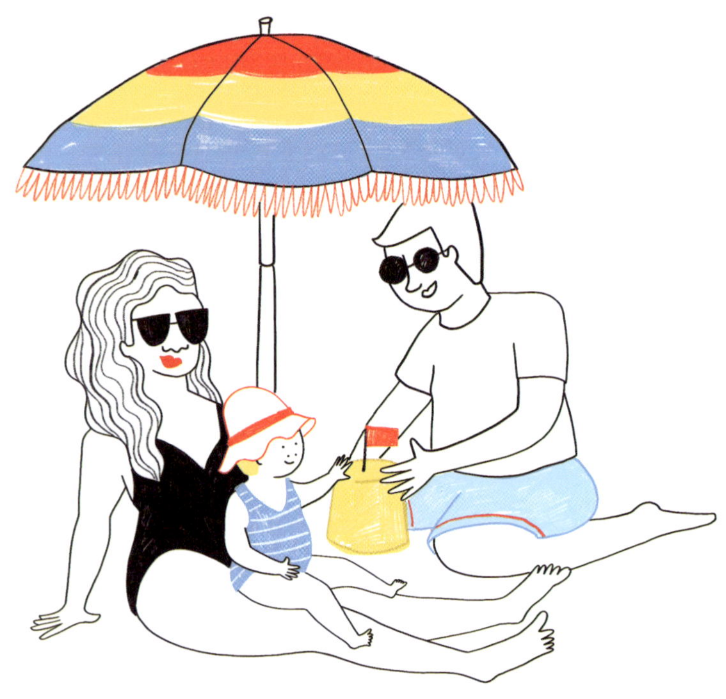

It's a glorious day and the beach is starting to fill up with people spending
a day out by the sea! Add more characters setting up camp for the day.
Do they have an umbrella or deck chair? Are children building sandcastles
or are there solo sunbathers quietly reading?

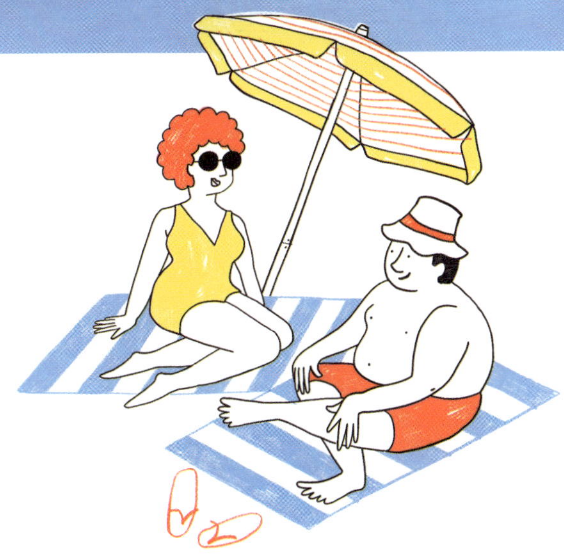

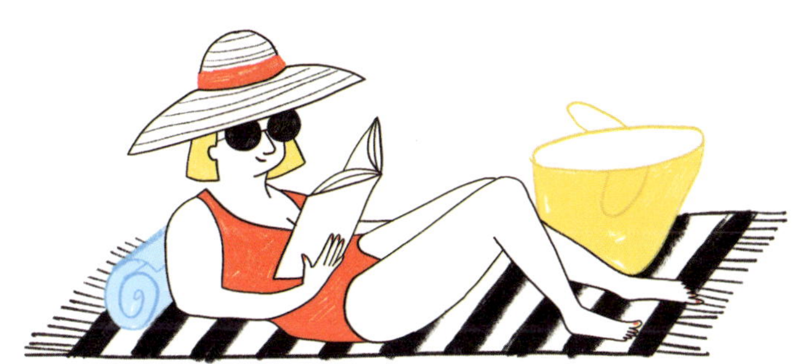

FAVORITE FACES

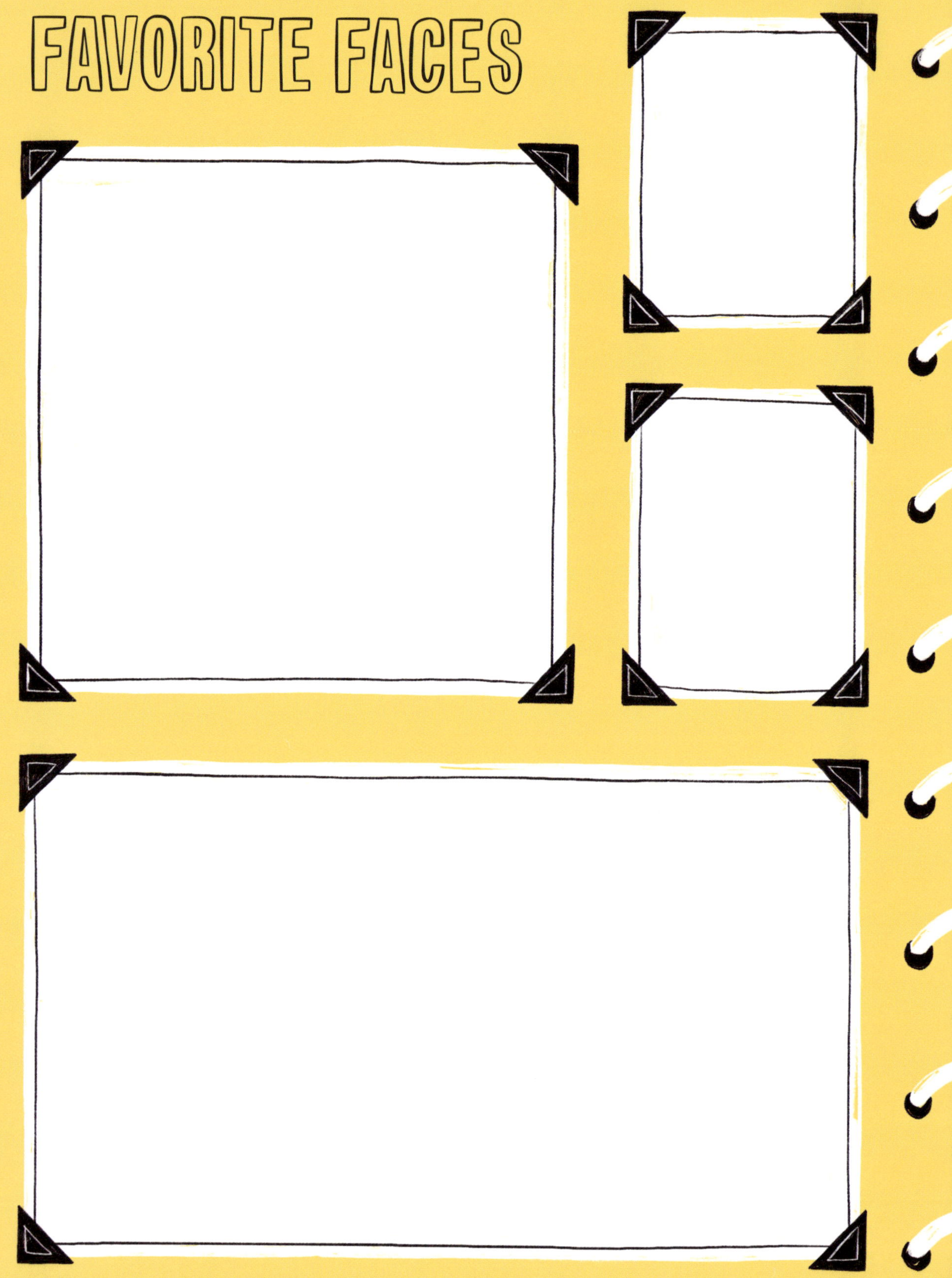

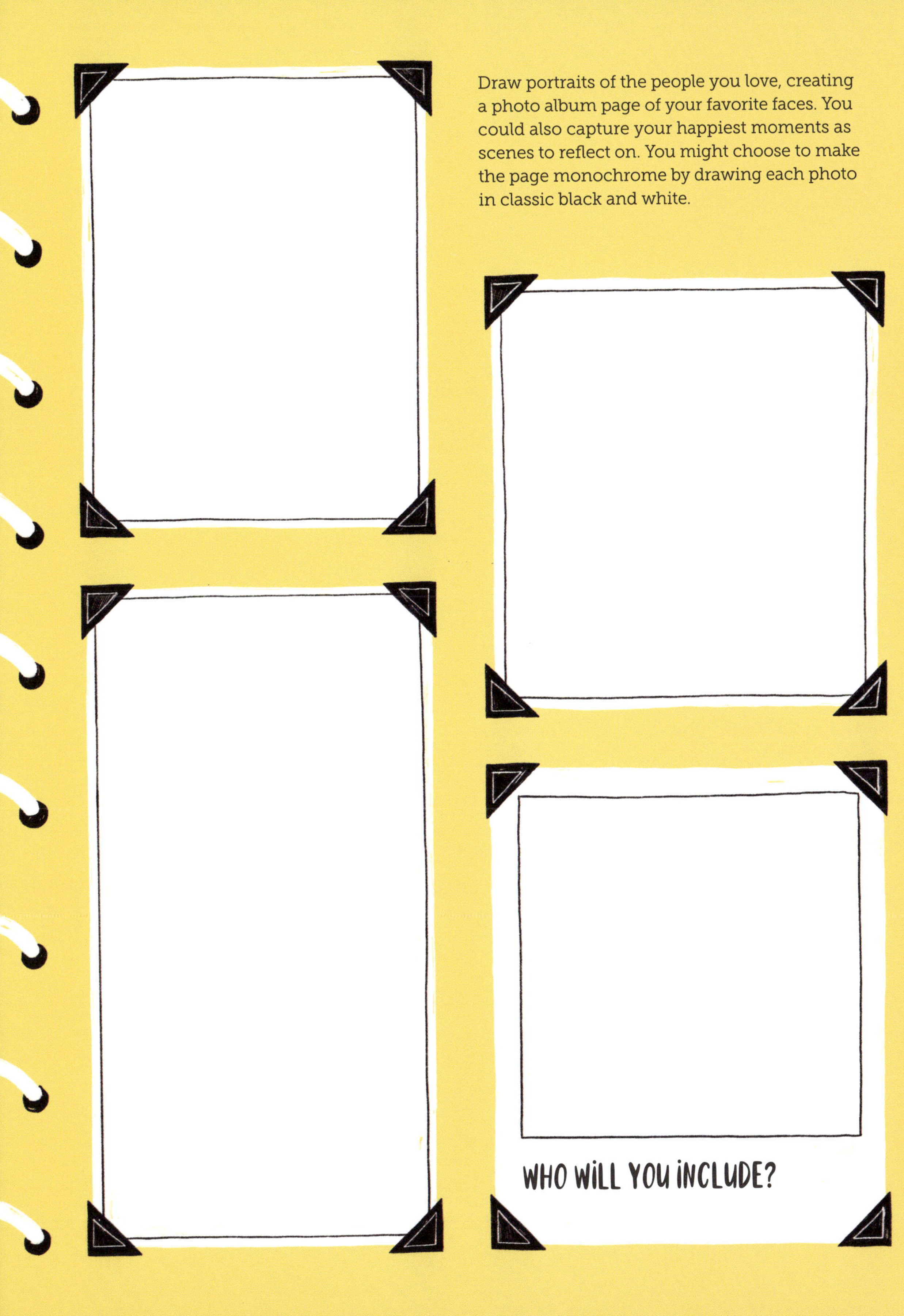

Draw portraits of the people you love, creating a photo album page of your favorite faces. You could also capture your happiest moments as scenes to reflect on. You might choose to make the page monochrome by drawing each photo in classic black and white.

WHO WILL YOU INCLUDE?

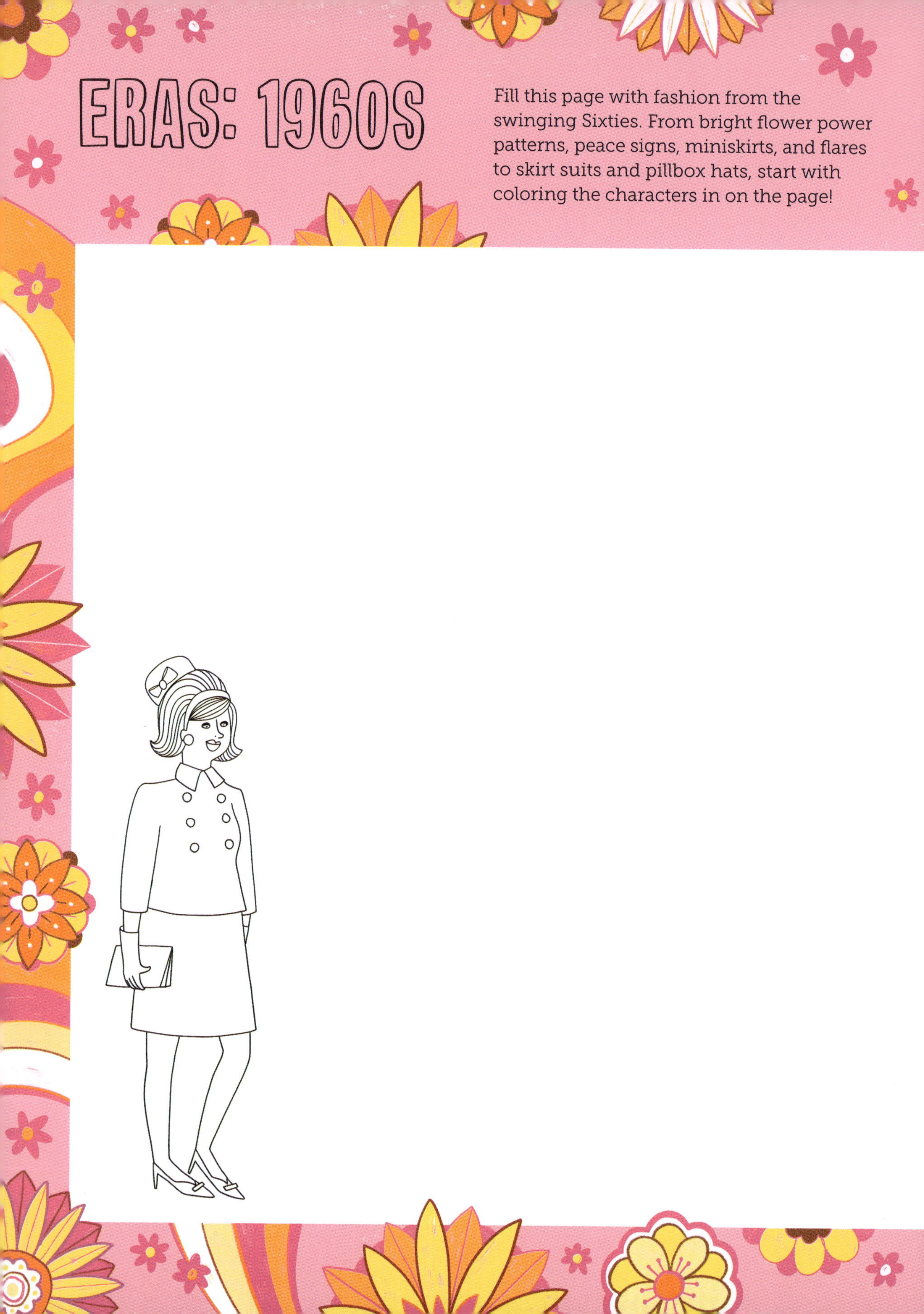

ERAS: 1960S

Fill this page with fashion from the swinging Sixties. From bright flower power patterns, peace signs, miniskirts, and flares to skirt suits and pillbox hats, start with coloring the characters in on the page!

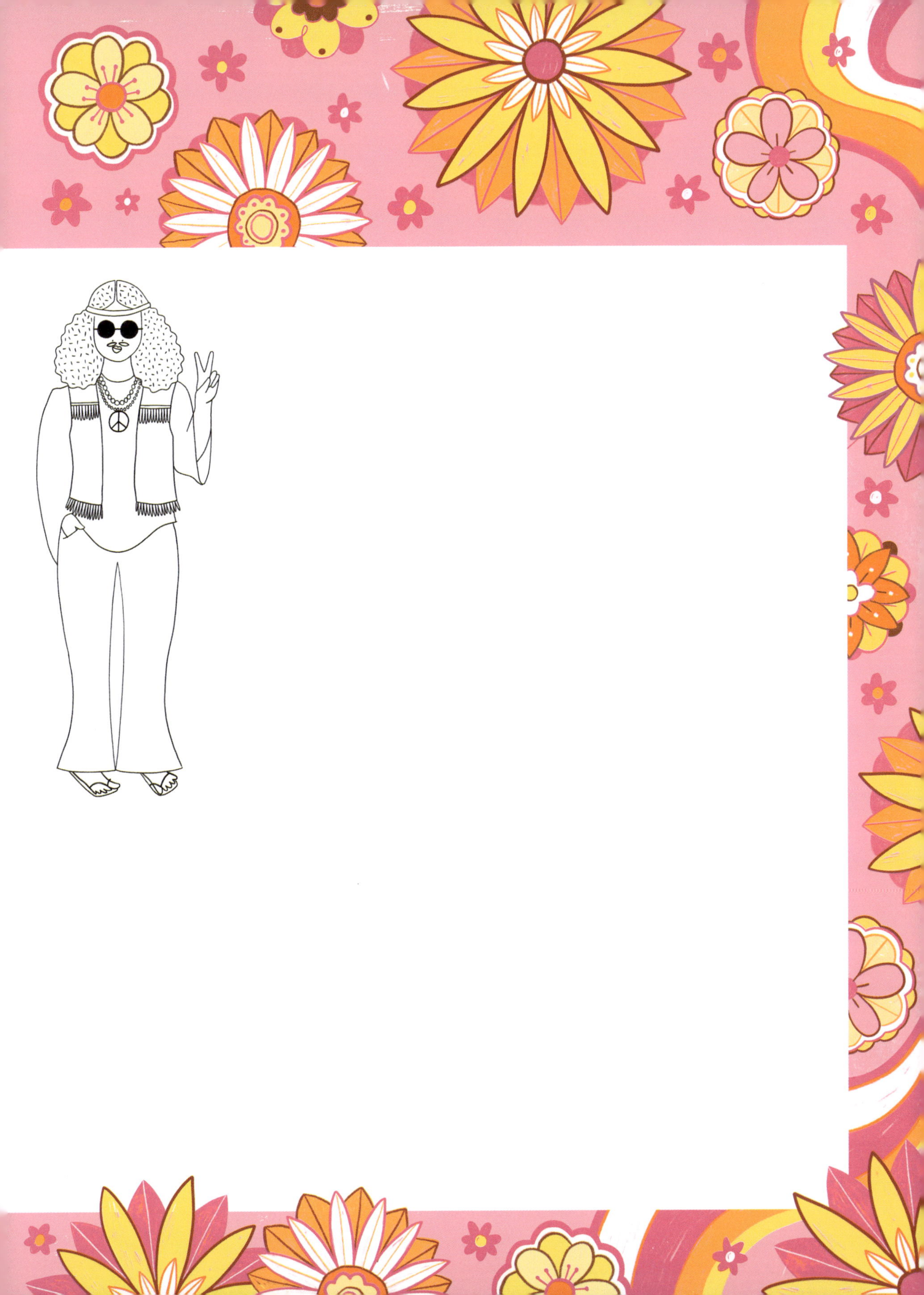

MAKING HAPPY FACES

Create a collection of joyful characters with smiles and round, open eyes. Imagine what brings you happiness and look at your expressions when you think about them in the mirror. Channel these feelings when filling in this page to create more authentic characters!

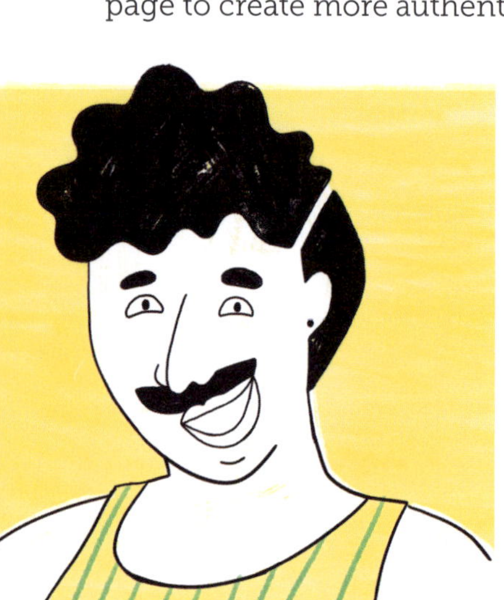
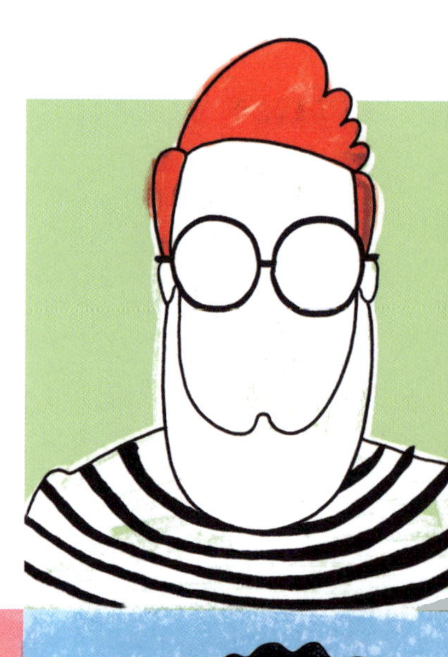
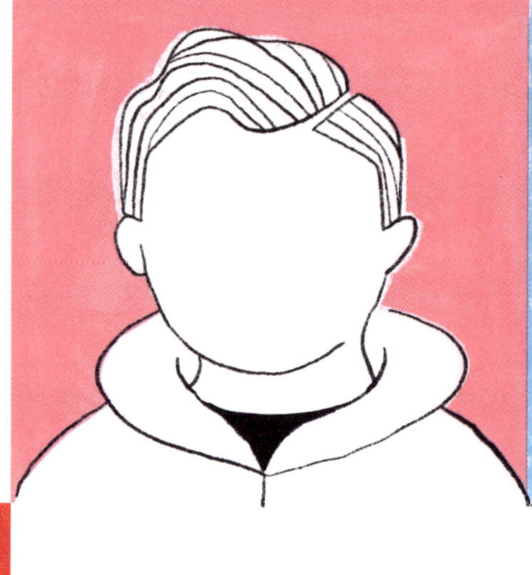
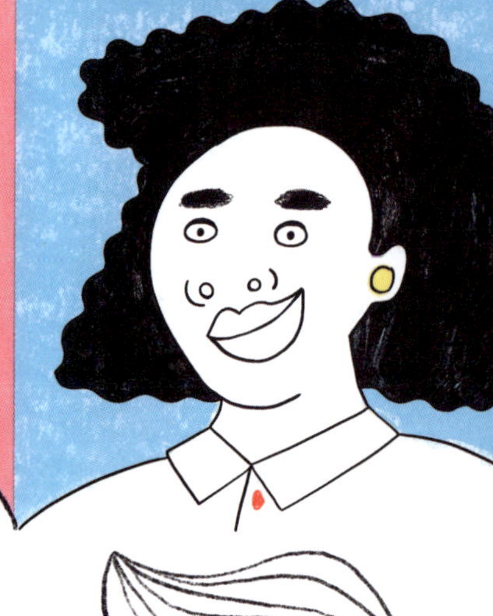
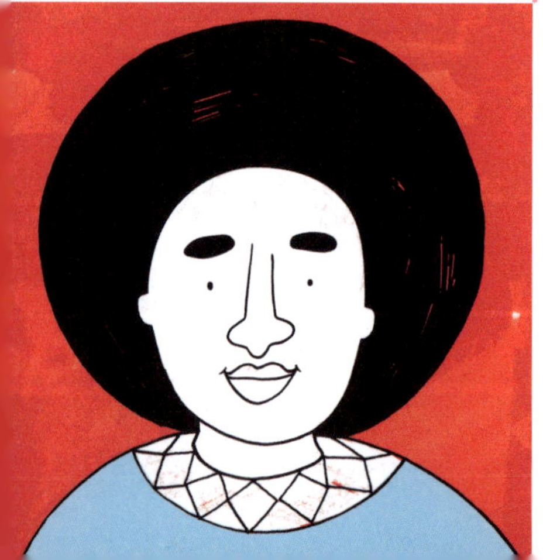
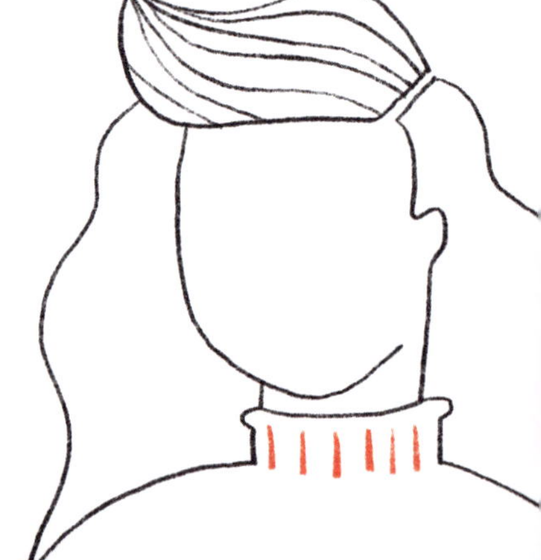

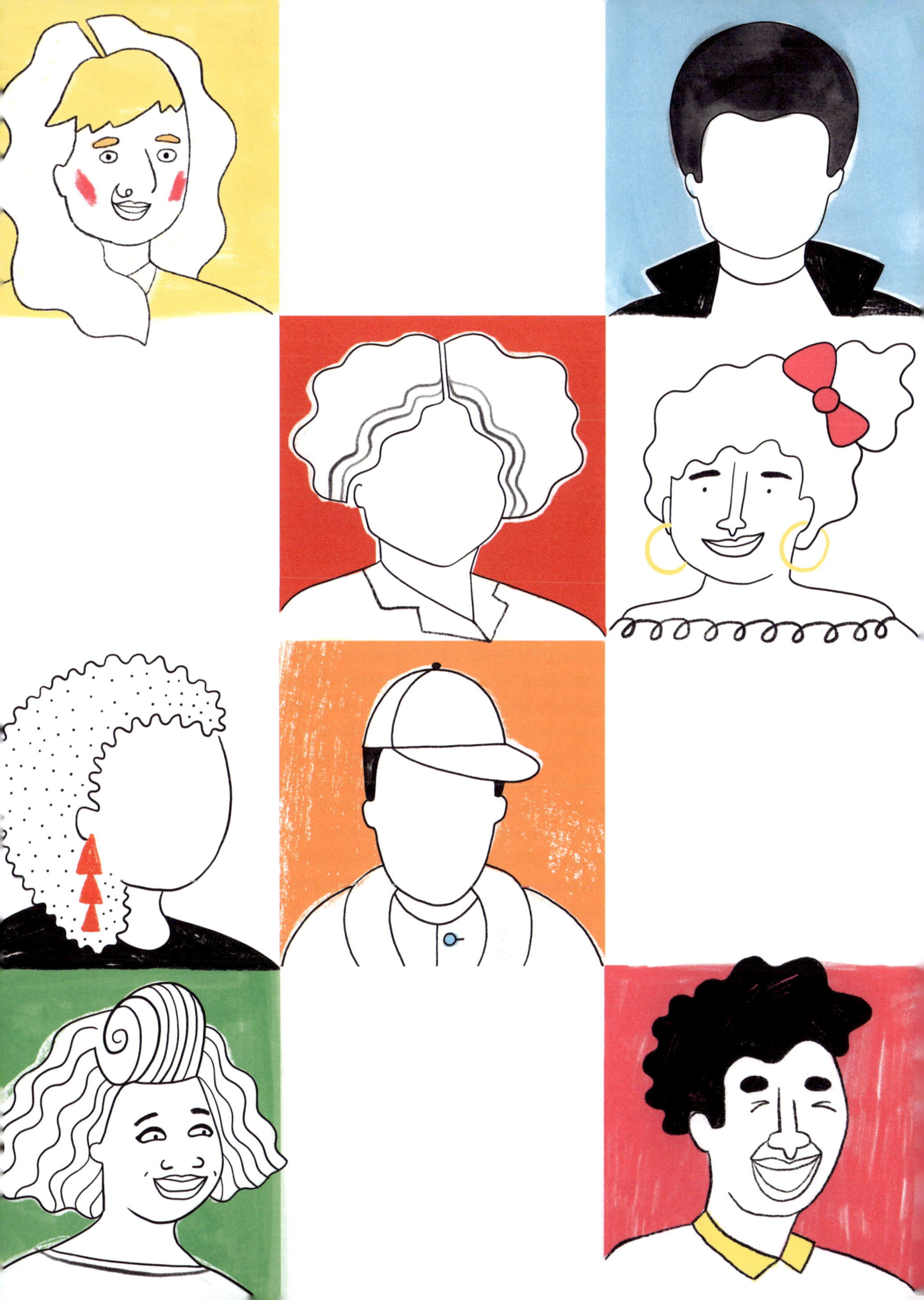

RUNNING SEQUENCE

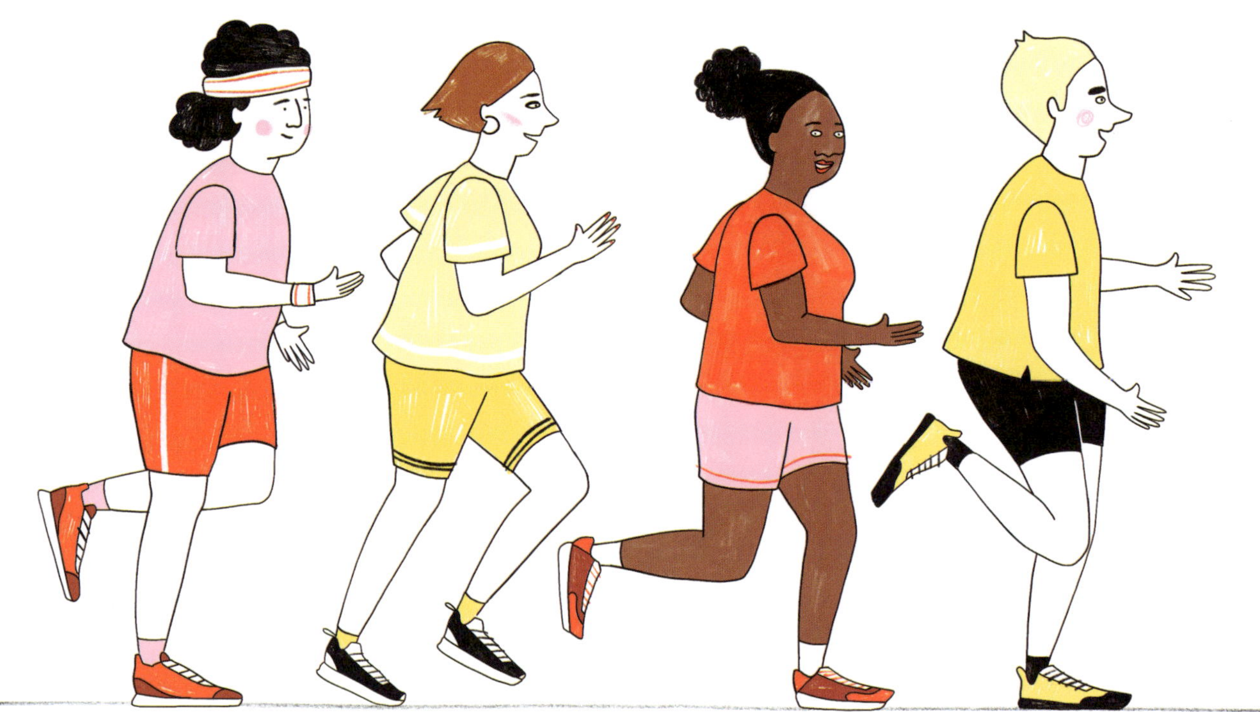

Practice illustrating the stages of someone running, shown in eight steps. Observe the movements of the people jogging on the top line, then draw your own characters running across the page on the line below.

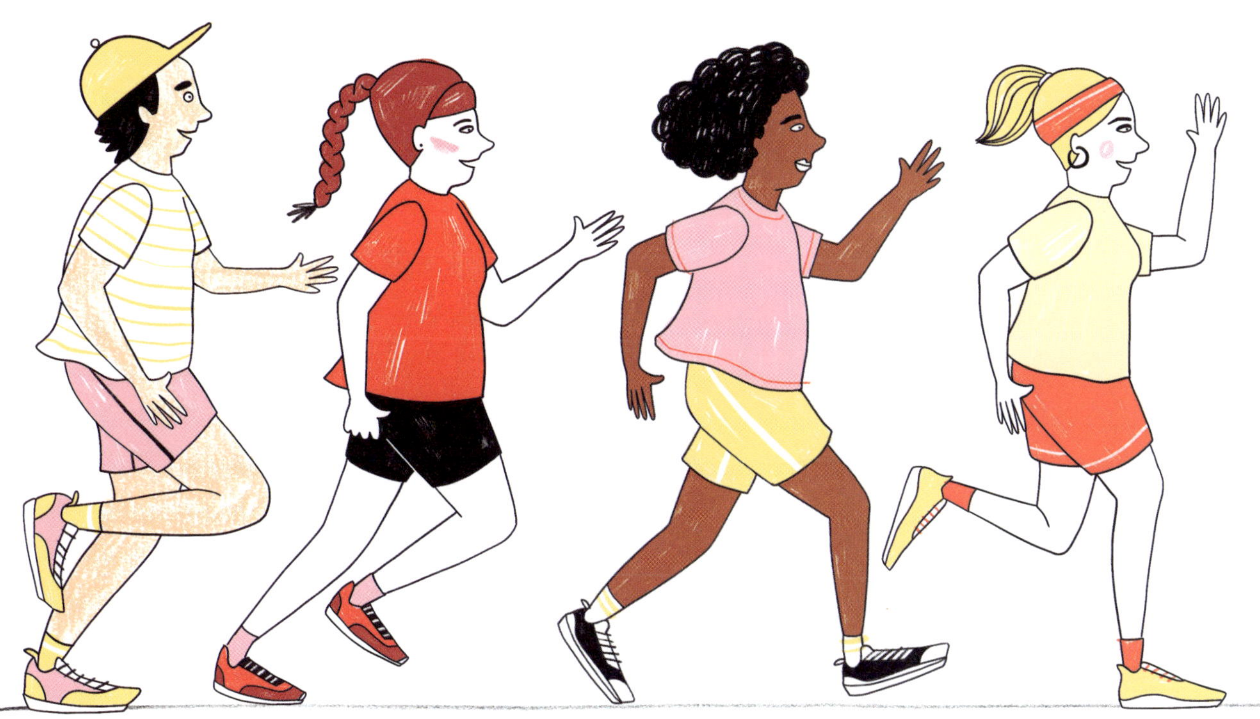

CARNIVAL SEASON

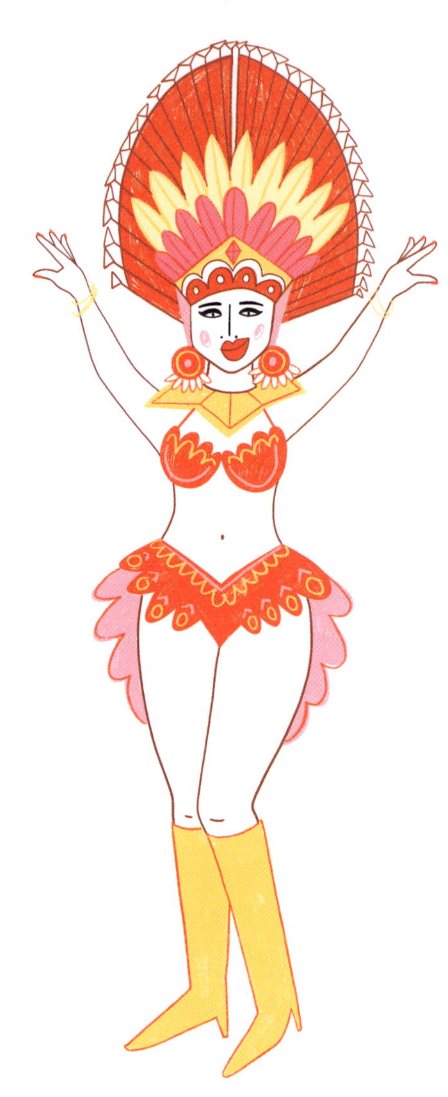

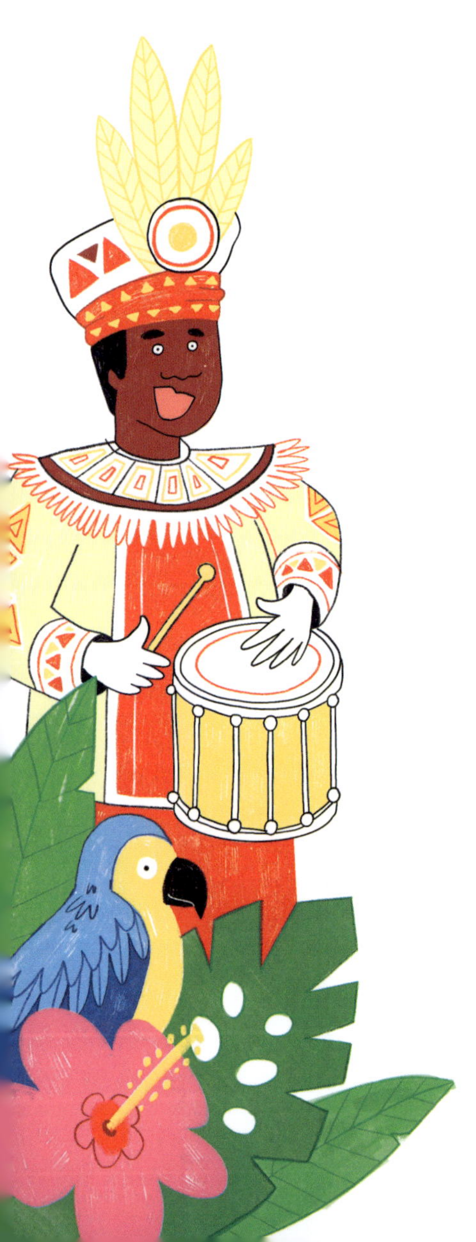

Celebrate the arrival of carnival season at the biggest parade in the world, Rio Carnival! Fill the page with people dancing samba in feathered headdresses, marching to the beat of the drums, and shaking maracas.

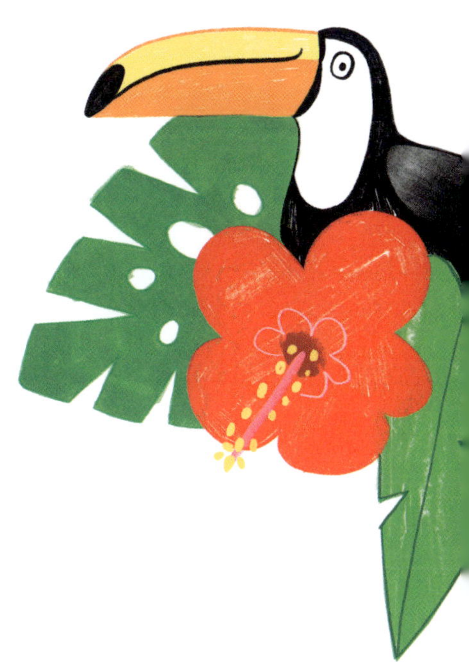

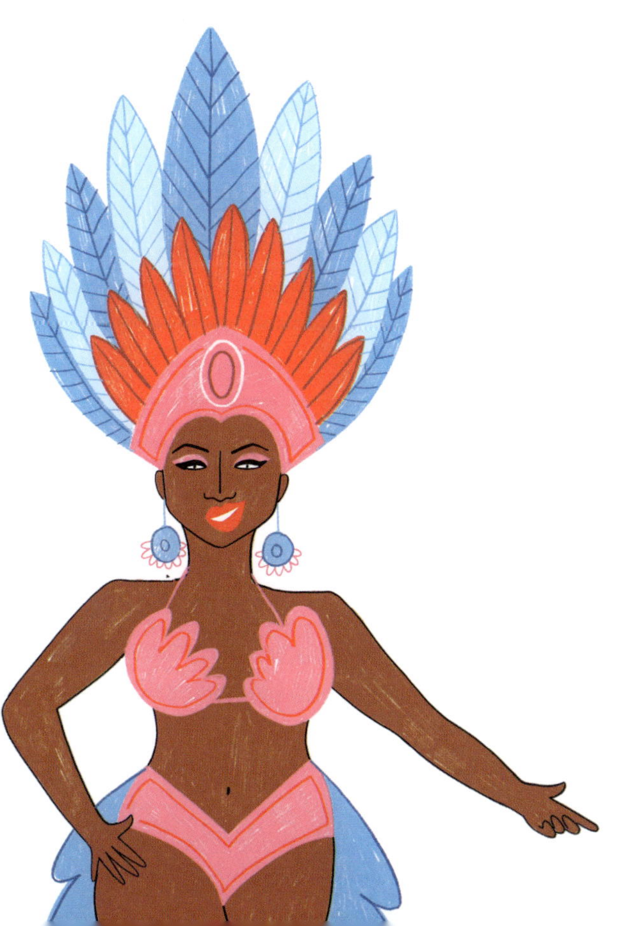

SPECTACULAR SPECTACLES

Glasses can change a person's face and give a strong sense of that character's style and personality. Give these faces glasses and these glasses owners. From flamboyant to conservative, think about what character you want to draw, then design glasses you think they would wear.

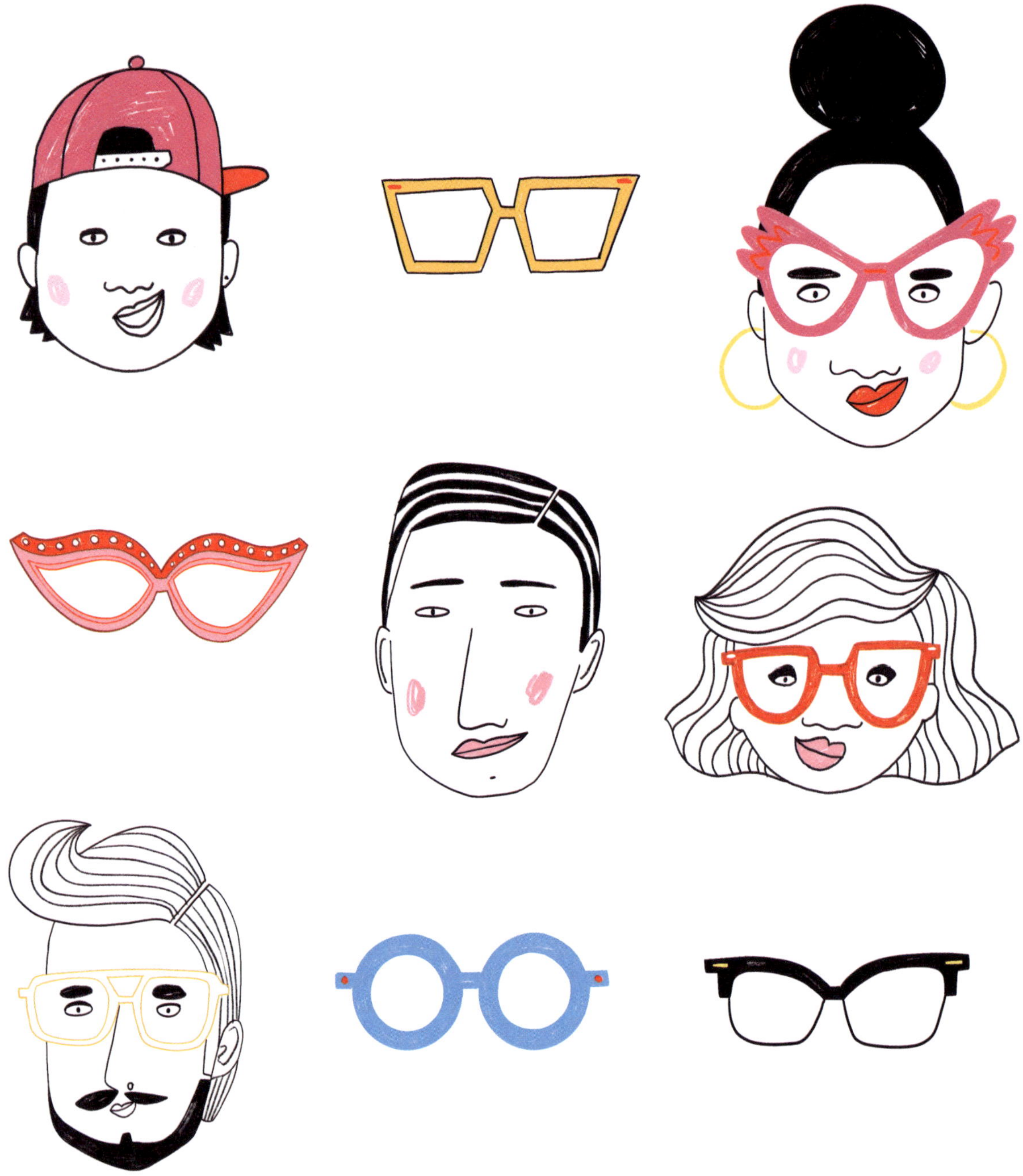

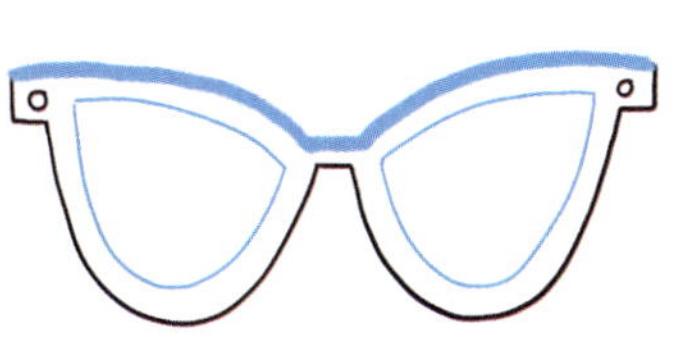

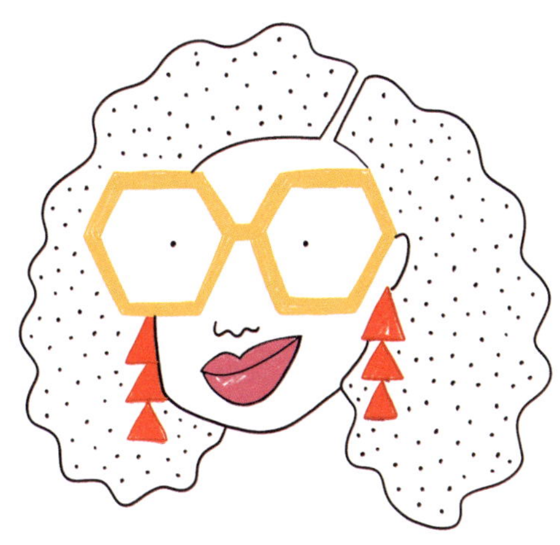

THEN, FILL THIS PAGE WITH
YOUR SPECTACLE DESIGNS!

SUBCULTURES: HIPSTER

Fill in the remainder of this page with characters following the 21st-century hipster look. Style them in skinny jeans, full beards, brimmed hats, and pushing a trademark fixed-gear bike.

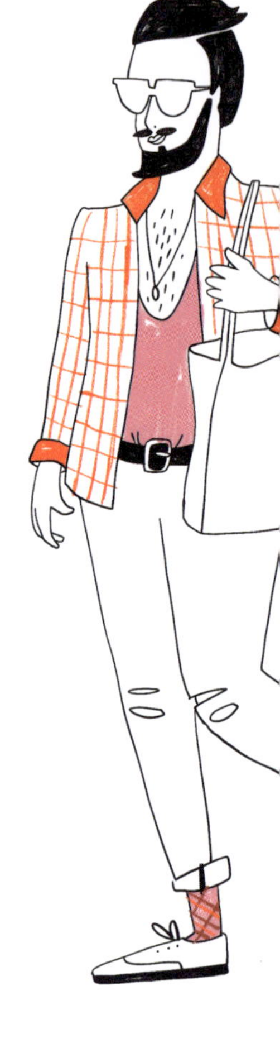

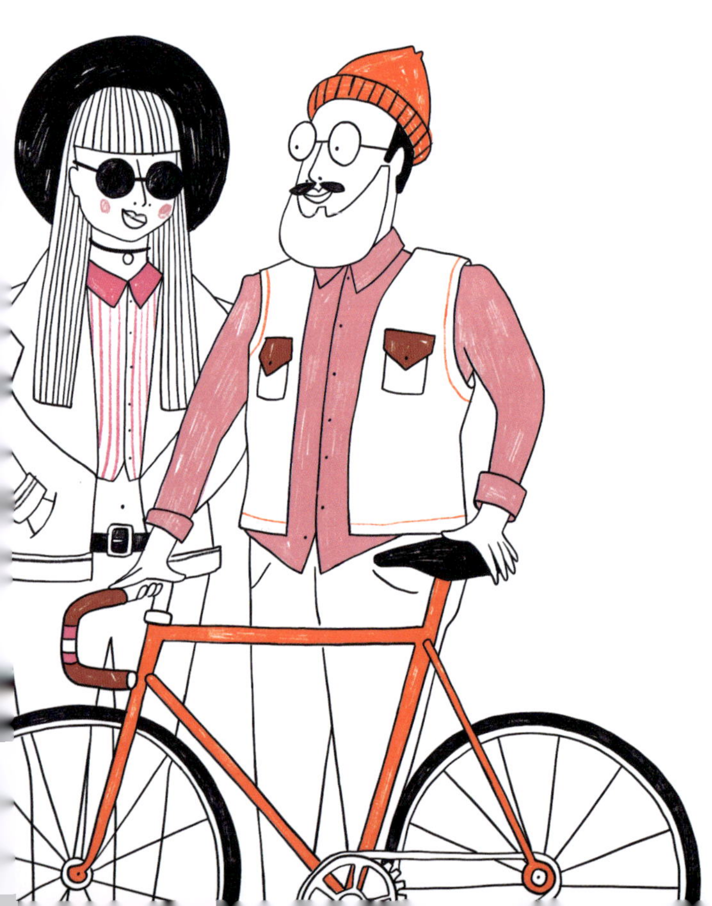

FINISH THE PORTRAIT

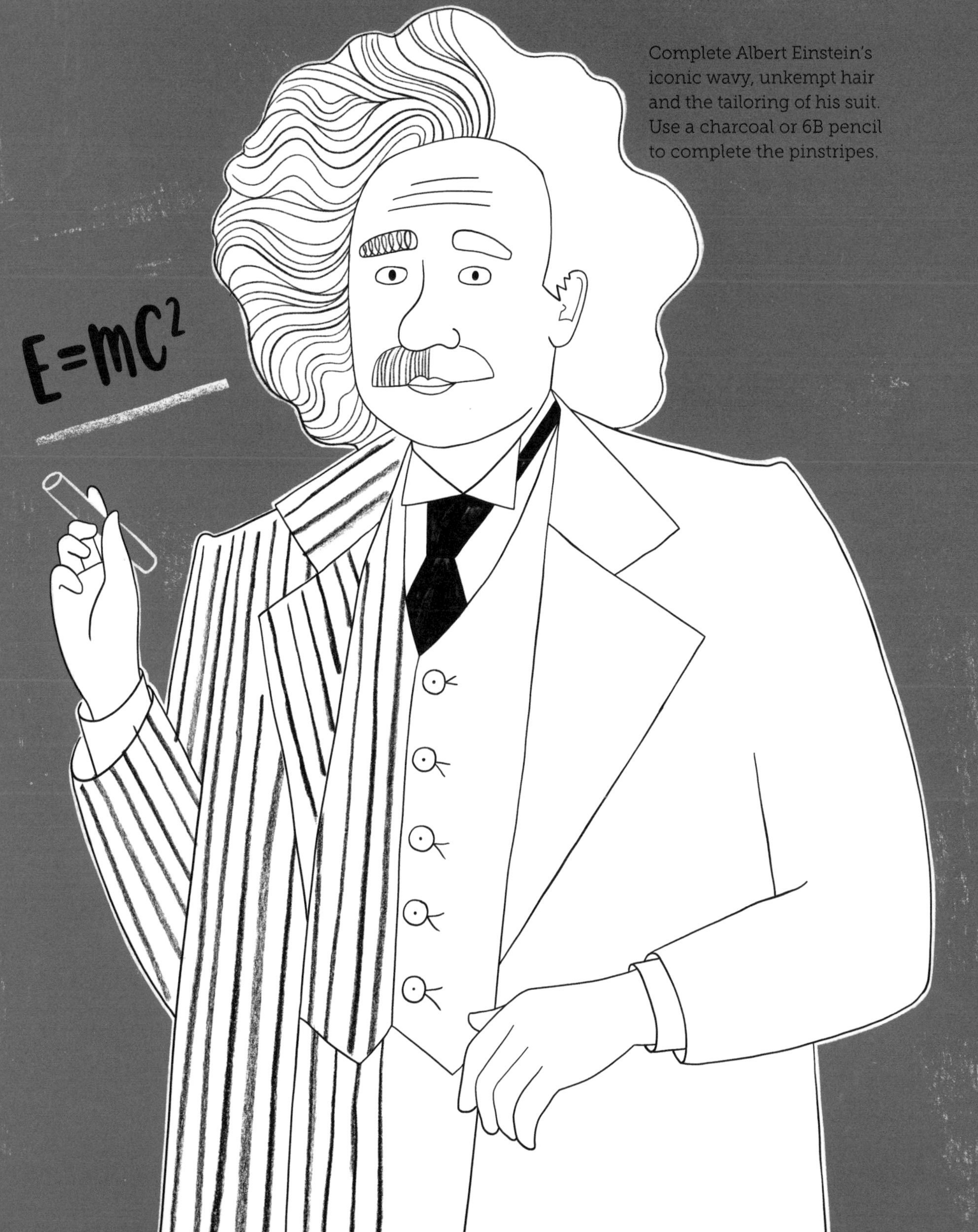

Complete Albert Einstein's iconic wavy, unkempt hair and the tailoring of his suit. Use a charcoal or 6B pencil to complete the pinstripes.

DRAWING PEOPLE IN MOTION

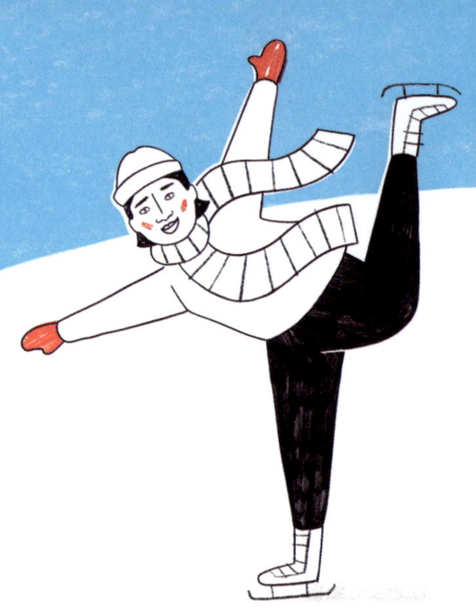

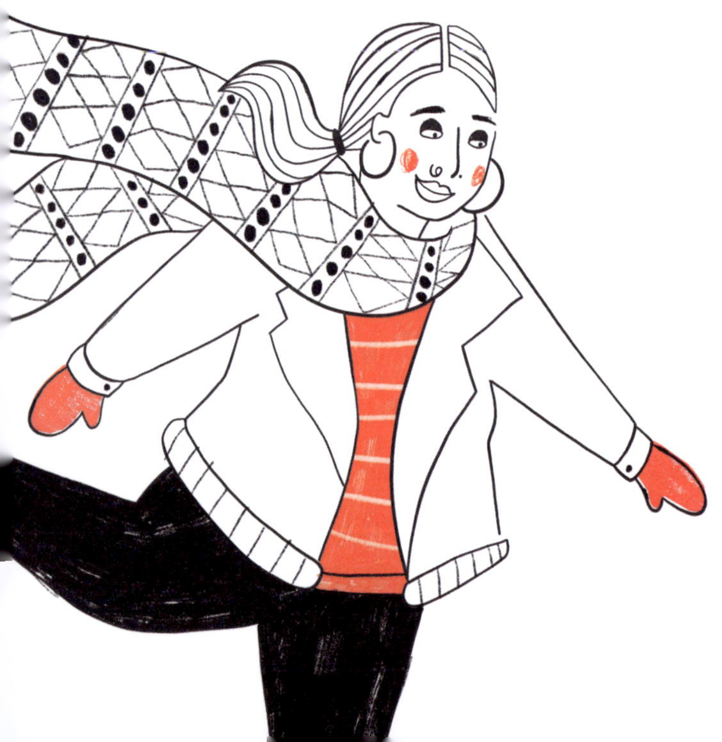

Fill this ice rink with people ice skating. Think about practicing movement and using perspective in your drawing by making the skaters larger up close and smaller toward the back.

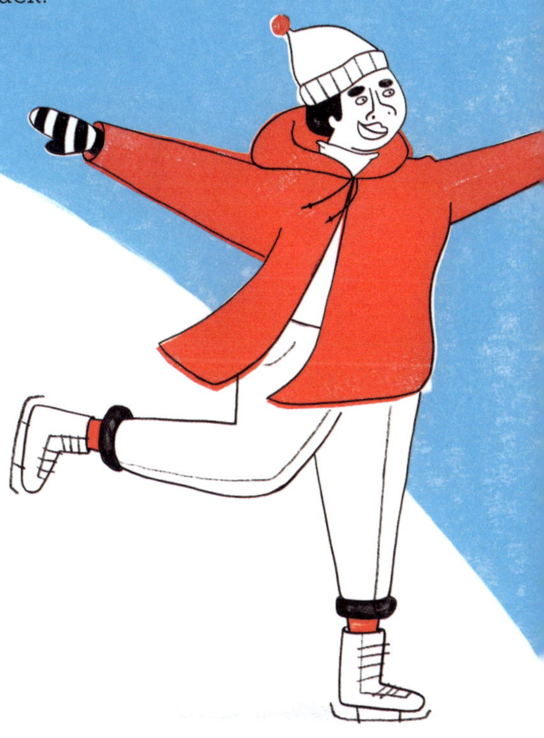

UPSIDE-DOWN DRAWING

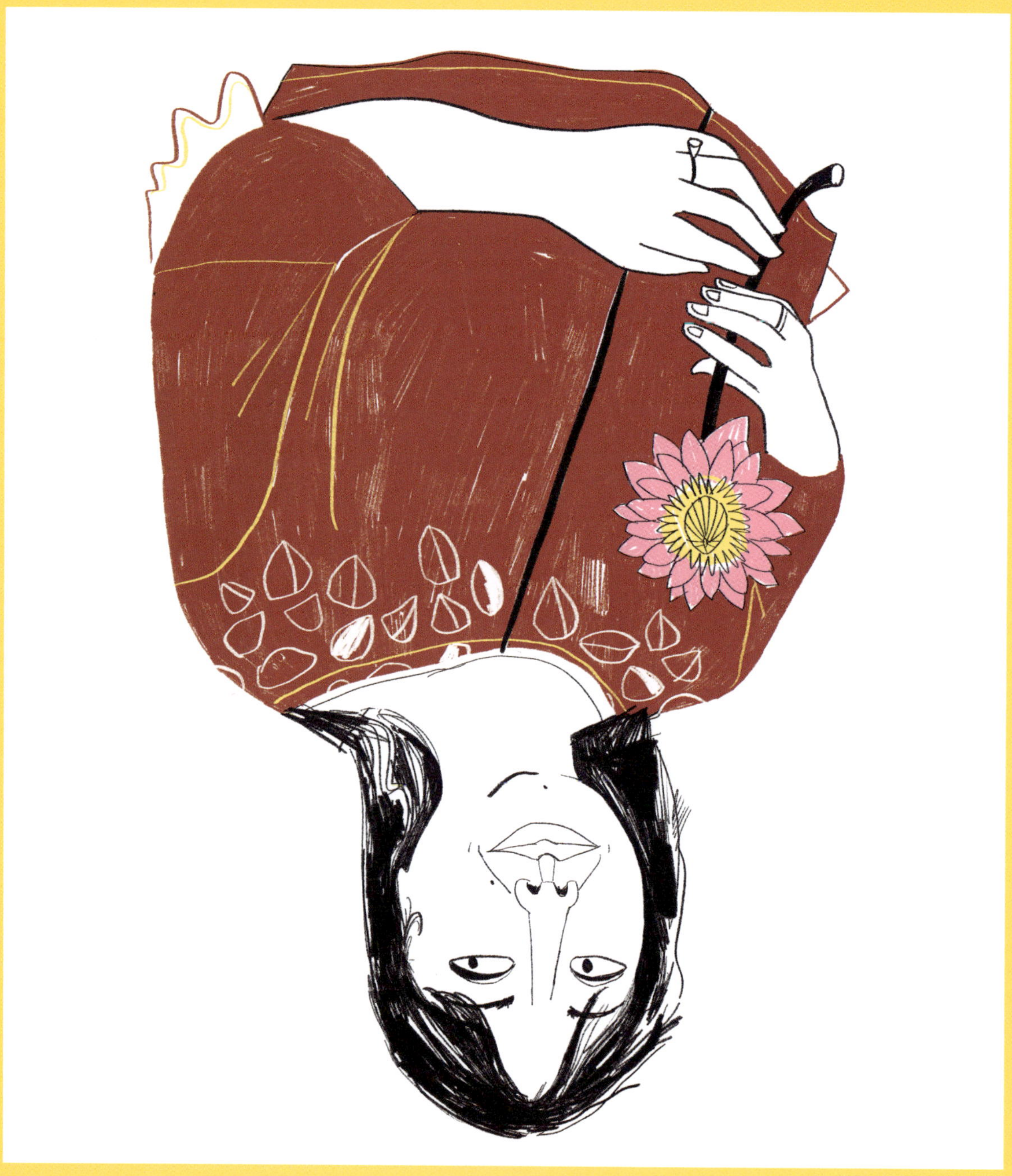

This person's portrait was drawn the right way
up, a few pages back on Timed Poses: Faces,
so you can compare!

This exercise was created by American artist Betty Edwards in the 1970s. Choose a portrait photo, but turn it upside down. This will encourage you to draw what you actually see in front of you, instead of what your brain thinks it sees!

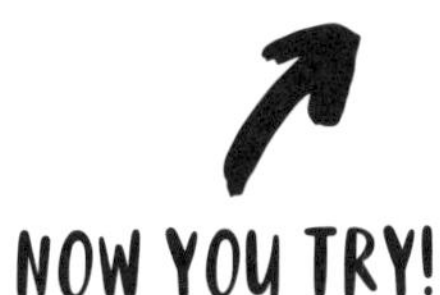

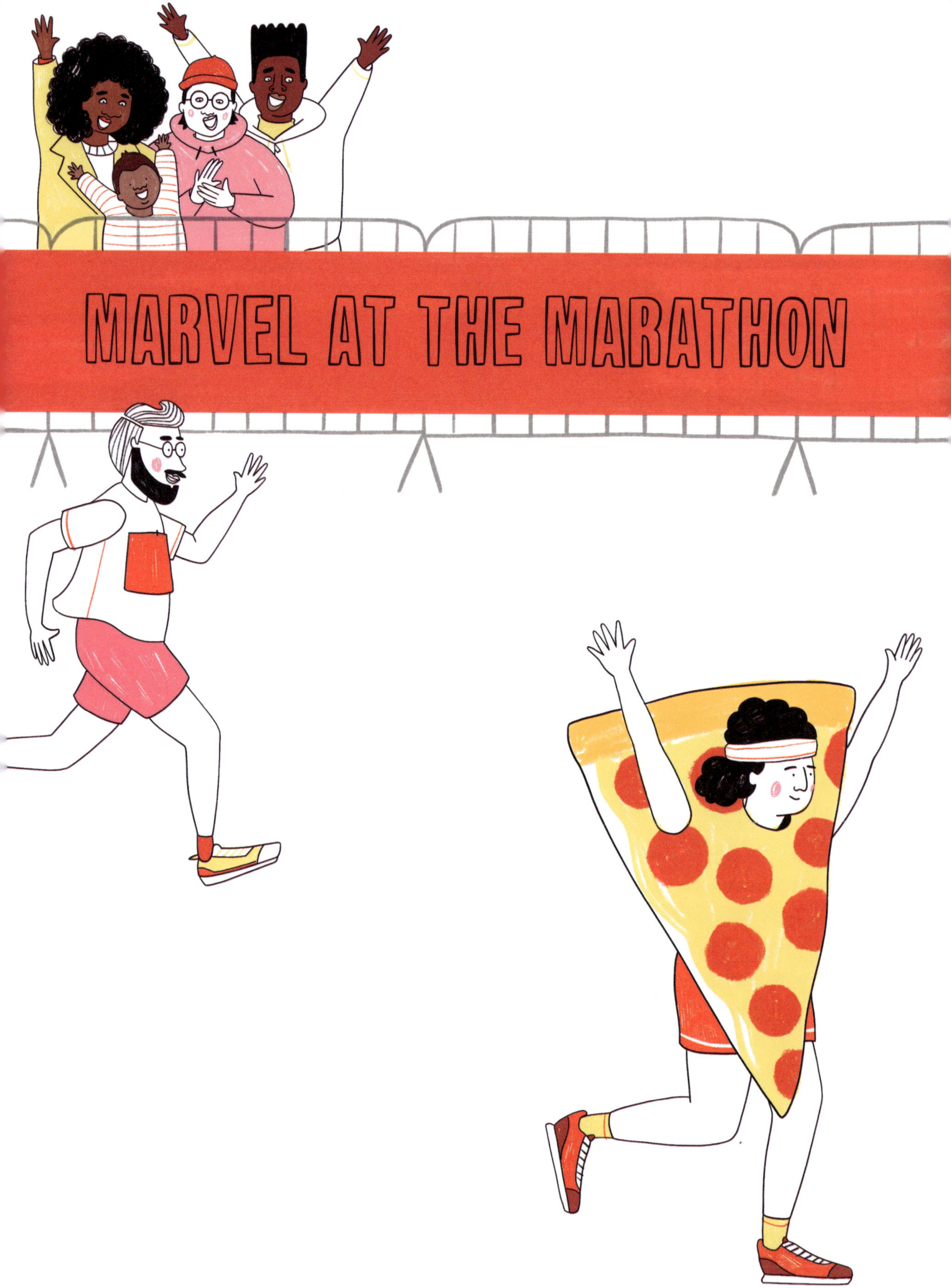

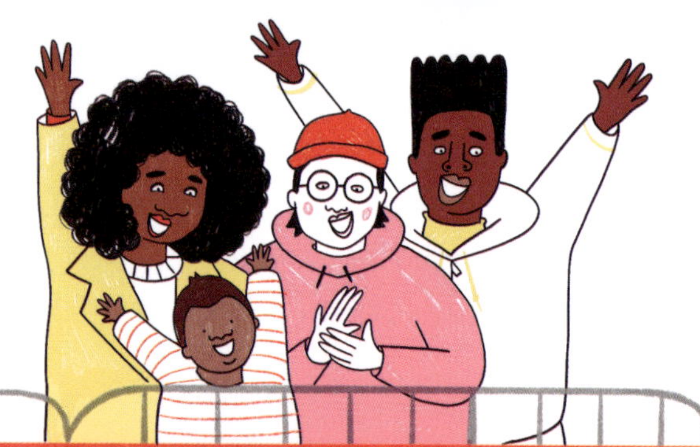

MARVEL AT THE MARATHON

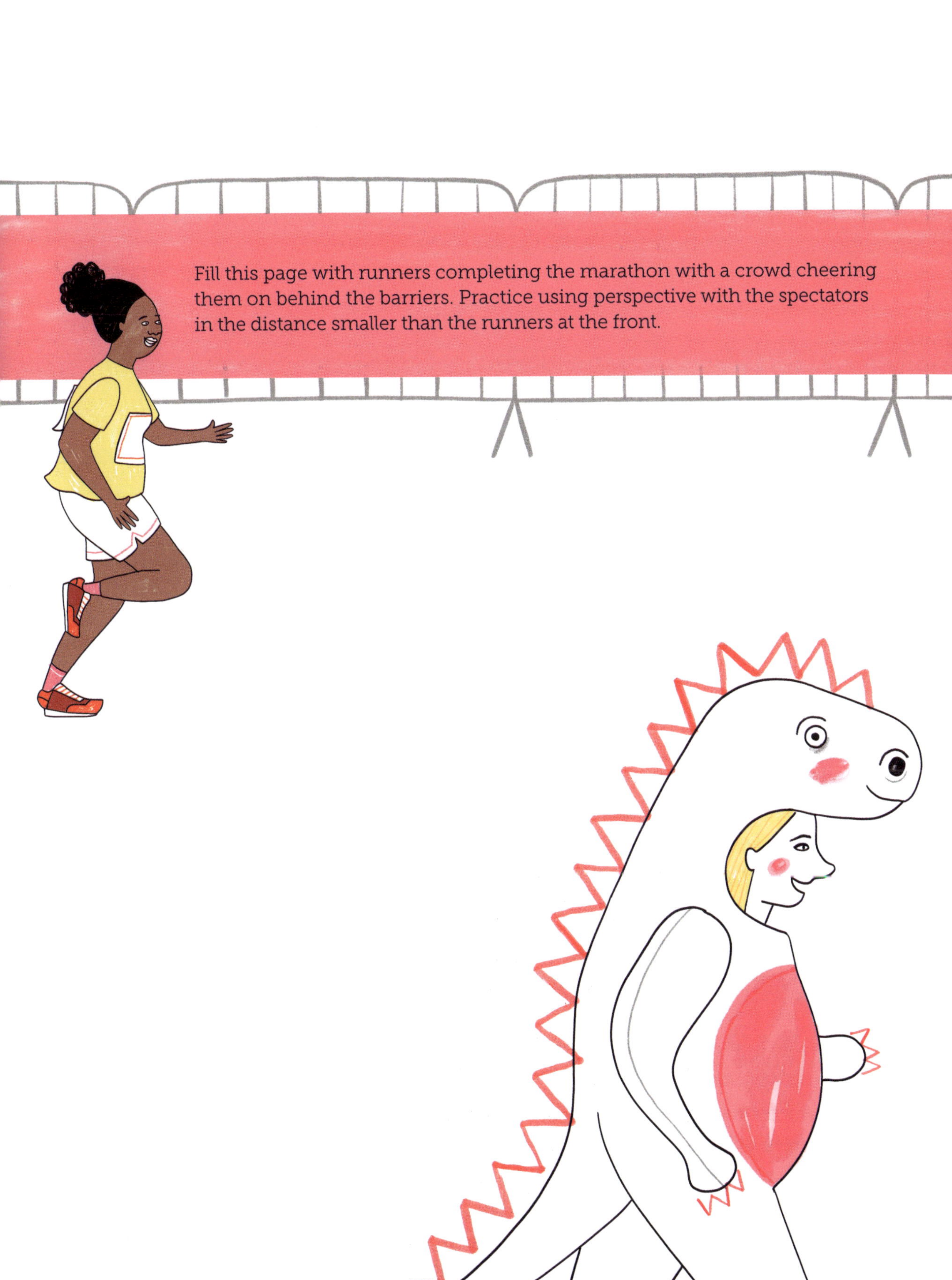

Fill this page with runners completing the marathon with a crowd cheering them on behind the barriers. Practice using perspective with the spectators in the distance smaller than the runners at the front.

UNDER THE SEA

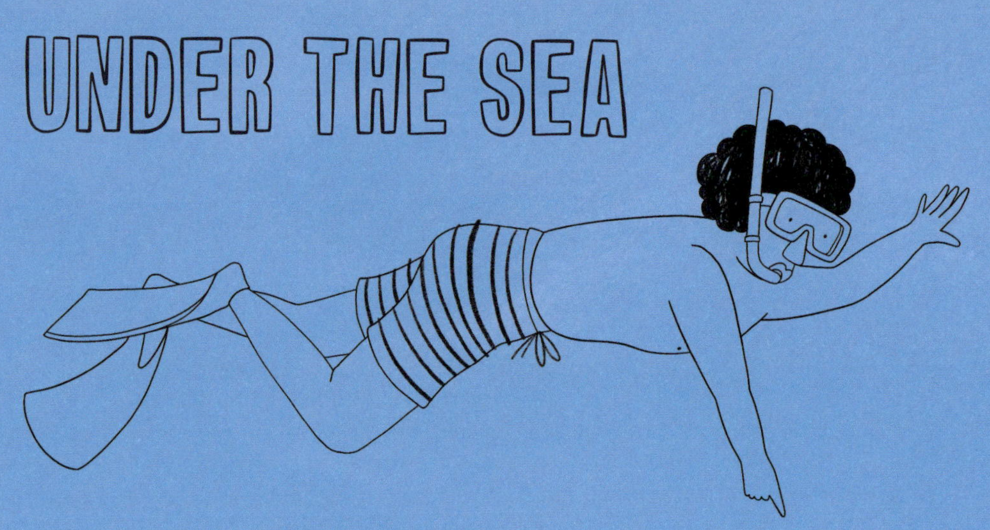

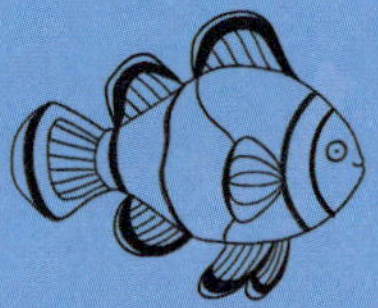

COLOR THE CORAL IN
BRIGHT VIVID COLORS!

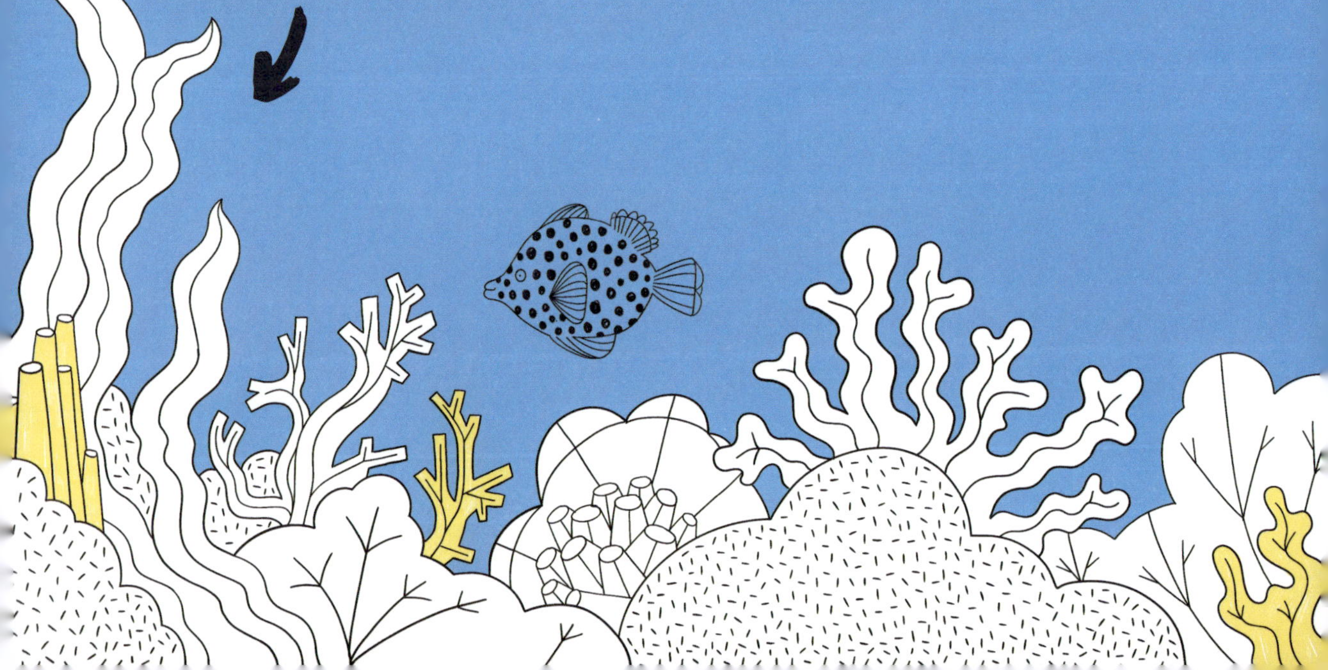

Using a black fineliner, fill the sea with colorful fish and people snorkeling. Draw the people as they dive to see what wonders are down there and as they swim back up to catch a breath.

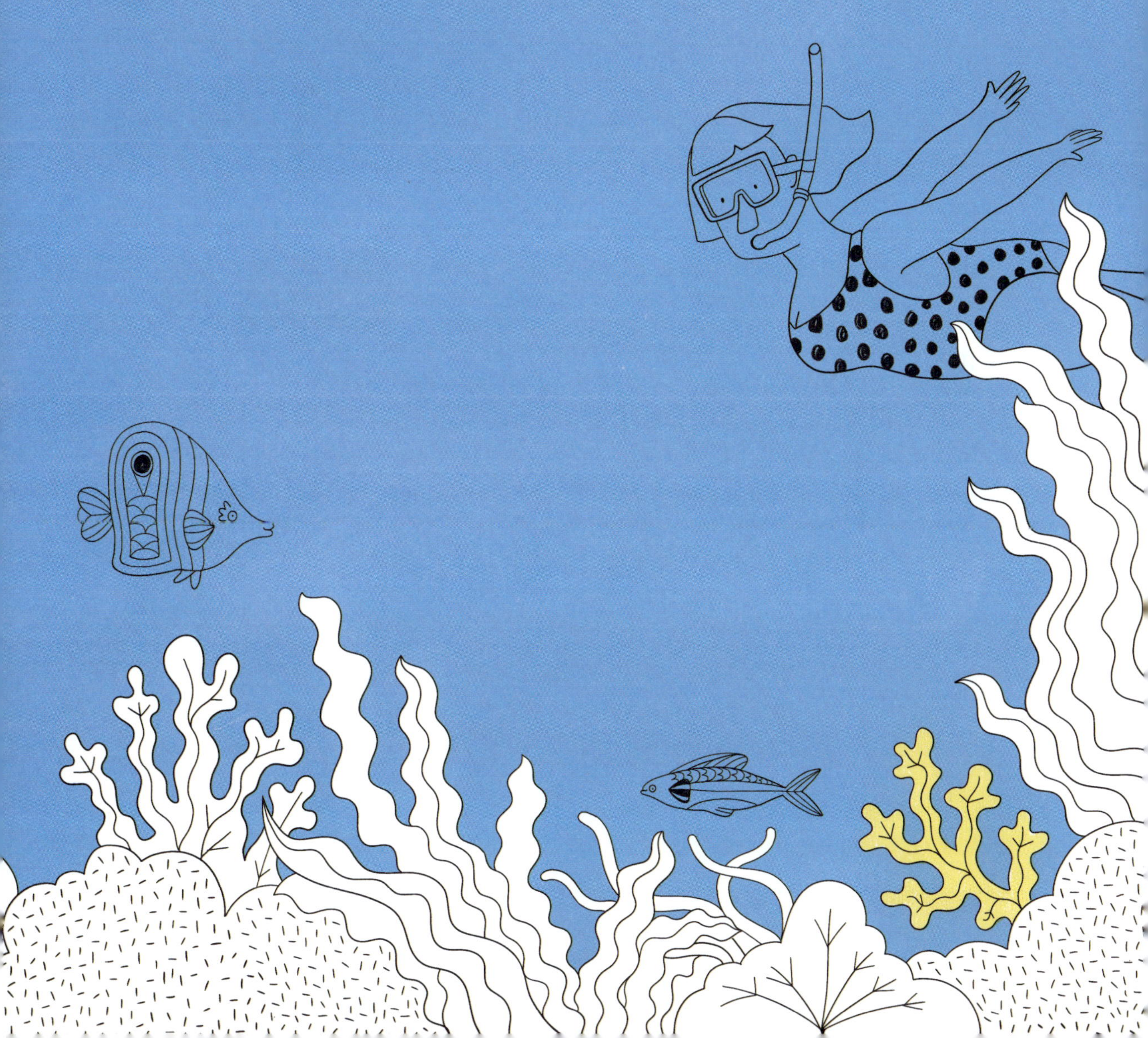

NEXT IN LINE

Take your characters out dancing to a nightclub—but first, they need to stand in line. Draw them waiting to get in. Who's going and what will they be wearing?

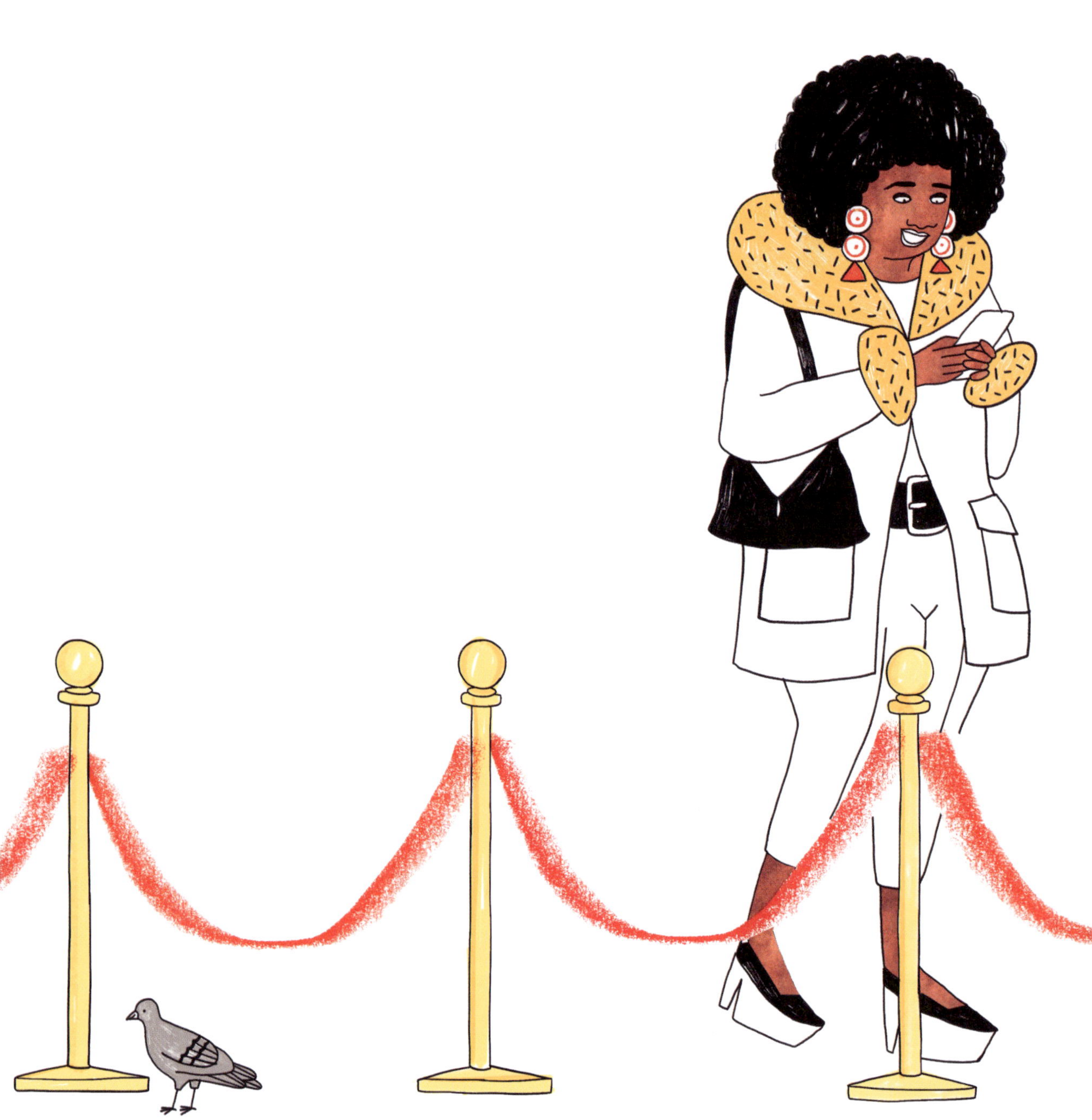

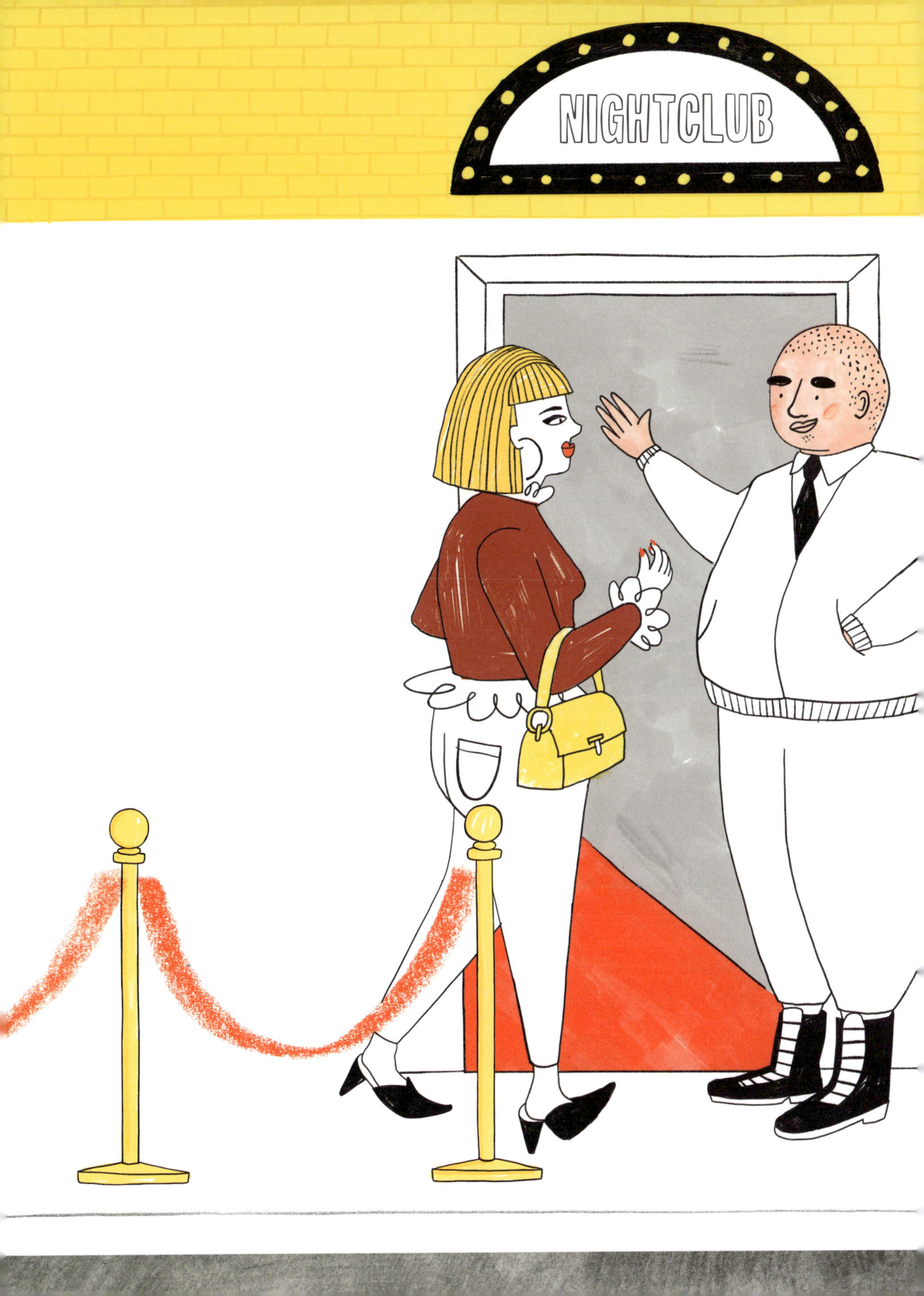

NIGHTCLUB

IN THE CLUB

You're in the club! Finish the scene by filling the page with characters dancing under the disco lights. Have the people you drew on the previous page entered the club yet?

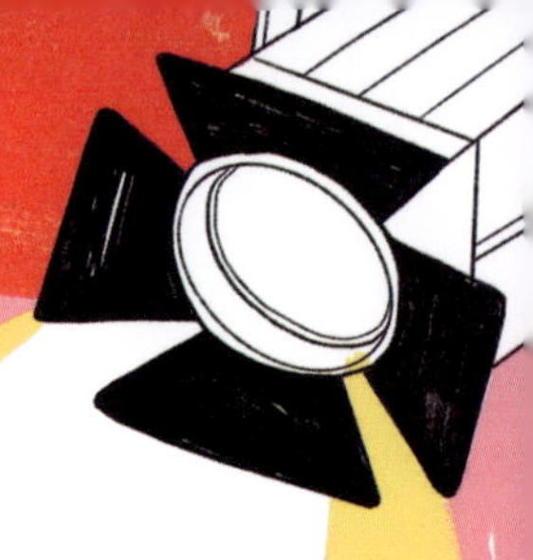

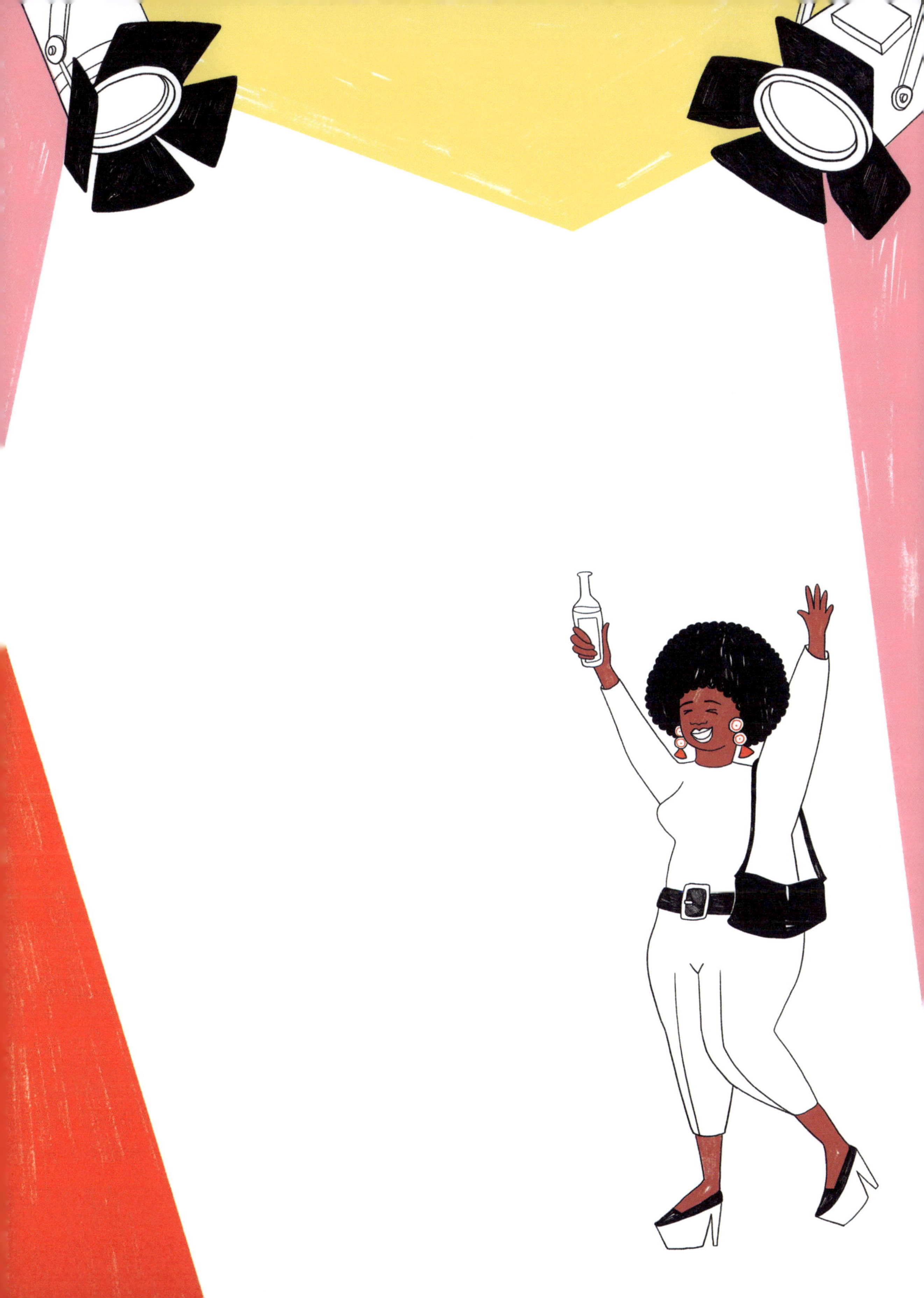

SEASONS: WINTER

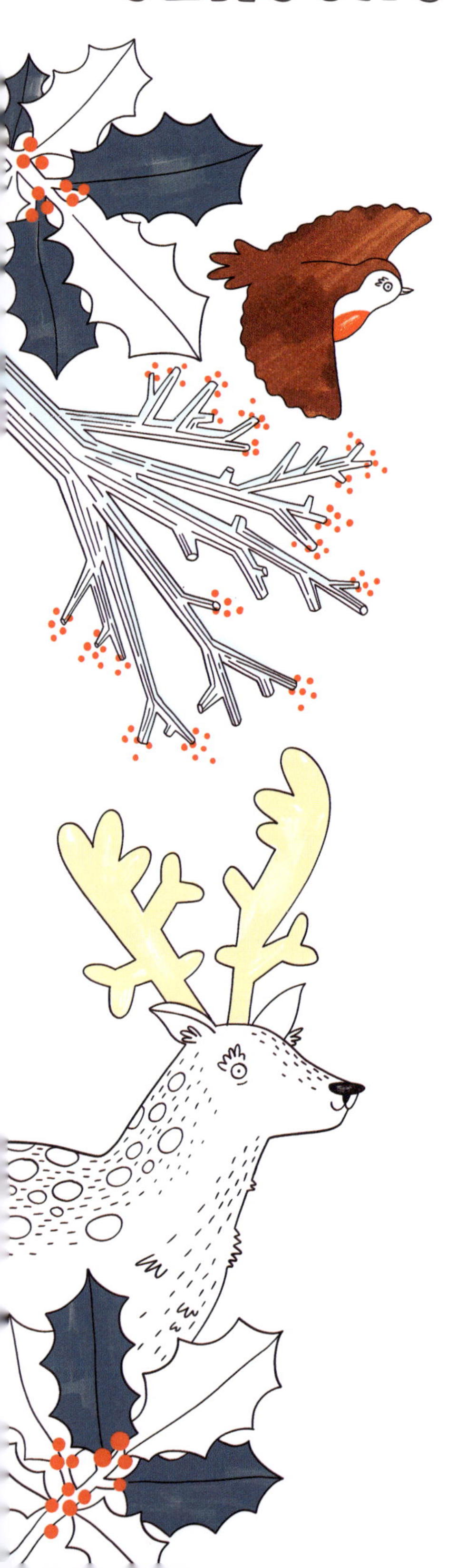

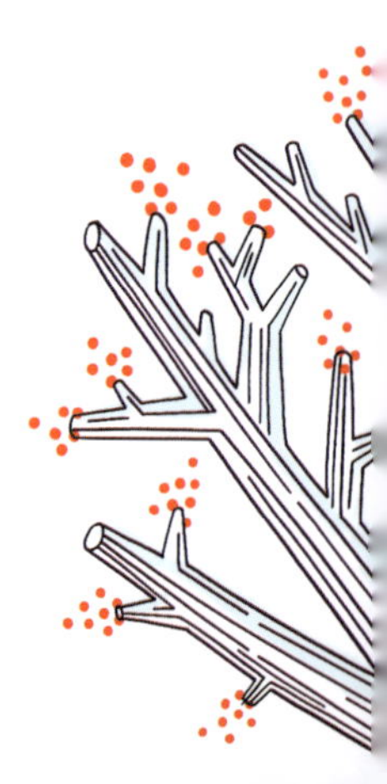

Using a cool color palette, draw people in the wintertime.
Wrap them up for the cold weather in bobble hats,
big chunky scarves, and a cozy, warm winter coat.

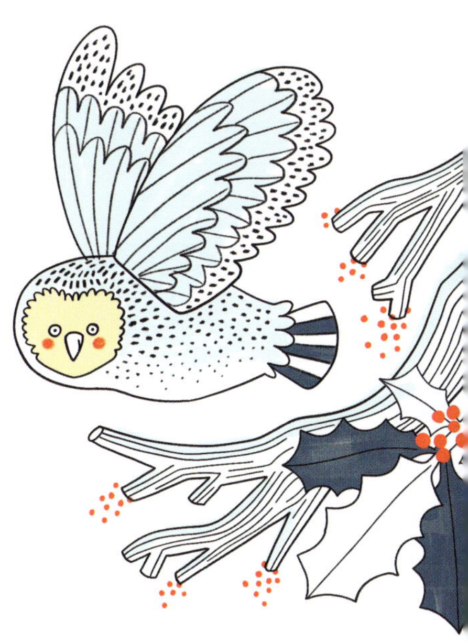

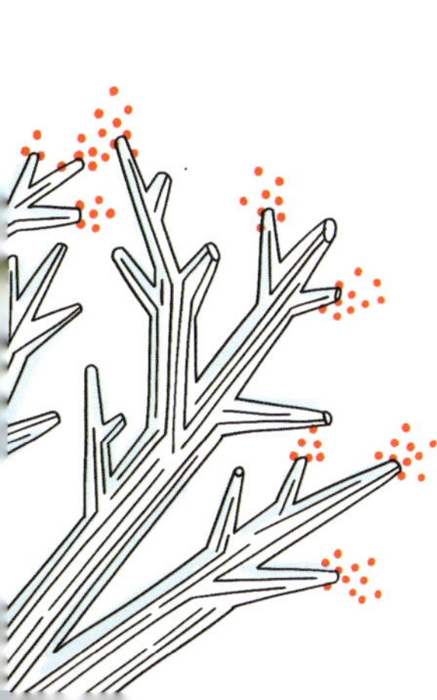

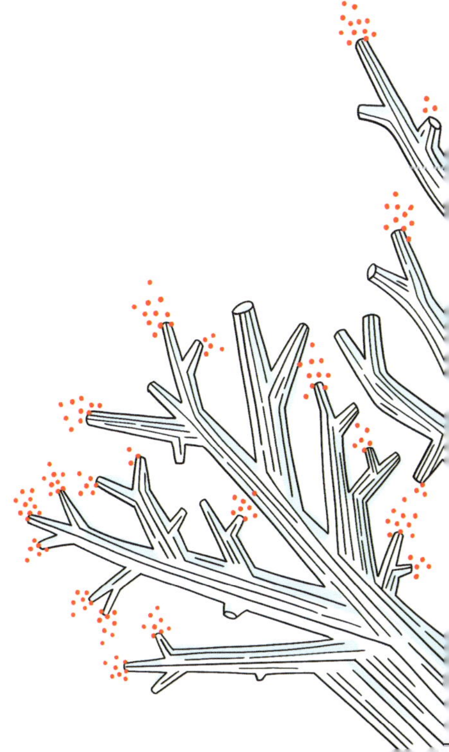

TIMED POSES: PEOPLE

Ask your friends and family to pose for you. Set a timer and draw them in the spaces provided. Focus on getting the lines and shapes down for the quick poses, then enjoy the finer details for the longer pose.

5 MINUTE POSE

15 MINUTE POSE

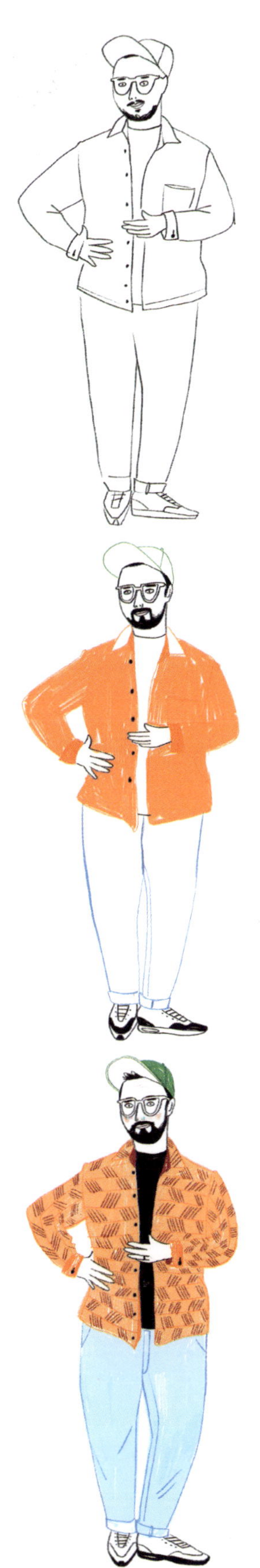

30 MINUTE POSE

CREATING CHARACTERS

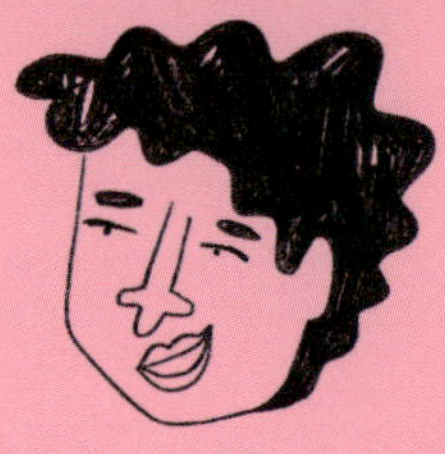

PERSONALITY TRAITS

HOBBIES AND INTERESTS

JOB

RELATIONSHIP STATUS

NAME

Learn to develop your characters further by building a narrative about who they are. Draw them in the boxes below, then fill out each section describing them as people, creating your own imaginary friends!

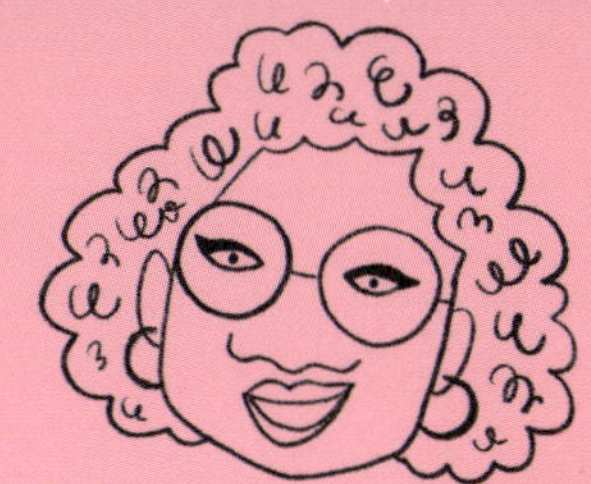

PERSONALITY TRAITS

HOBBIES AND INTERESTS

JOB

RELATIONSHIP STATUS

NAME

FUN ON THE FUNICULAR

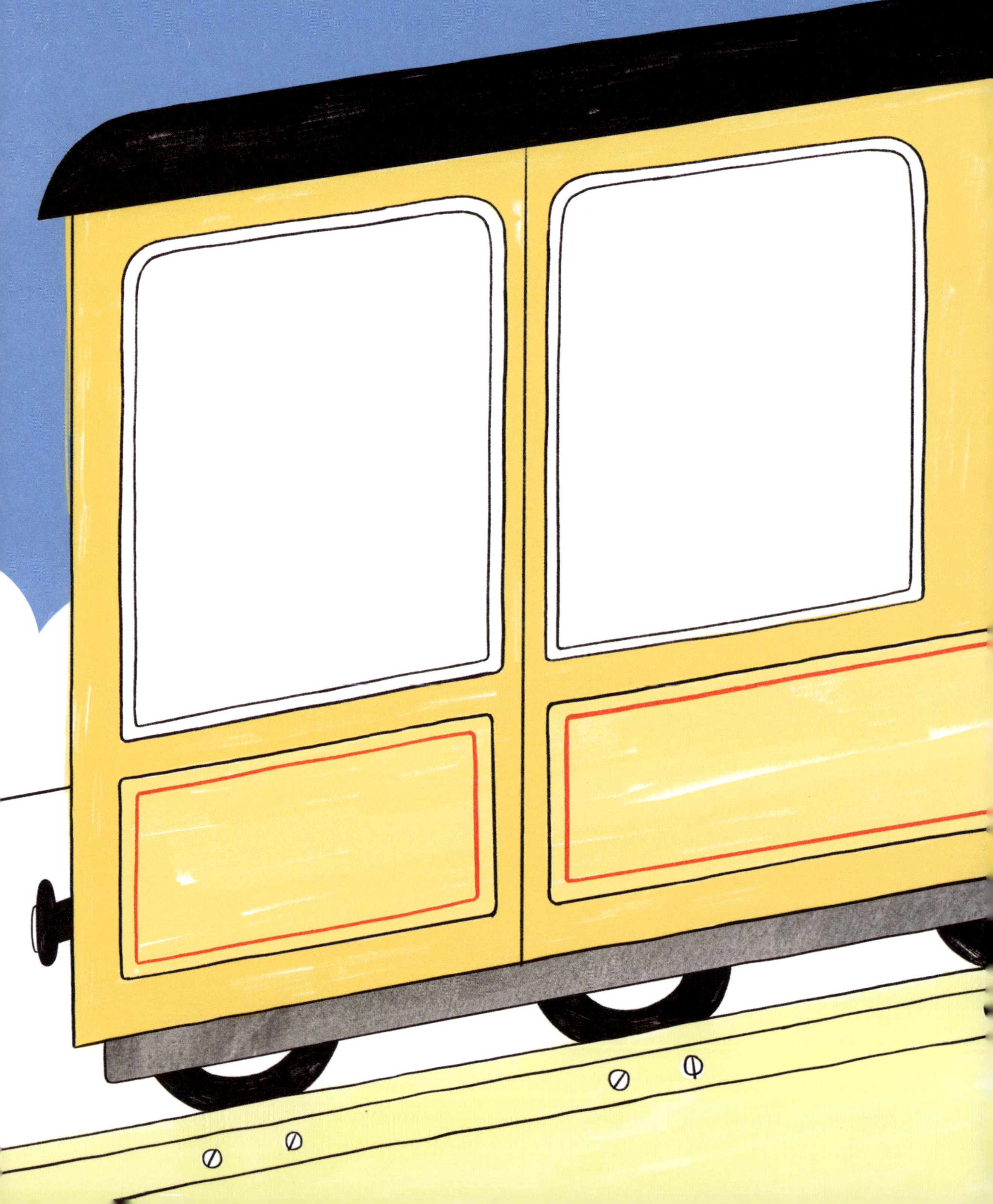

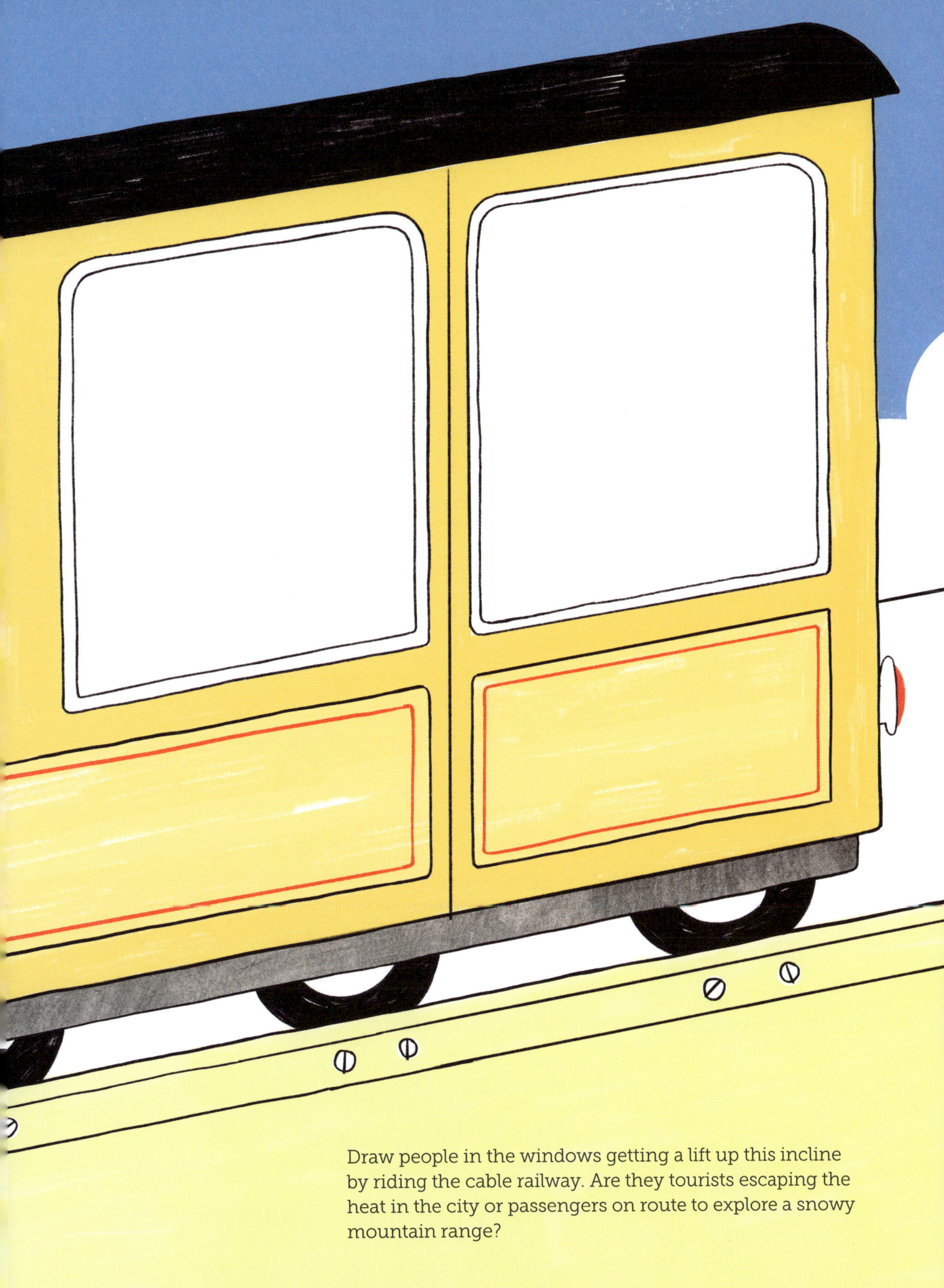

Draw people in the windows getting a lift up this incline by riding the cable railway. Are they tourists escaping the heat in the city or passengers on route to explore a snowy mountain range?

BIRDERS

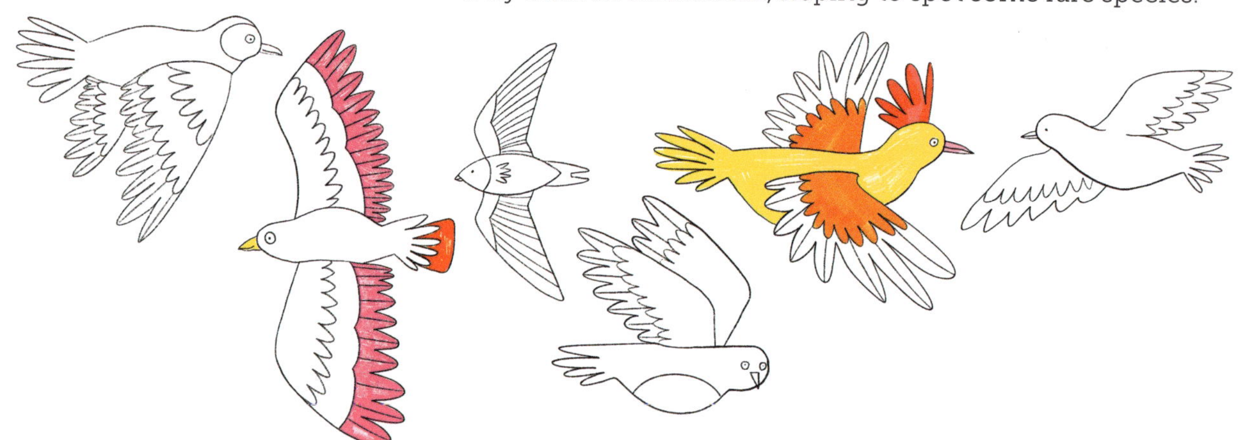

The sky is full of beautiful birds and a crowd of bird watchers, affectionately known as birders, are gathering to see what they can spot. Fill the page with more watchers as they flock in excitement, hoping to spot some rare species!

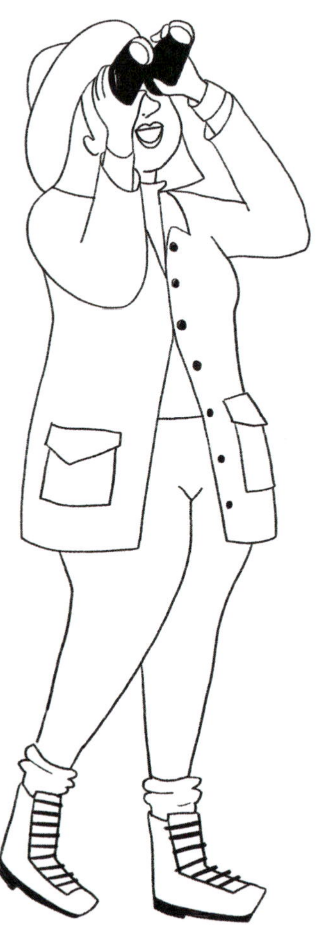

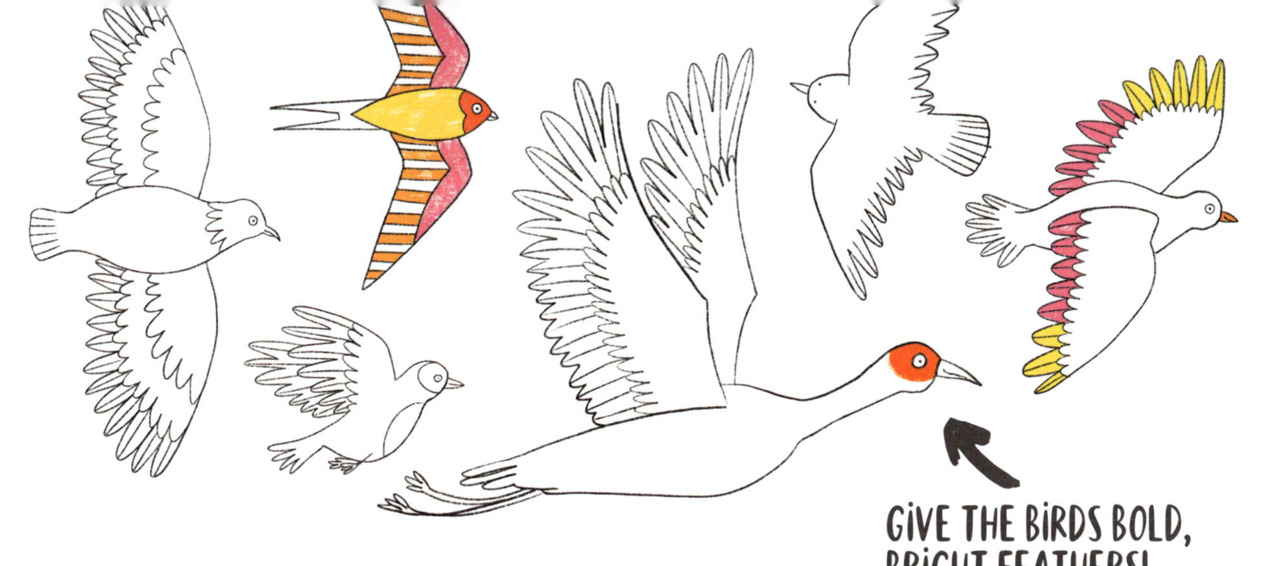
GIVE THE BIRDS BOLD, BRIGHT FEATHERS!

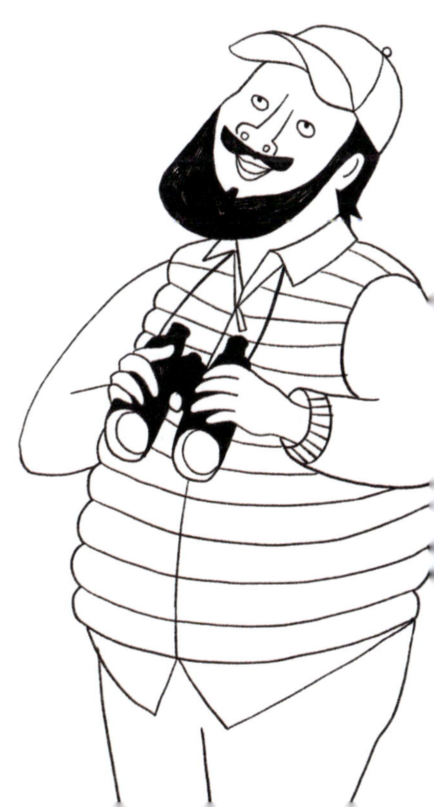

FUTURE FASHION

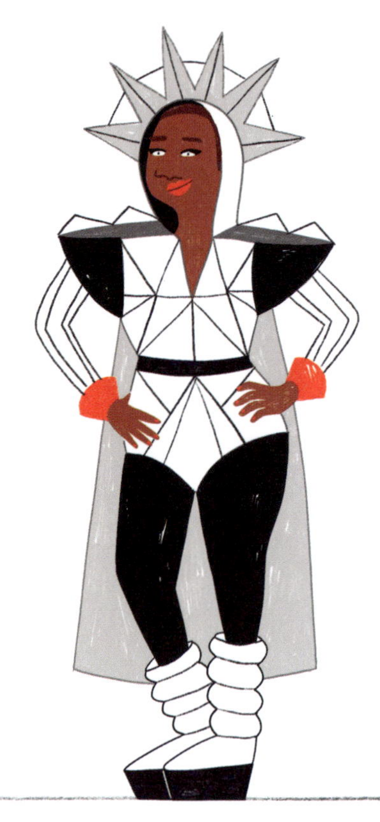

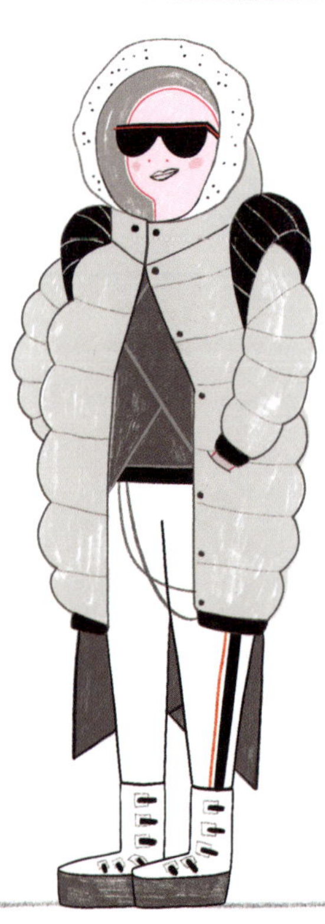

What will we look like in fifty years? Will we follow a futuristic
space-age style with metallic dresses or something different?
Imagine what style you'd like to see and add them to the collection.

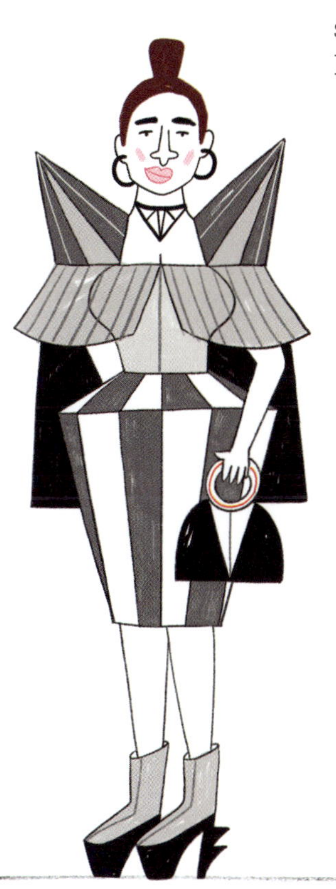

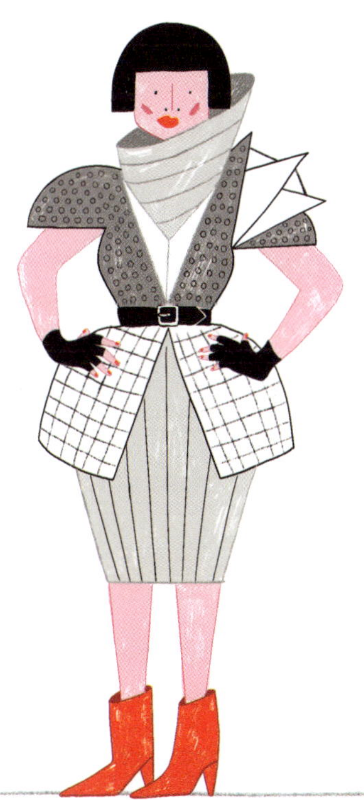

JOIN A CHOIR

The choirmaster is leading this group of singers, but they need more people to join. Fill the remaining rows behind them with characters singing their hearts out.

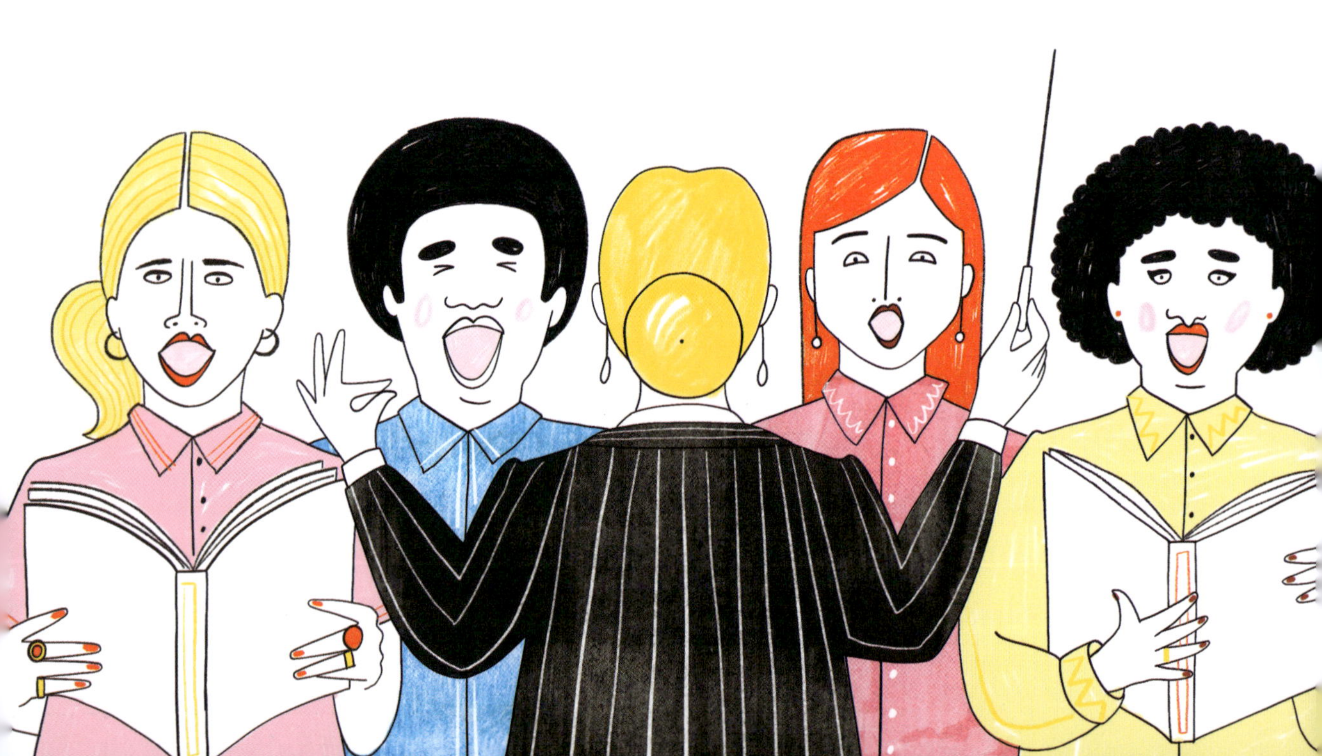

WISH YOU WERE HERE

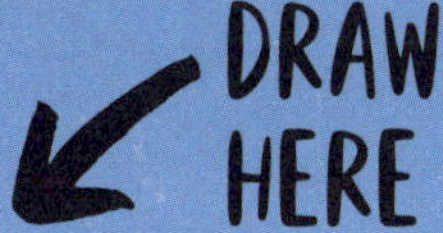

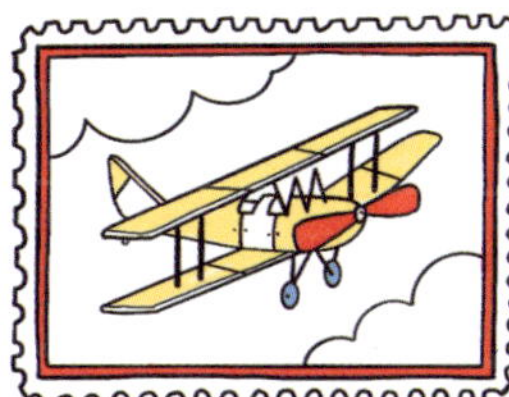

POSTCARD

Draw yourself at your dream vacation destination. On the back, write about what you would be doing, then address the postcard to whom you wish was there with you.

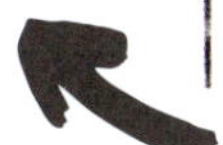

MAKING SHADOWS

Observe where the shadows fall depending on where the figures are and the direction of the sunbeams. Fill the rest of the page with characters, giving each one their own shadow.

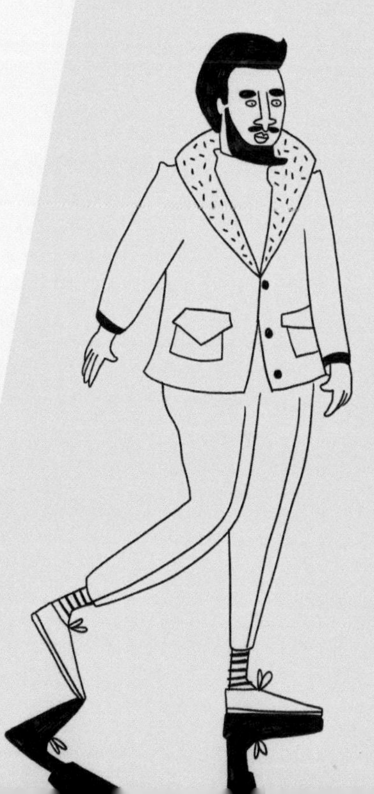

ERAS: 1980S

Fill this page with fashion from the Eighties. From power suits and shoulder pads to Lycra, rara skirts, and legwarmers, design characters in your favorite styles of this era. Start by coloring in the people below.

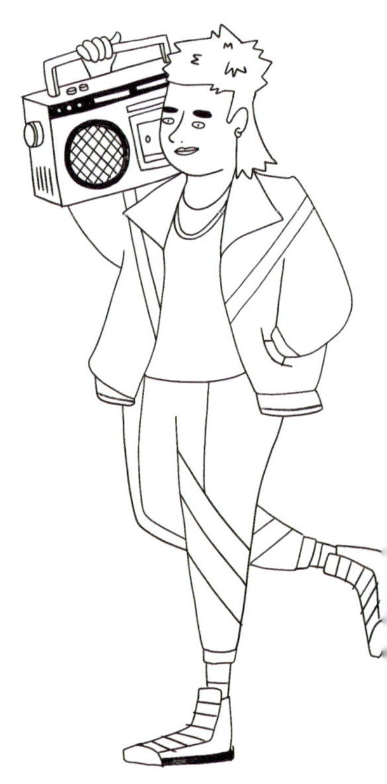

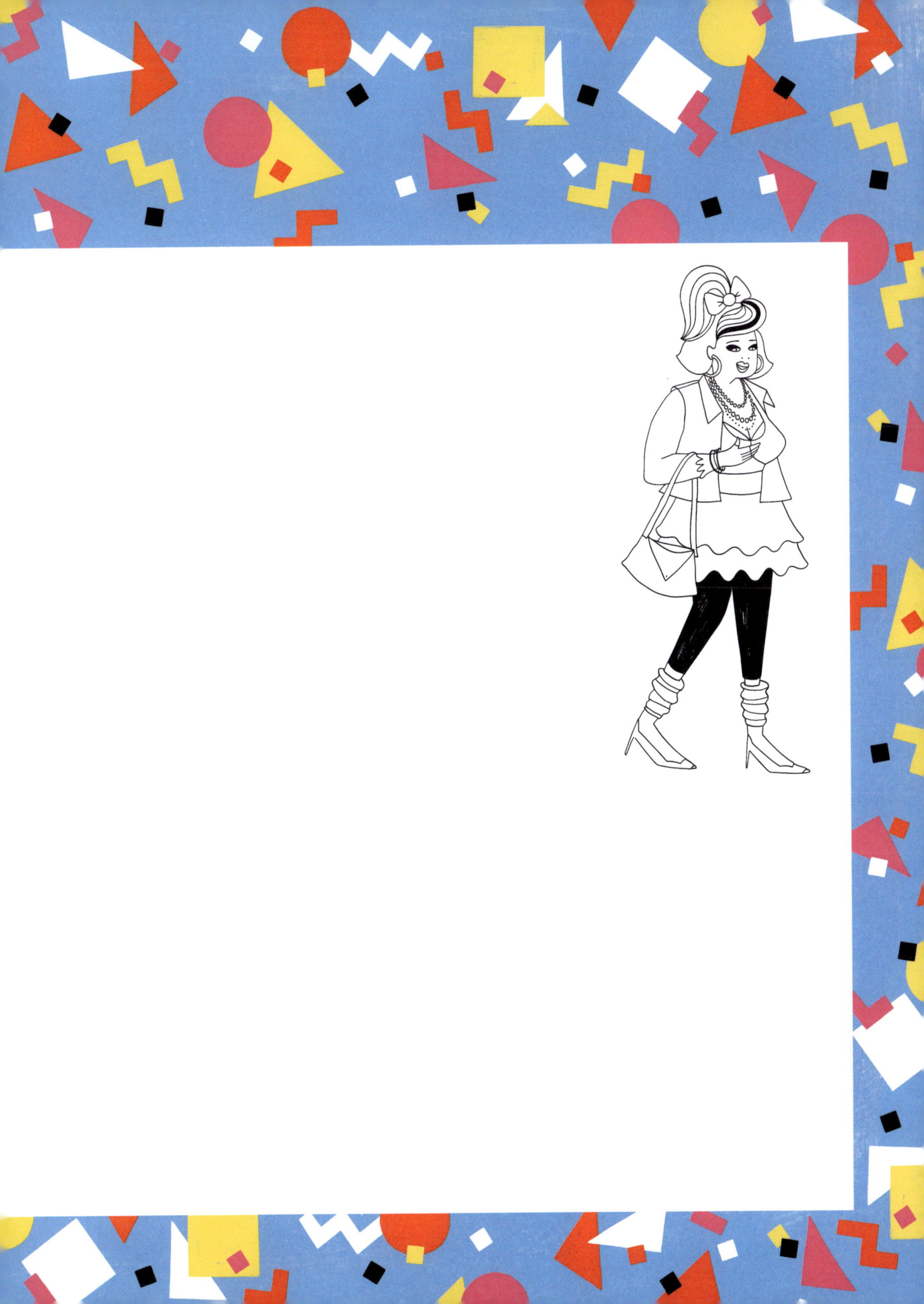

SNOW DAY!

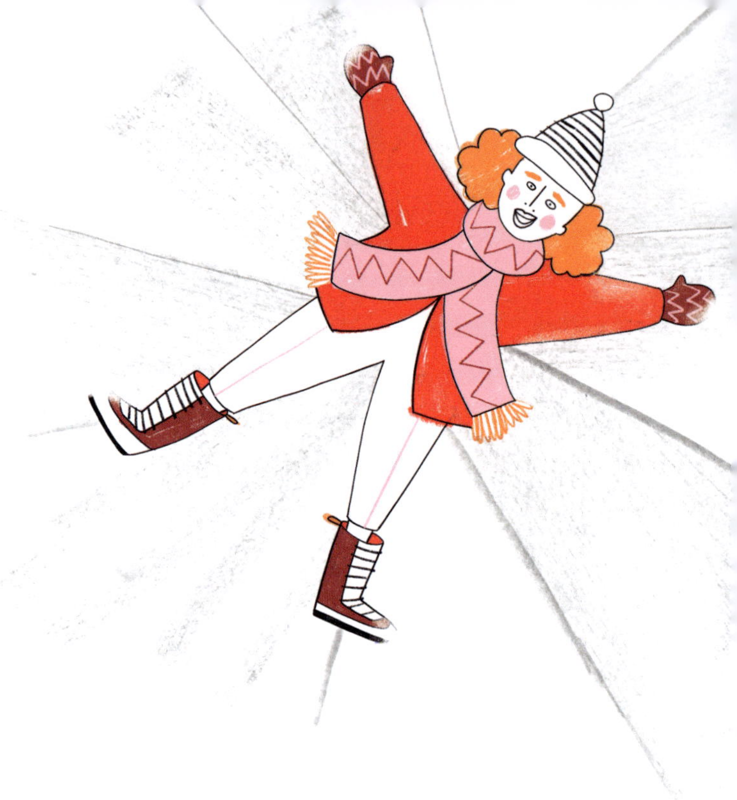

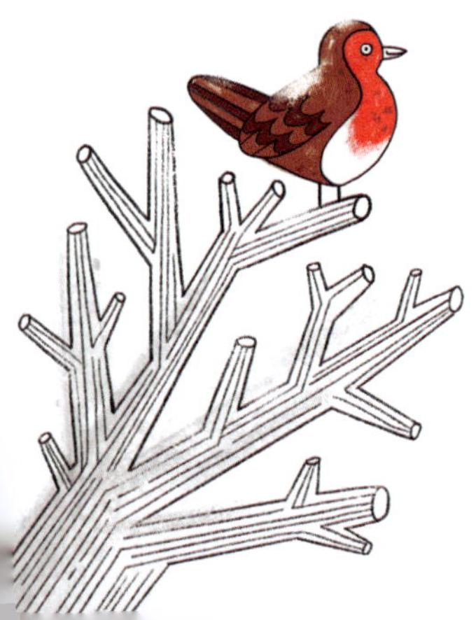

Fill the page with people making snow angels, throwing snowballs, and racing down the page in a toboggan! Have fun with texture and experiment with different materials, such as pastels, to illustrate the snow.

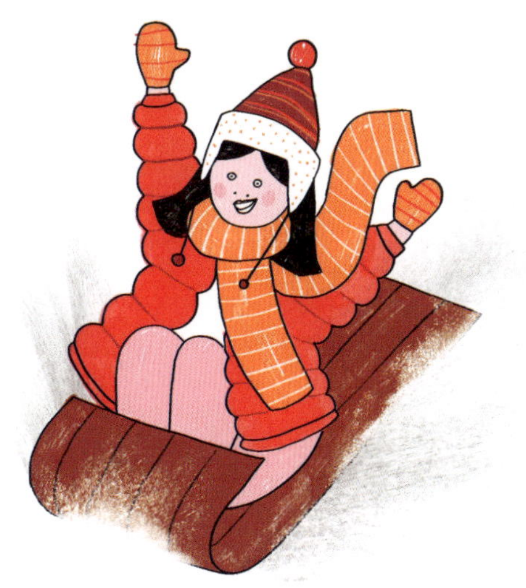

DRAWING TECHNIQUES

Try experimenting with fun ways of making marks and drawing with these four exercises using different techniques. Work from real life, either creating self-portraits or use the same face for reference, to show the differences more clearly.

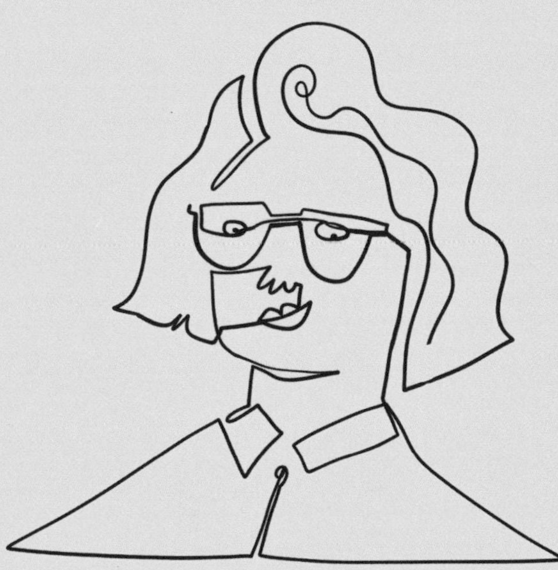

Continuous line: Draw without taking your pen off the paper.

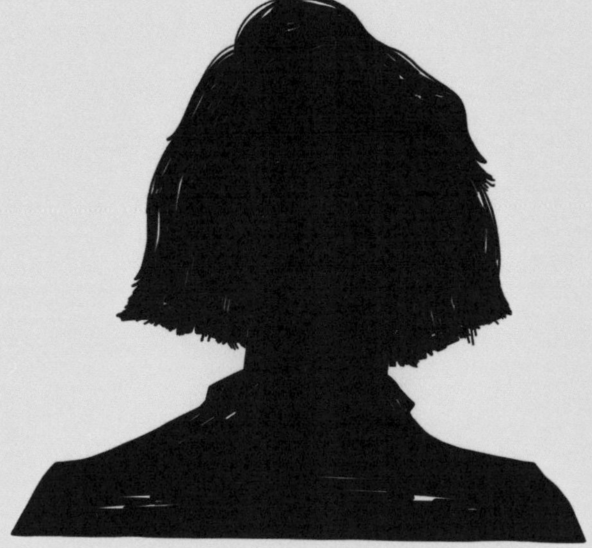

Silhouette: A simple, quick exercise using solid color to define the shape.

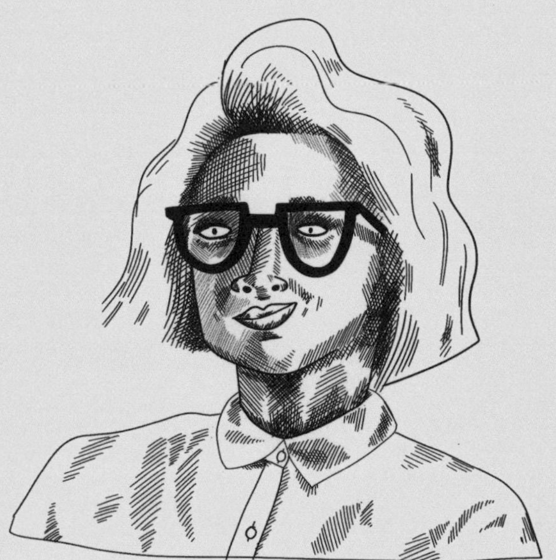

Cross hatching: Use overlapping lines to show light and shadow in your portrait.

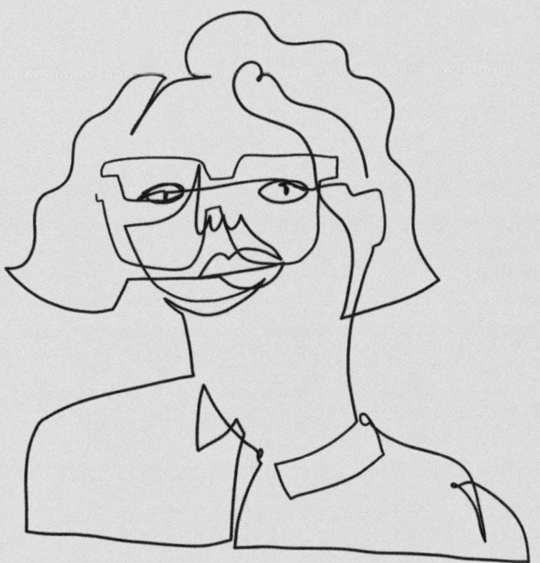

Blind contour: Draw what you see without looking or lifting up your pen.

CONTINUOUS LINE

SILHOUETTE

CROSS HATCHING

BLIND CONTOUR

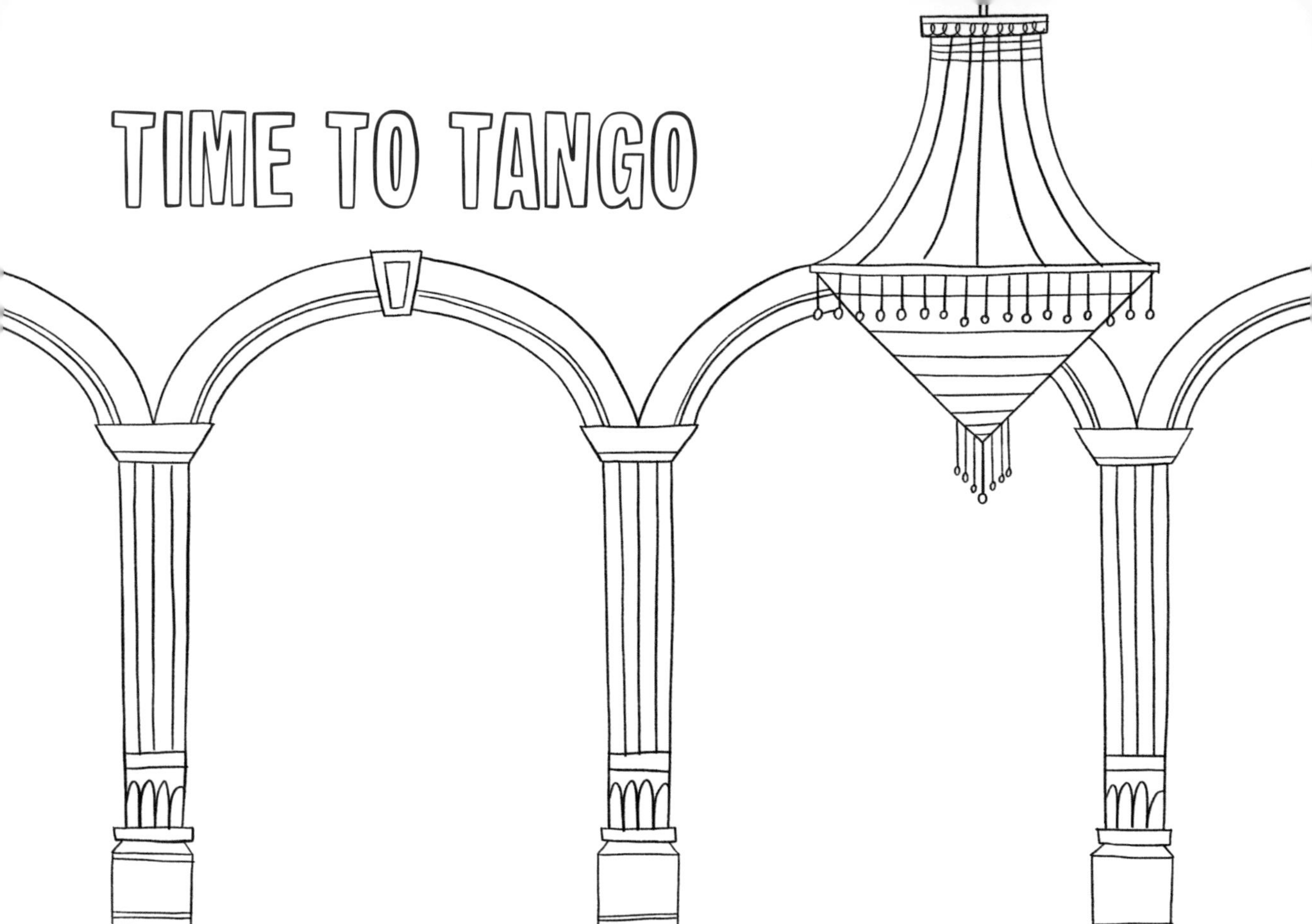

TIME TO TANGO

Fill this ballroom with duos showcasing their dance skills. Dress
them for the occasion with suits and asymmetrical dresses.
Limit your color palette to the traditional red and black.

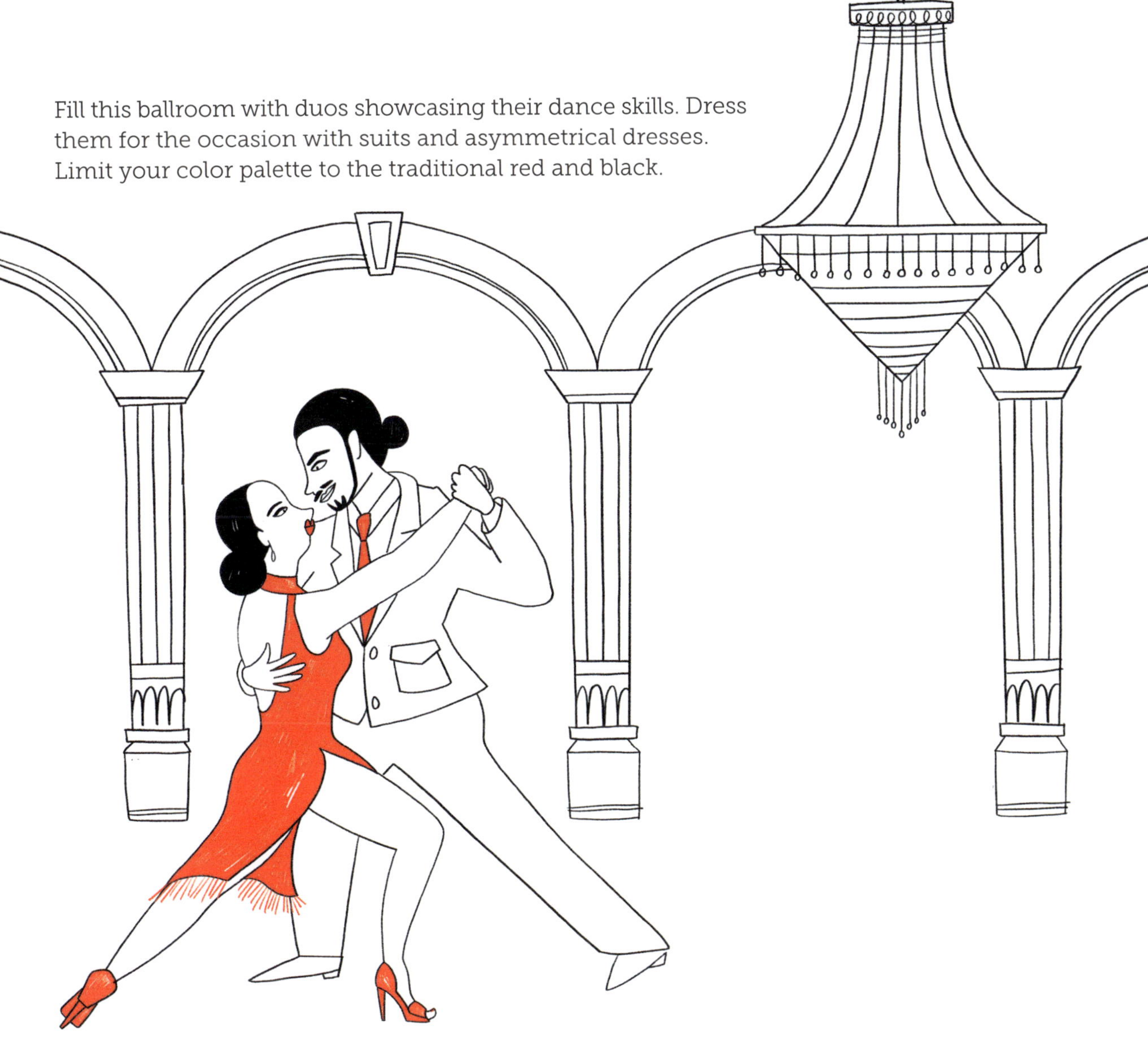

PEACEFUL PURSUITS

Choose two hobbies that make you feel happy, then draw scenes of yourself, friends, or characters from your imagination enjoying them. Perhaps you find joy in drawing (in this book!), love sports, or being out in nature?

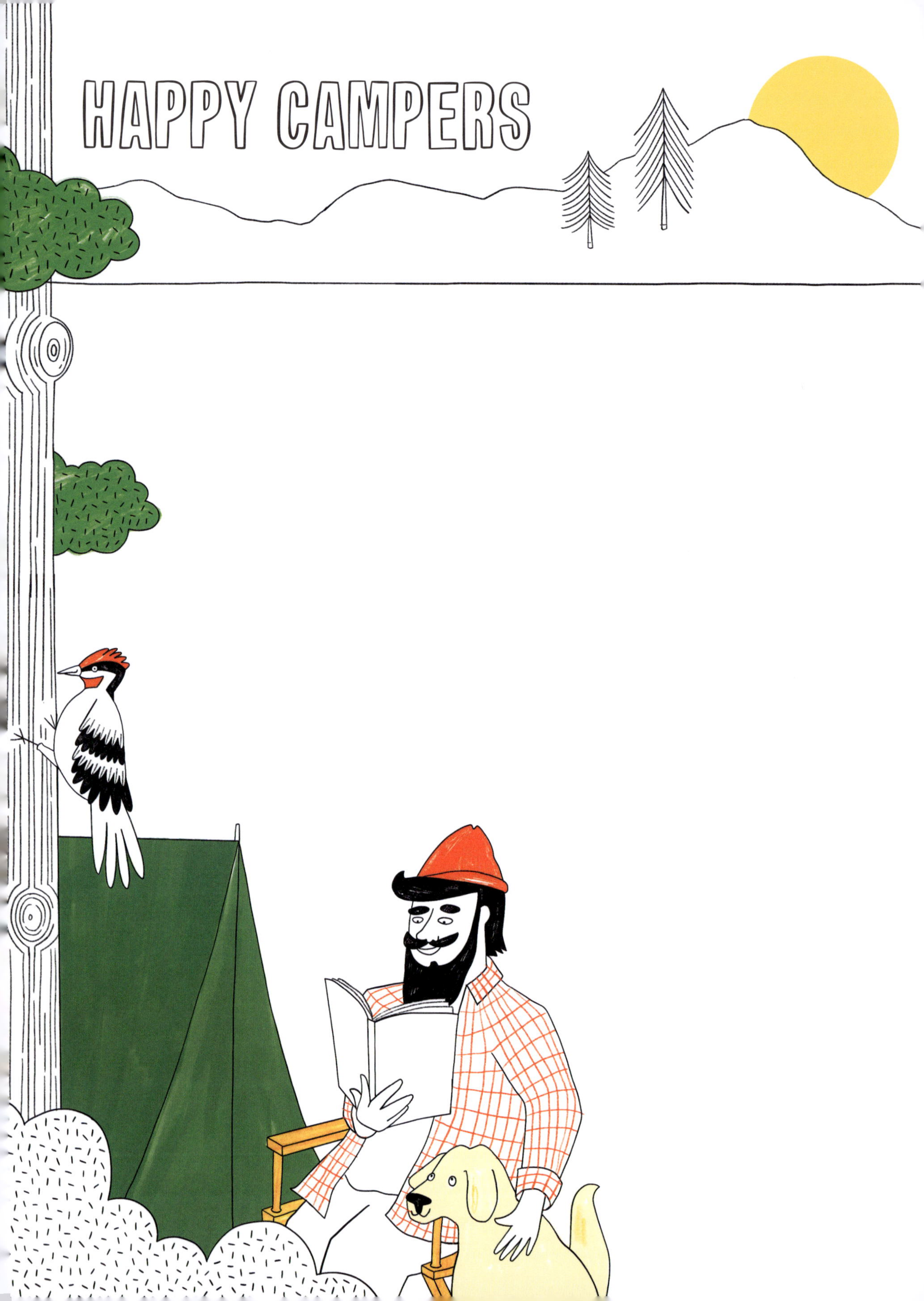

HAPPY CAMPERS

Fill this field with happy campers. It's peak summertime and this campsite is fully booked! Start by adding more people to the camps that are set up already, then bring new holidaymakers to the scene.

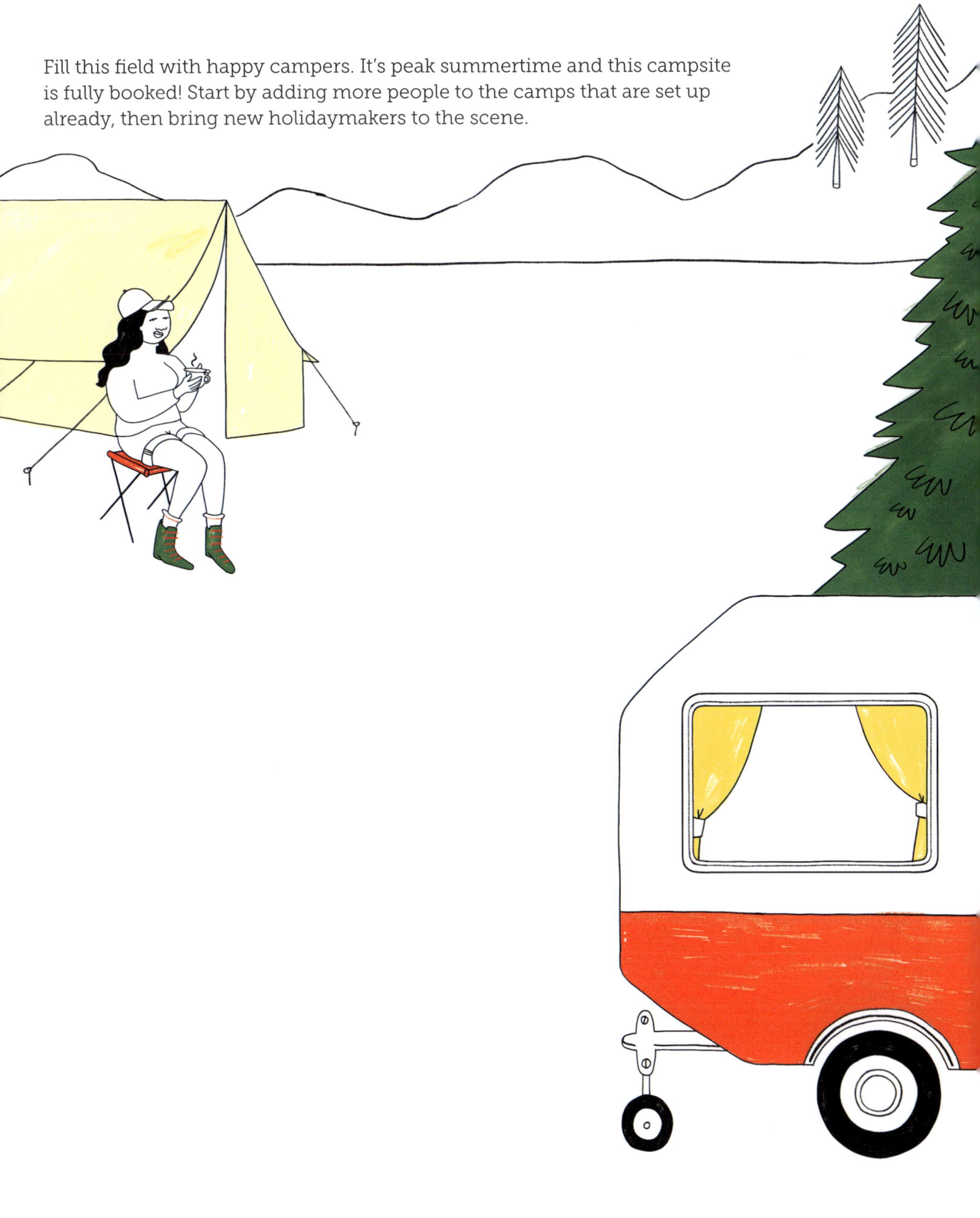

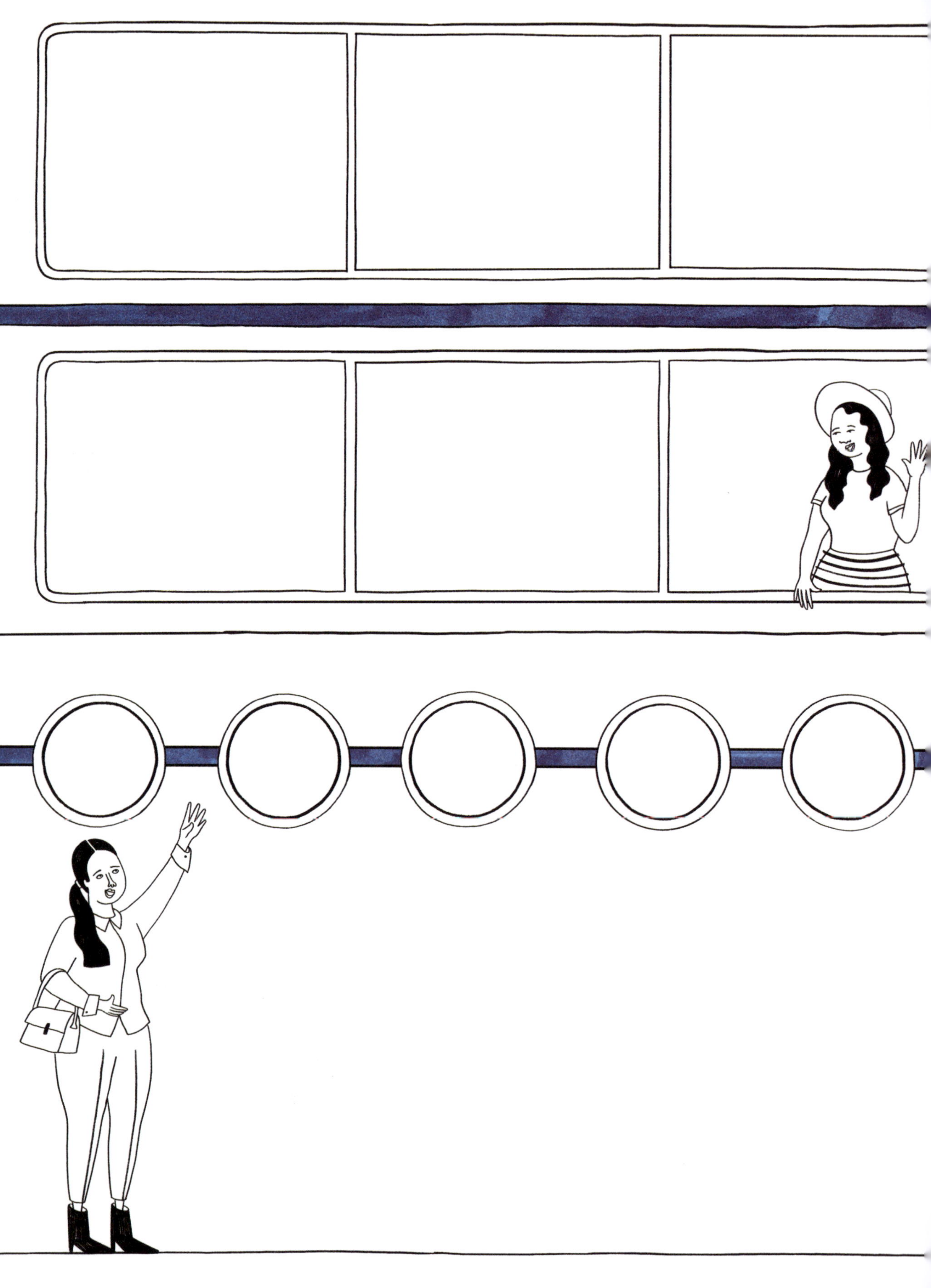

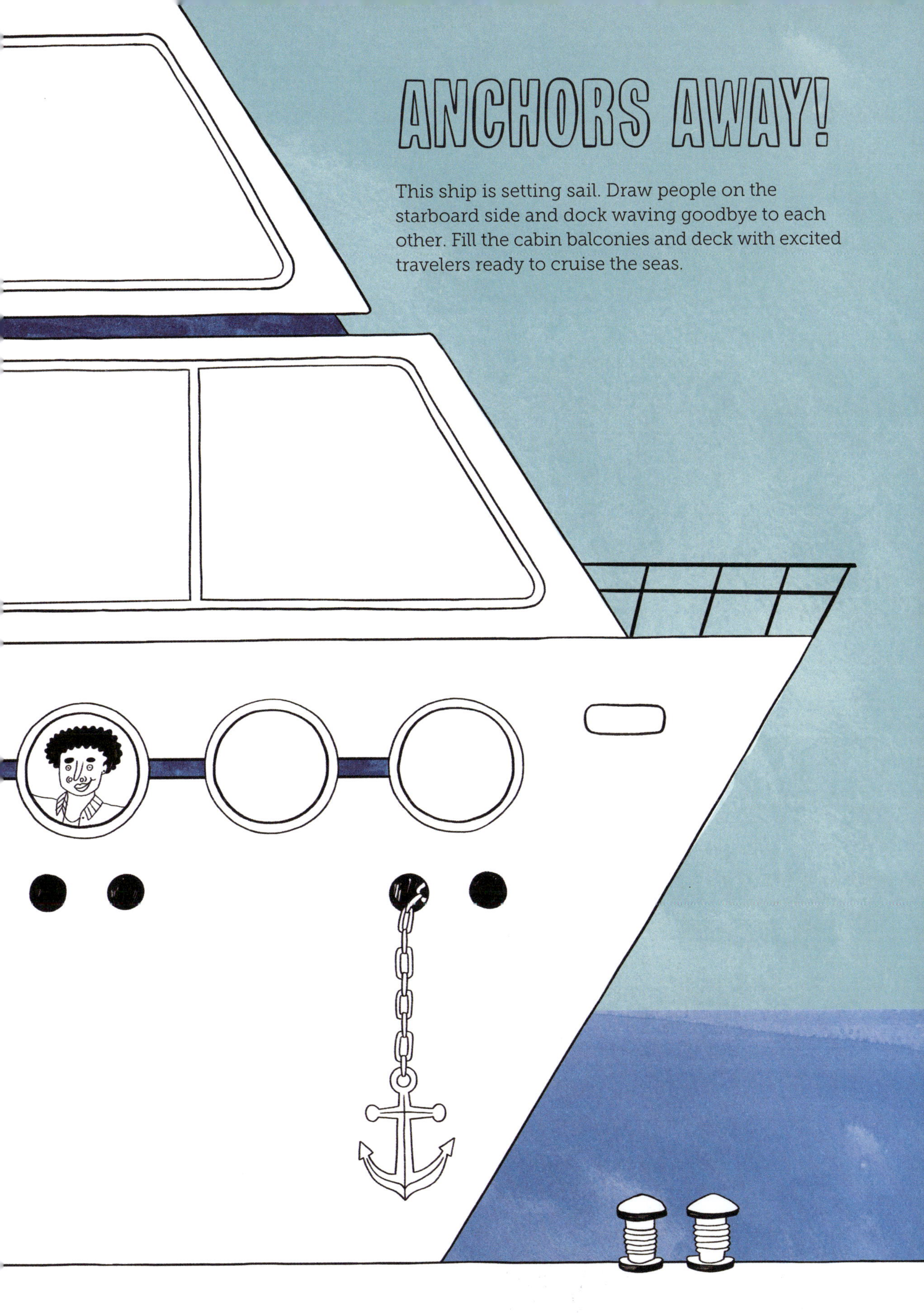

ANCHORS AWAY!

This ship is setting sail. Draw people on the starboard side and dock waving goodbye to each other. Fill the cabin balconies and deck with excited travelers ready to cruise the seas.

COSTUME PARTY

These people are having a costume party; any theme goes. Fill the rest of the page with characters dressed in fun, fabulous fancy dress!

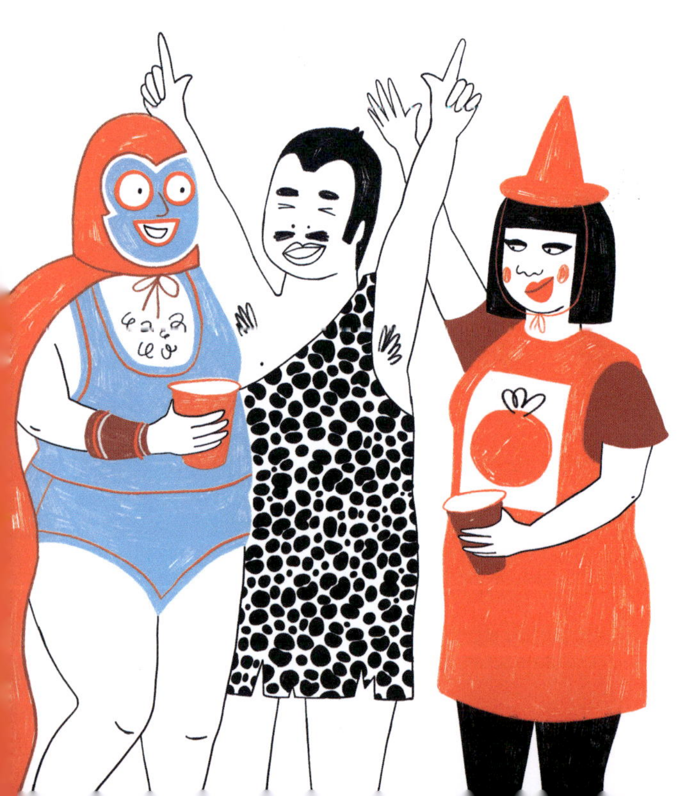

DANCE FLOOR FILLER

This trio are showing us their breakdancing skills. Bring more people to the dance floor with characters practicing their energetic dance moves!

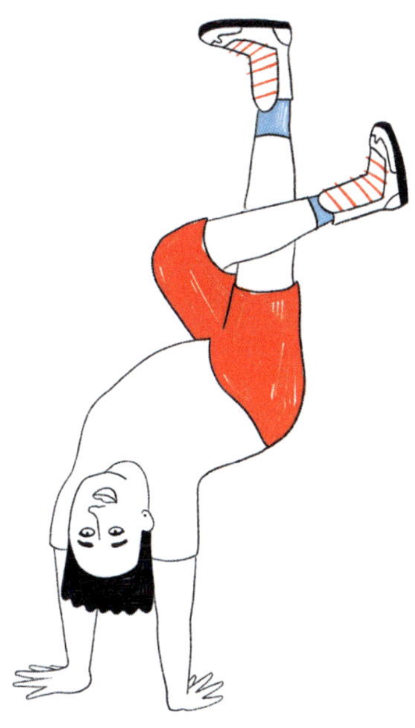

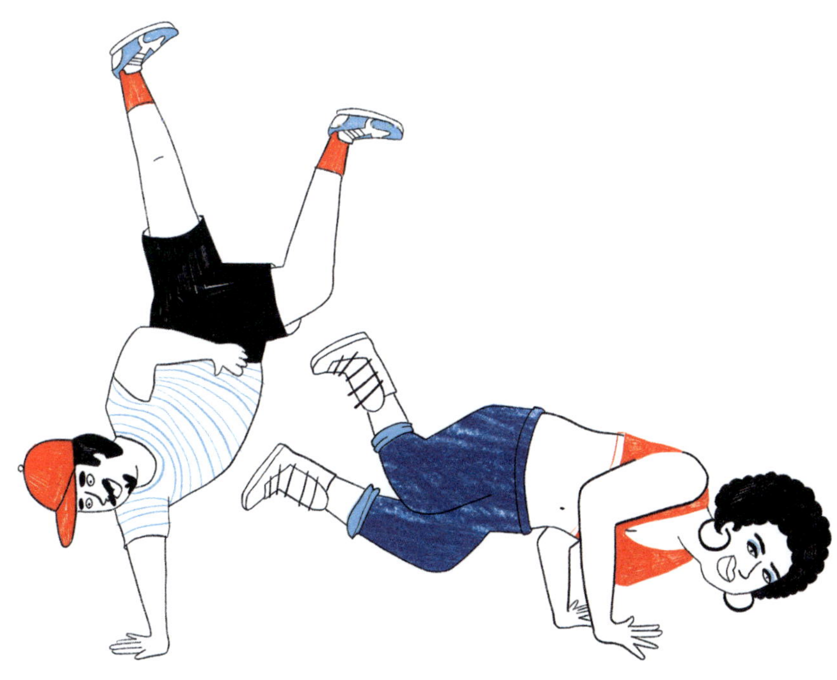

MY FAVORITE DRAWINGS

Have a look back at what projects and characters you loved drawing the most in this book. Grab your tools and enjoy revisiting your favorites and developing some of them a little further.

Who was your favorite person to draw? Draw them again but wearing a hat or glasses.

What material did you love using the most? Sketch a profile portrait using that material.

Draw a character from your favorite celebration in the book, but doing something different.

Which drawing technique did you enjoy the most? Have another go here.

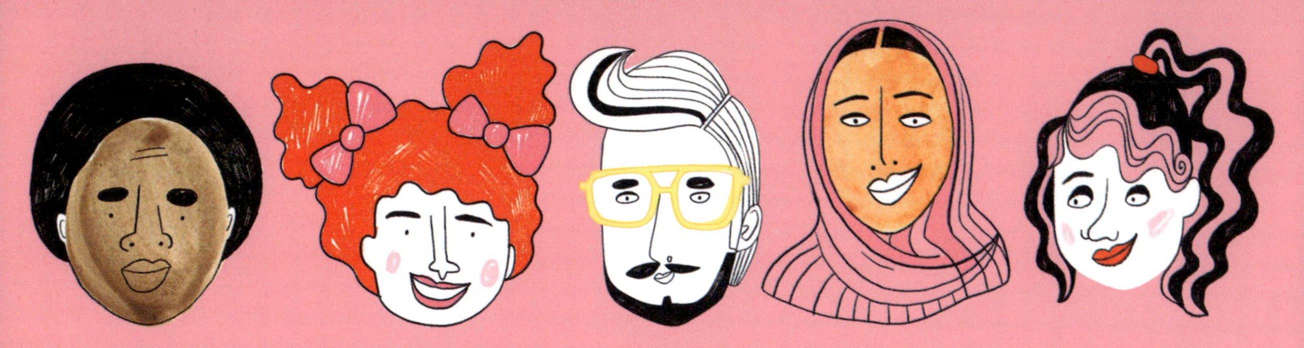

Pick a character you enjoyed drawing but this time give them a different expression!

Which of your portraits brought you the most joy? Draw it again using a different material.

Which was your favorite subculture to draw? Draw a portrait in that style with only two colors.

What color palette did you enjoy using the most? Create a character using those colors.

ARTISTIC DISCOVERIES

Reflect on the skills you want to develop further, thinking about when and where you felt the most inspired while using this book, as well as how you worked through times of frustration or creative blocks.

1.

2.

3.

4.

5.

Five things I want to practice. List them with the intention of drawing more of them.

If you experienced frustration or a creative block what helped inspire you? Draw or write it here.

Where did you create your best work? Draw your favorite workspace.

Draw what time of day you create your best work.

CREATIVE OBSERVATIONS

At the start of this book, you were asked to write your goals. Do you feel you met or perhaps exceeded what you originally hoped to achieve? How do you plan to continue your creative practice?

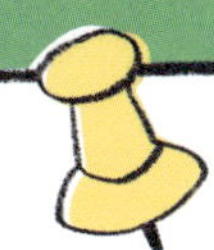
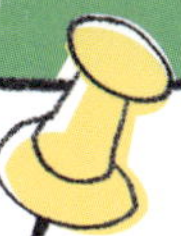

WRITE HERE

SKETCHBOOK PAGES

The next few pages are somewhere to practice, explore, test new materials, and try things out. Enjoy any imperfections: it's all in the process!

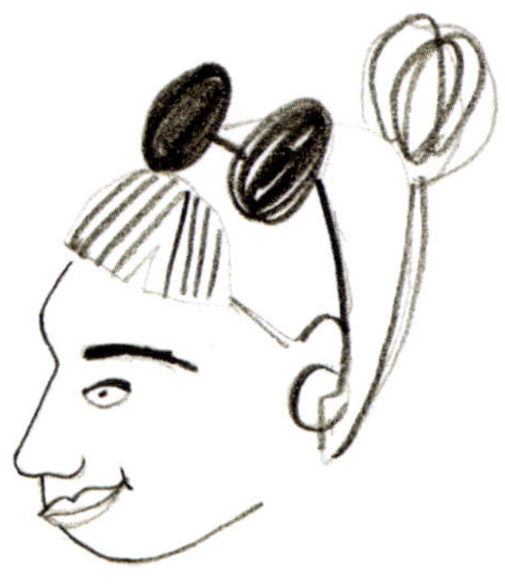

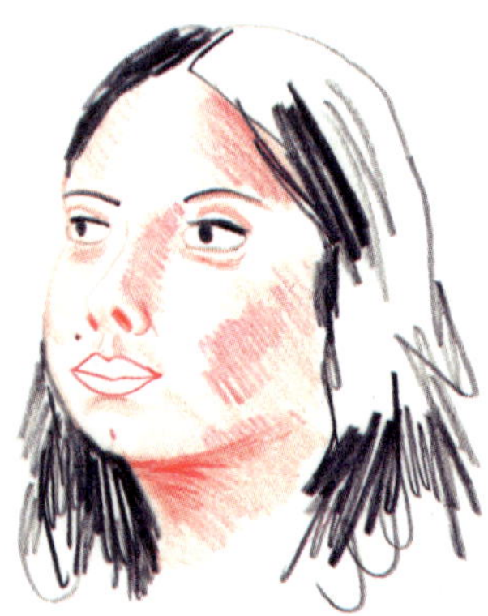

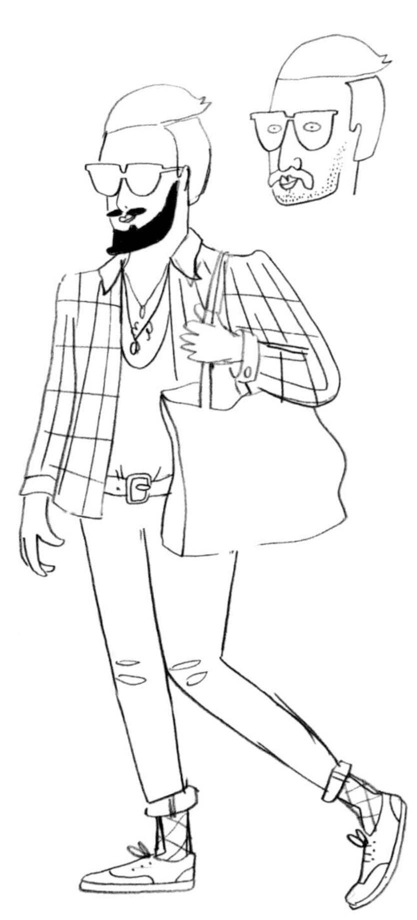

KEEP ON SKETCHING, KEEP ON PRACTICING!

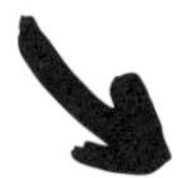

PLAY, CREATE, AND MOST
IMPORTANTLY HAVE FUN!

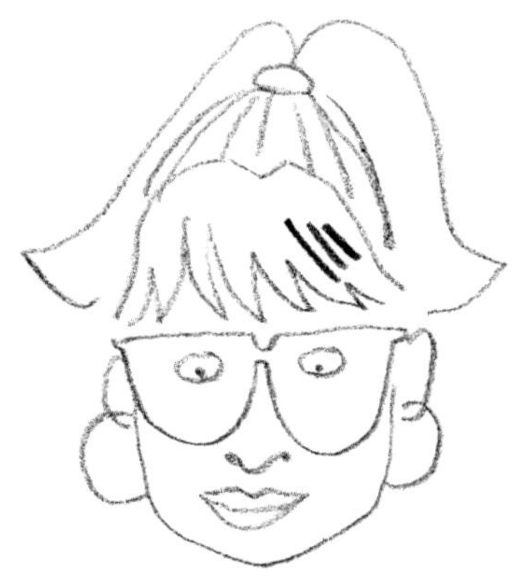

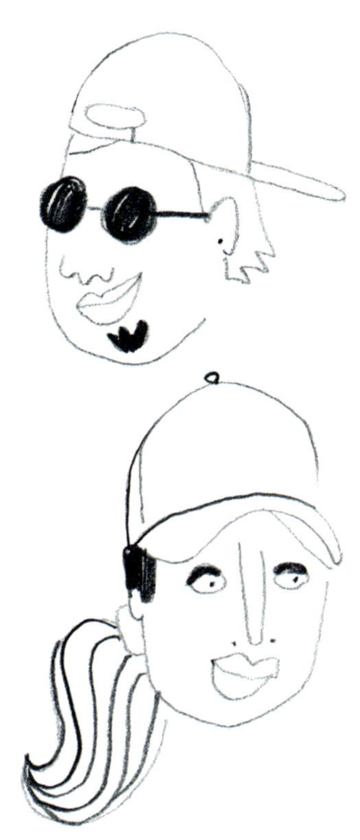
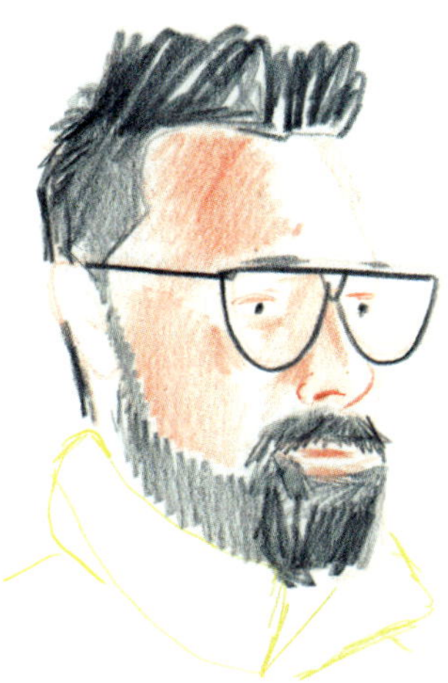

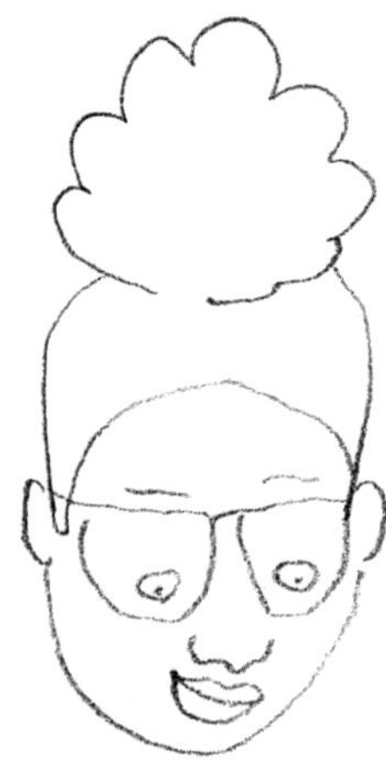

FILL THE PAGE WITH IMPERFECT SKETCHES!

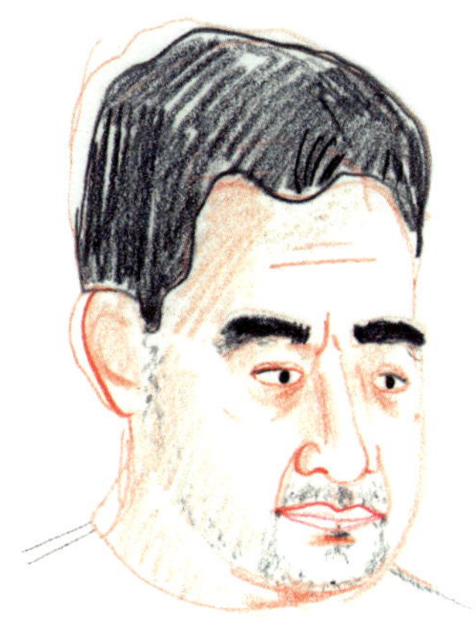

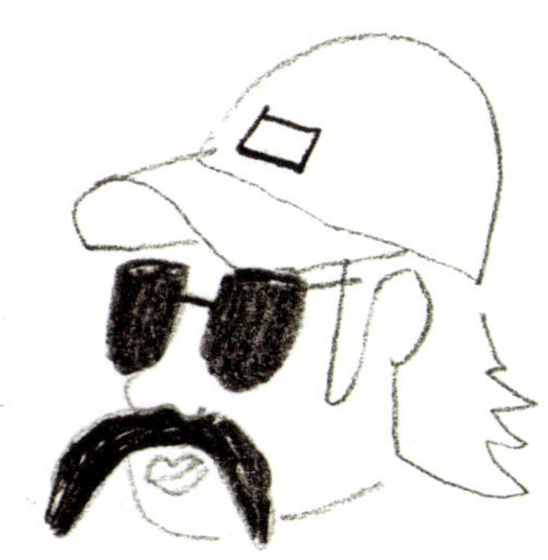

ABOUT THE AUTHOR

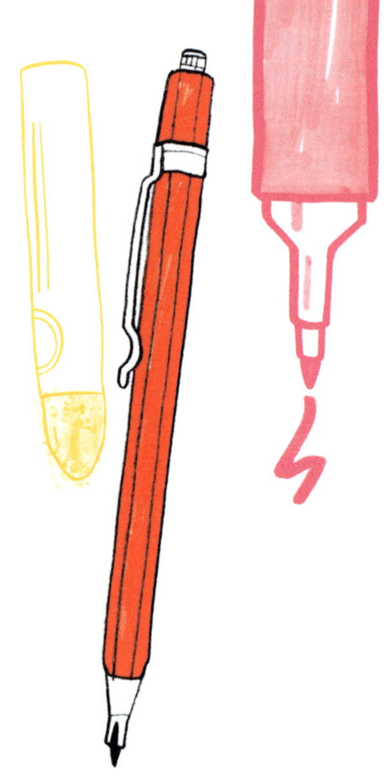

Tilly, also known as Running For Crayons, is an illustrator and book designer whose studio is just a stone's throw from the sea in Brighton, UK. She draws inspiration from the every day and the odd and enjoys creating characters based on the folks around her. Since graduating with an MA in Sequential Illustration and Design in 2006, she has worked with clients worldwide in editorial, advertising, and publishing including *The Wall Street Journal*, *The Guardian*, *National Geographic Traveller*, the BBC, and Wembley Park, along with multiple publishers for whom she has illustrated and designed dozens of books.

She is passionate about the power art has to bring meaning, joy, and connection into people's lives and that art should be accessible to all, having facilitated art sessions in acute mental health hospitals and inclusive groups for individuals facing isolation or physical and mental disabilities. She believes anyone can draw and experience the benefits art can bring in improving wellbeing, happiness, and enhancing their quality of life.

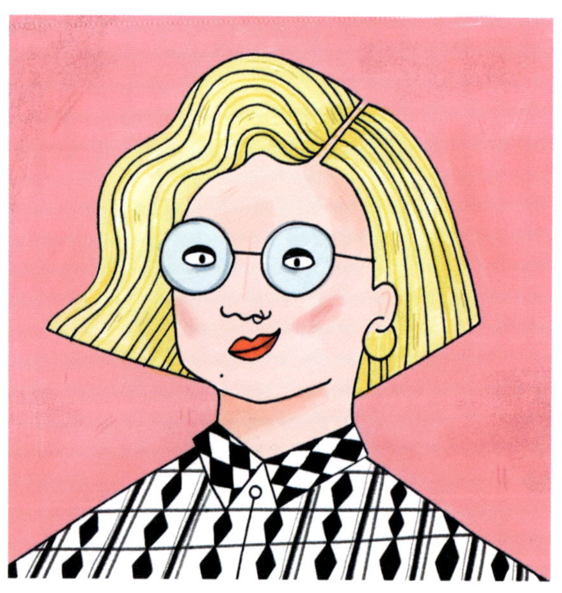

YOU CAN FIND HER ONLINE AT:

www.runningforcrayons.co.uk
instagram/runningforcrayons

ACKNOWLEDGMENTS

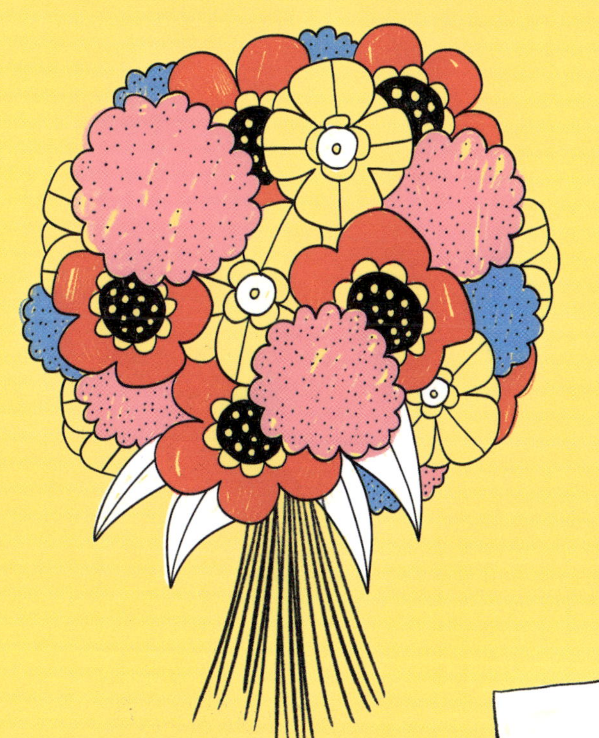

A big thank you to Catie for commissioning me to create another book in this series. Giving me such creative freedom, with feedback that always made for a better page. A huge thanks to Charles and the team at Rizzoli for publishing another in the series and asking me to create it. And to Kathy for always being the best editor anyone could wish for!

Thank you to my studio buddies Ant and Dan for being great inspiration and being brilliant at bouncing ideas. Along with my amazing husband and friends Claire, KT, and Eugénie for being my sitters and posing at a drop of a hat.

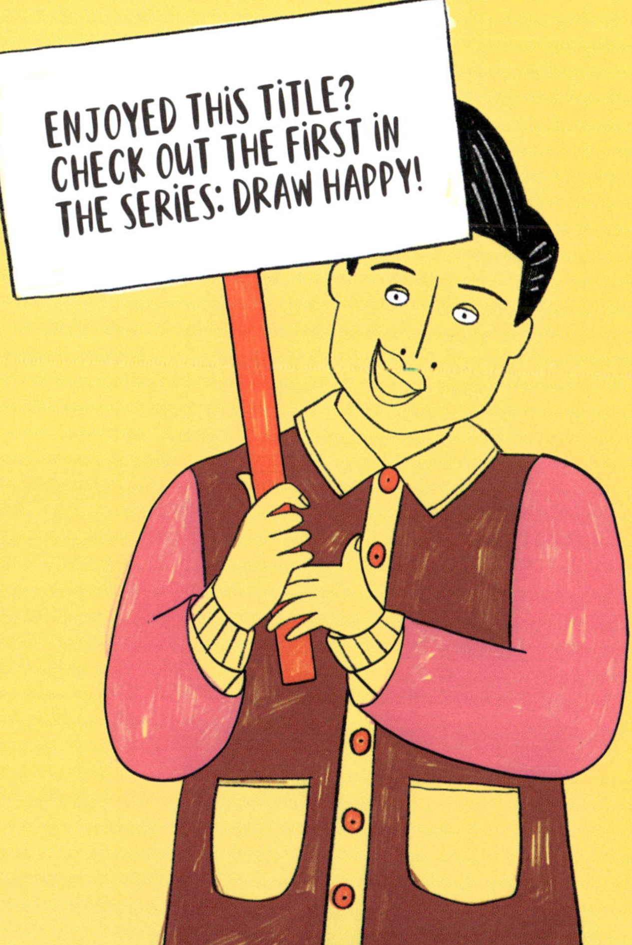

Published in 2026 by Rizzoli Universe,
a division of Rizzoli International Publications

Rizzoli International Publications Inc
49 West 27th Street
New York, NY 10001

Rizzoli International Publications UK Ltd
Somerset House, West Wing
Strand, London WC2R 1LA

www.rizzoliusa.com

Copyright © 2026 Rizzoli Universe UK

Text and illustrations copyright © 2026 Tilly,
Running For Crayons Ltd

Publisher: Charles Miers
Associate Publisher: Tina Persaud
Acquisitions Editor: Catie Ziller
Designer: Tilly
Copy Editor: Kathy Steer

All rights reserved. No part of this publication may be
reproduced, stored in a retrieval system, or transmitted
in any form or by any means, electronic, mechanical,
photocopying, recording, or otherwise, without prior
consent of both the copyright owner and the publisher
of this book.

A CIP catalogue record for this book is available from
the British Library.

ISBN: 9780789344267

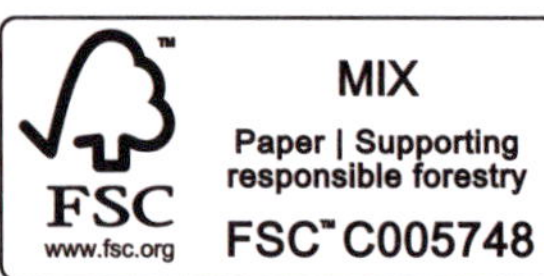

2026 / 1

Printed in China

The authorized representative in the EU for safety and
compliance is Mondadori Libri S.p.A., via Gian Battista Vico
42, Milan, Italy, 20123, www.mondadori.it

Visit us online: Instagram.com/RizzoliBooks
Facebook.com/RizzoliNewYork
Youtube.com/user/RizzoliNY

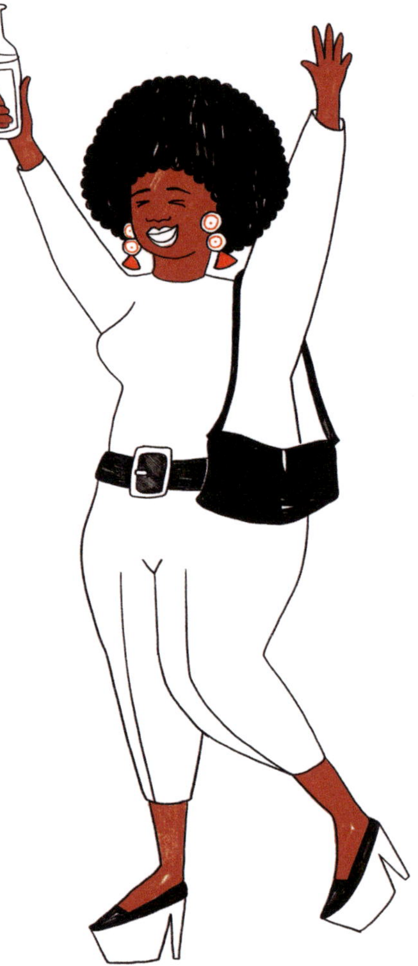

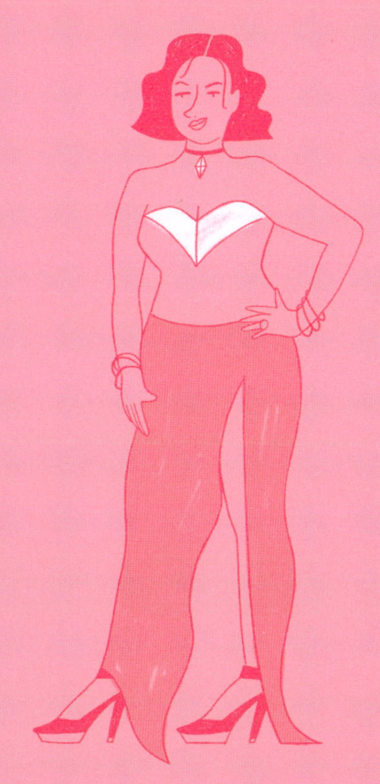

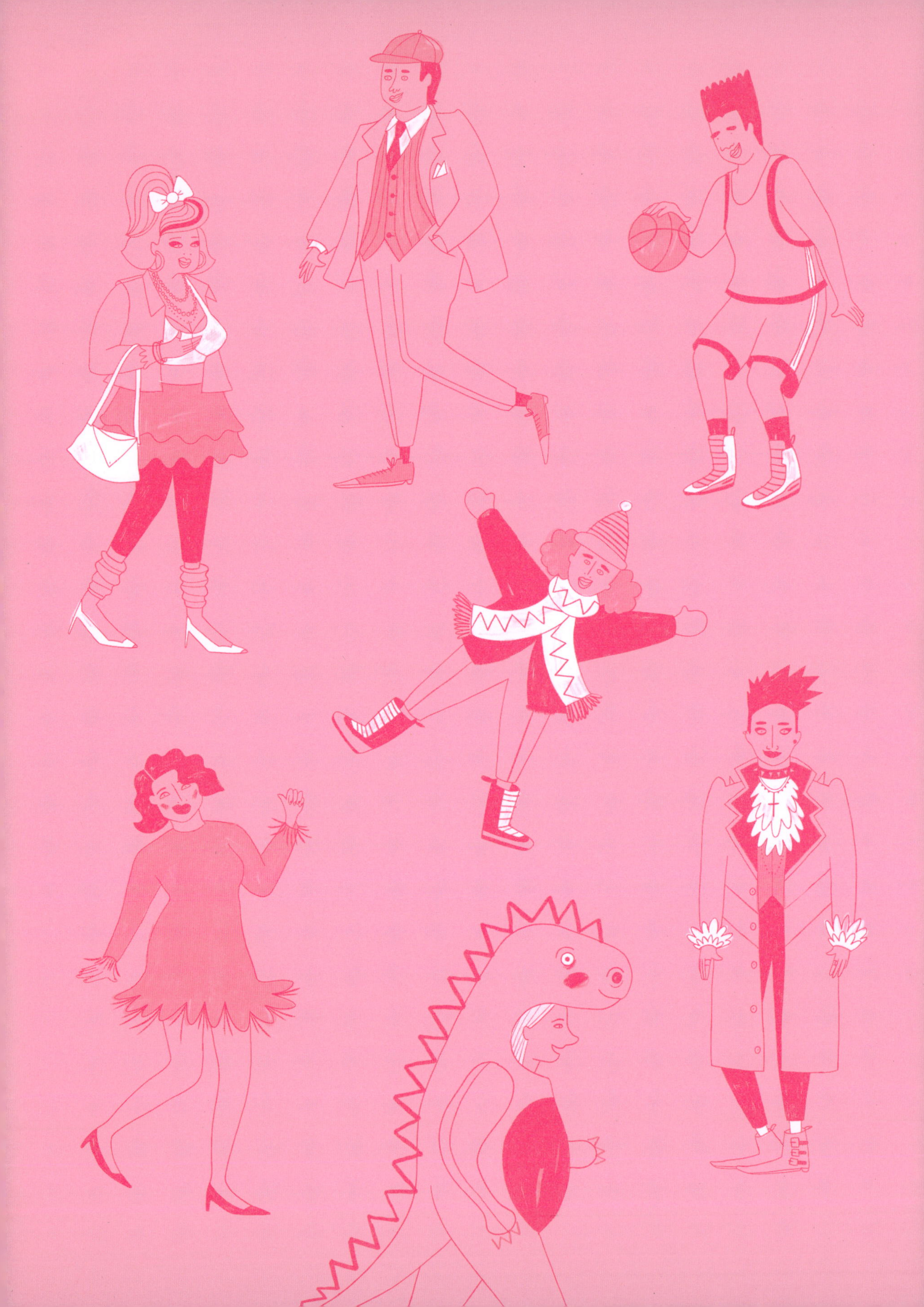